MAJOR PROBLEMS IN INTERNAL MEDICINE

Published

Cline: Cancer Chemotherapy (second edition by Cline and Haskell now available separately)
Shearn: Sjögren's Syndrome
Cogan: Ophthalmic Manifestations of Systemic Vascular Disease
Williams: Rheumatoid Arthritis as a Systemic Disease
Cluff, Caranasos and Stewart: Clinical Problems with Drugs
Fries and Holman: Systemic Lupus Erythematosus
Kass: Pernicious Anemia
Braude: Antimicrobial Drug Therapy
Bray: The Obese Patient
Zieve and Levin: Bleeding Disorders
Gorlin: Coronary Artery Disease
Sleisenger and Brandborg: Malabsorption
Beeson and Bass: The Eosinophil

MAJOR PROBLEMS IN INTERNAL MEDICINE

In Preparation

Krugman and Gocke: Viral Hepatitis
Potts: Disorders of Calcium Metabolism
Felig: Diabetes Mellitus
Havel and Kane: Diagnosis and Treatment of Hyperlipidemias
Siltzbach: Sarcoidosis
Scheinberg and Sternlieb: Wilson's Disease and Copper Metabolism
Atkins and Bodel: Fever
Lieber and De Carli: Medical Aspects of Alcoholism
Merrill: Glomerulonephritis
Goldberg: The Scientific Basis and Practical Use of Diuretics
Laragh: Reversible Hypertension
Kilbourne: Influenza
Deykin: Diseases of the Platelets
Schwartz and Lergier: Immunosuppressive Therapy
Cohen: Amyloidosis
Salmon: Multiple Myeloma
Seegmiller: Gout
Weinstein: Infective Endocarditis
Sasahara: Pulmonary Embolism
Smith: Renal Lithiasis
Remington: Toxoplasmosis
Swartz: Meningitis
Raskin and Appenzeller: Headache
Sparling: Venereal Diseases
Brooks: Diseases of the Exocrine Pancreas
McLees: Critical Care
Hurwitz, Duranceau, and Haddad: Disorders of Esophageal Motility
Mason: Oral Manifestations of Systemic Disease
Engel: Psychosocial Problems in Medical Practice
Utz: Systemic Mycotic Infections
Solomon and Chopra: Graves Disease and Hyperthyroidism
Galambos: Cirrhosis

H. FRANKLIN BUNN, M.D.
Associate Professor of Medicine,
Harvard Medical School;
Chief of Hematology Section
Peter Bent Brigham Hospital, Boston

BERNARD G. FORGET, M.D.
Associate Professor of Medicine,
Chief of Hematology Section,
Yale University School of Medicine, New Haven

HELEN M. RANNEY, M.D.
Professor and Chairman Department of Medicine,
University of California, San Diego

HEMOGLOBINOPATHIES

VOLUME
XII
IN THE SERIES
MAJOR PROBLEMS IN INTERNAL MEDICINE
Lloyd H. Smith, Jr., M.D., *Editor*

W. B. SAUNDERS COMPANY • PHILADELPHIA • LONDON • TORONTO

W. B. Saunders Company: West Washington Square
Philadelphia, PA 19105

1 St. Anne's Road
Eastbourne, East Sussex BN21 3UN, England

1 Goldthorne Avenue
Toronto, Ontario M8Z 5T9, Canada

Library of Congress Cataloging in Publication Data

Bunn, Howard Franklin

Hemoglobinopathies

(Major problems in internal medicine; v. 12)

1. Hemoglobinopathy. 2. Hemoglobin. I. Forget, Bernard G., joint author. II. Ranney, Helen M., joint author. III. Title. [DNLM: 1. Hemoglobinopathies. 2. Hemoglobins, Abnormal. W1 MA492T v. 12 / WH150 B942h]

RC641.7.H35B86 616.1′5 76–14678

ISBN 0–7216–2179–1

Hemoglobinopathies ISBN 0–7216–2179–1

Last digit is the print number: 9 8 7 6 5 4 3 2

FOREWORD

Aerobic metabolism requires molecular oxygen as the final receptor of hydrogen atoms (protons) filtering down the cascade of energy release. In picking up its cargo of protons, oxygen forms water, so that although it enters the body through the lung, it is largely excreted by the kidney. The delivery of oxygen to tissues depends on its diffusing capacity. Dissemination by diffusion is inherently limited despite elaborate networks of capillaries which supply a large permeable surface, low resistance to flow, and proximity to the site of delivery.

In the adult approximately 250 ml (11 m mole) of O_2 per minute is utilized at rest and up to 15 times that amount during exercise. Perhaps 3 per cent of the resting O_2 requirement is supplied to tissues from that absorbed in plasma. To deliver all O_2 in this primitive fashion would be unacceptable hemodynamically. It was necessary to evolve a molecular sponge for the selective transport of oxygen, one that could be finely tuned for rapid absorption of oxygen in the lung and its rapid release in peripheral tissues. A "sponge" has evolved which is complex in structure but elegantly adapted to the task. In the simplest statement: (1) Oxygen is bound at the sixth coordination position of iron in its bivalent state. (2) This iron is embedded in the tetrapyrrol ring of heme, the animal equivalent of chlorophyll. (3) Four hemes rest in specific clefts produced by the tertiary structure of globin. (4) The globin normally consists of four polypeptide chains, two pairs of unlike chains, coiled in α helical segments and shaped to produce the heme sites. (5) Hemoglobin is packaged in high concentration in the biconcave disks of erythrocytes. The integration could be further extrapolated to the cardiovascular and pulmonary systems in increasing complexity of the mechanisms necessary to supply atmospheric oxygen for intracellular proton acceptance.

Hemoglobin is the most available of human proteins and consequently that most intensively studied. The biochemistry of heme synthesis and catabolism has been well elucidated over the past 25 years, stimulated by the genetic disorders collectively called the porphyrias. Although heme may be limiting for hemoglobin synthesis, no "abnormal hemes" have been found. Much more attention has been directed toward the globin, the structure of which may have varied remarkably little over the past 500 million years (Romero-Herrera et al., 1973). The structure of hemoglobin has been unraveled in great detail by analysis of amino acid sequences and by x-ray crystallography. The synthesis of globin also has been studied extensively in vitro as a prototype of the control of protein synthesis in eucaryotic cells. From these studies globin has been found to be far more than a convenient but passive vehicle for transporting heme molecules. The molecule itself undergoes major conformational changes during a respiratory cyle from its T structure ("tense" when unliganded with O_2, for example) to its R structure ("relaxed" when liganded with O_2 or CO). These reversible contortions uniquely modify the affinity of the associated heme molecules for oxygen: (1) This is the presumed mechanism for what has been called the heme-heme interaction, i.e., the increased affinity for oxygen with increasing saturation with oxygen giving the sigmoid shape to the oxygen dissociation curve. (2) The role of 2,3-diphosphoglycerate (DPG) as an adaptive regulator in increasing oxygen unloading in the tissues results from its stabilization of the β chains of hemoglobin A in the T state. (3) The Bohr effect—the long-known effect of acidosis to shift the oxygen dissociation curve to the right and thereby enhance tissue unloading—results from the effect of pH on the salt bridges between globin chains and therefore from conformational changes.

It has been said that hemoglobin "breathes" in its structural changes during oxygen uptake and release (Winterhalter, 1973), and that each molecule might take appropriately 10^8 breaths during the lifetime of the individual erythrocyte (Desforges, 1976). If this figure of speech is valid, it is now clear that abnormal hemoglobins may result in "molecular dyspnea." Amino acid substitutions, or rarely deletions, may increase or decrease oxygen affinity because of dysmorphic molecules. Heme clefts may be abnormal or, rarely, missing. An abnormal hemoglobin may undergo polymerization or molecular stacking. Fortunately many abnormalities may occur in relatively silent areas of the molecule with little or no effect on overall function.

The study of hemoglobins in health and in disease has been one of the most productive areas in the application of protein chemistry and molecular biology to human physiology. Drs. Bunn, Forget, and Ranney have been in the forefront of these developments. They have written a monograph that spans the stretch between laboratory investigation and clinical application. The result of this exciting chapter in biology is a new understanding of some important hematological disorders and a model for studies of other genetic diseases in man.

LLOYD H. SMITH, JR., M.D.

REFERENCES

Desforges, J. F.: Hemoglobin—a working molecule. N. Engl. J. Med. *295*:164, 1976.

Romero-Herrera, A. E., Lehmann, H., Joysey, K. A., et al.: Molecular evolution of myoglobin and the fossil record: A phylogenetic synthesis. Nature *246*:389, 1973.

Winterhalter, K. H.: Does hemoglobin breathe, and if so, how?—The T and R state of hemoglobin. N. Engl. J. Med. *289*:41, 1973.

ACKNOWLEDGMENTS

We are indebted to many individuals for their valuable help at all stages of this project.

Individual chapters were thoroughly reviewed by the following colleagues: Arthur Arnone, Philip Bromberg, George Buchanan, William Eaton, Stuart Edelstein, Alan Keitt, Philip Pulsinelli, Ronald Rieder and Vijay Sharma.

Edward Benz contributed immensely to the literature search and organization of material related to the sections on the biosynthesis of hemoglobin and the molecular genetics of the thalassemias.

Philomena Morrison and Kathy Strutz provided expert secretarial assistance. Their patience, good humor and conscientious attention to detail continued throughout the book's long gestation. We are also indebted to the library staff at UCSD School of Medicine for their painstaking check of all the references, and to Betsy Bunn for extensive proofreading of both typescript and page proofs.

Diane Forti has been an exceptionally able copy editor, providing invaluable advice on style, usage and organization as well as an unfailing eye for inconsistencies, omissions, redundancies, etc. We also thank the senior editors at Saunders, John Dusseau and Jack Hanley, for their sound advice and enthusiastic cooperation.

Finally, we thank those friends and colleagues with whom our interest in hemoglobin began:

The Benesches	Irving London
Robin Briehl	David Nathan
James Jandl	Sherman Weissman

CONTENTS

Chapter 1

STRUCTURE AND FUNCTION OF HUMAN HEMOGLOBIN

The determination of the structure of hemoglobin is one of the milestones of molecular biology. This information has provided an intimate understanding of the way in which the molecule functions physiologically. Study of hemoglobin has proved relevant to a number of biomedical disciplines. This protein is a prototype of a general class of allosteric enzymes whose function depends upon transition from one conformation to another. Recently, attention has been focused on environmental factors, including 2,3-DPG, hydrogen ion concentration, and CO_2, which can modify and perhaps regulate the behavior of hemoglobin within the red cell. Comparisons of primary amino acid sequences of animal hemoglobins have provided new and independent phylogenetic insights. Furthermore, surveys of human hemoglobin phenotypes have been of considerable utility in the study of population genetics. Finally, certain variants are responsible for specific clinical syndromes. As we shall discuss in detail, in most cases the clinical features can be directly attributed to lesions at a submolecular level. This chapter will first present a detailed account of interrelationships between hemoglobin structure and function. Secondly, we will consider the various factors in health and disease which can modify hemoglobin's physiologic role. This background information will be useful in the consideration of inherited and acquired disorders of hemoglobin structure and function.

HEMOGLOBIN STRUCTURE

Hemoglobin is a tetramer approximately $50 \times 55 \times 64$ Å, with a molecular weight of 64,400. It consists of two pairs of unlike polypeptide chains. A heme group, ferroprotoporphyrin IX, is linked covalently at a specific site to each globin polypeptide chain. When heme iron is in the reduced (ferrous) state, it can bind reversibly with gaseous ligands, such as oxygen or carbon monoxide. The ferrihemes of methemoglobin are incapable of oxygenation but can bind tightly to anionic ligands, such as cyanide. Such modifications of hemoglobin cause specific alterations in its color and absorption spectrum.

Human Hemoglobin Phenotypes

There are at least six genes which govern globin synthesis in developing human erythroblasts, resulting in the formation of structurally different globin polypeptide chains, designated as α, β, γ, δ, ϵ, and ζ. There is evidence in man (Lehmann and Carrell, 1968; Chap. 2) and primates (Barnicot et al., 1970) that the α-chain gene is duplicated. Furthermore, structural heterogeneity in the γ chain can be best explained by the presence of more than one gene (Schroeder et al., 1968). The β, γ, and δ genes are probably closely linked. In the thalassemia syndromes there is a defect in the synthesis of one (or rarely two) globin subunit(s) (Chapter 2).

Hemoglobin A

The various normal human hemoglobins are listed in Table 1–1. In adult red cells, Hb A ($\alpha_2\beta_2$) makes up over 90 per cent of the total. The structure and function of this molecule will be described in detail later.

Hemoglobin A_2

About 2.5 per cent of the hemoglobin is A_2 ($\alpha_2\delta_2$). This minor component is evenly distributed among red cells (Heller and Yakulis, 1969). Its functional behavior is probably the same as that of Hb A (Bunn and Briehl, 1970). The amino acid sequence of the δ chain differs from that of the β chain in 10 out of 146 residues (Dayhoff, 1969). The increased percentage of Hb A_2 in beta thalassemia is a useful diagnostic aid (see Chapter 2). In addition, Hb A_2 may be increased in megaloblastic anemia (Josephson et al., 1958). In contrast, Hb A_2 is decreased in iron deficiency (Chernoff, 1964) and sideroblastic anemias (Reed and Mollin, 1968; White et al., 1971). The relative rate of synthesis of this minor component is markedly curtailed in the final stages of erythroid development (Rieder and Weatherall, 1965).

TABLE 1–1. *Human Hemoglobins*

Hemoglobin	Structure	% of Normal Adult Hemolysate	Increased In	Decreased In
A	$\alpha_2\beta_2$	92		
A_2	$\alpha_2\delta_2$	2.5	β thalassemia; Megaloblastic anemia	Iron deficiency; Sideroblastic anemia
A_{Ia}	Not known	< 1	Diabetes mellitus	Hemolytic anemia
A_{Ib}	" "	2		
A_{Ic}	$\alpha_2(\beta\text{-N-glucose})_2$	5		
F	$\alpha_2\gamma_2$	< 1	Fetal red cells; β thalassemia; Marrow "stress": Sickle cell anemia, pernicious anemia, etc.	
F_I	$\alpha_2(\gamma\text{-N-acetyl})_2$	< 1		
Gower 1	$\zeta_2\epsilon_2$	0	Early embryo	
Gower 2	$\alpha_2\epsilon_2$	0		
Portland	$\zeta_2\gamma_2$	0		
H	β_4	0	α thalassemias	
Bart's	γ_4	0		

Hemoglobin F

The main component during fetal development is Hb F ($\alpha_2\gamma_2$). Many other mammalian species which have been tested appear to have structurally different fetal hemoglobin(s). The γ chain differs from the β chain in 39 of 146 residues (Dayhoff, 1969). The oxygen equilibrium of purified Hb F is nearly identical to that of Hb A. However, fetal red cells have a considerably higher oxygen affinity than do adult red cells. This phenomenon has been observed in a number of mammalian species (Novy and Parer, 1969) and may facilitate the transport of oxygen across the placenta. In the human, this discrepancy in relative oxygen affinities is due to the diminished interaction of Hb F with red cell organic phosphates (Bauer et al., 1968) (see below). Hemoglobin F has the special property of being remarkably resistant to denaturation at extremes of pH. The measurement of alkali-resistant hemoglobin (Jonxis and Visser, 1956; Singer et al., 1951) has proved to be a very useful, although indirect, way of estimating the content of Hb F within a hemolysate. However, this approach tends to underestimate Hb F (Schroeder et al., 1970).

The red cells of the newborn contain about 80 per cent Hb F, 20 per cent Hb A, and less than 0.5 per cent Hb A_2. Occasionally, Hb Bart's (γ_4) may be detected in trace amounts in a normal neonate. Shortly before birth there is a switch from γ-chain to β-chain synthesis. Hemoglobin F falls steadily following birth, approaching a nadir at about age six months. However, the rate of fall of fetal hemoglobin is quite variable. Fetal hemoglobin persists longer in infants born prematurely (Garby et al., 1962). Conversely, there is a more rapid decline of Hb F in neonates having increased red cell turnover, such as in erythroblastosis fetalis. Although alkali denaturation is not sensitive enough to detect Hb F in normal adults, recent fluorescent labeling has demonstrated this hemoglobin distributed rather unevenly among red cells (Boyer et al., 1975; Hosoi, 1965). Hemoglobin F is increased to a variable extent in several hereditary disorders, including beta thalassemia, hereditary persistence of fetal hemoglobin, and sickle cell anemia. In addition, increased levels of fetal hemoglobin may be seen in a variety of acquired hematologic disorders, including megaloblastic anemia, aplastic anemia, and leukemias. This subject will be considered in more detail at the end of this chapter (pp. 26 and 27). The mechanism underlying this return to γ-chain synthesis is unknown.

Embryonic Hemoglobins

The Gower hemoglobins ($\zeta_2\epsilon_2$ and $\alpha_2\epsilon_2$) and Hb Portland ($\zeta_2\gamma_2$) (Kamuzora, 1974) are detectable only in the first three months of fetal development. Epsilon and zeta chains are probably synthesized in the yolk sac. Only minute amounts of these hemoglobins can be obtained. For this reason their structure and function have not been fully evaluated.

Hemoglobin H and Hb Bart's

Hemoglobin H and Hb Bart's are tetramers of β chains and γ chains, respectively. In order for hemoglobin to function physiologically, a tetramer must consist of pairs of α and non-α chains. In contrast, Hb H and Hb Bart's have very high oxygen affinity and absent heme-heme interaction and Bohr effect. These hemoglobins are found to a variable extent in patients with the different types of alpha thalassemia (see Chapter 2).

Hemoglobins A_{Ia}, A_{Ib}, A_{Ic}

When the hemoglobin from normal adult red cells is carefully analyzed by column chromatography (Allen et al., 1958; Huisman and Meyering, 1960), several minor components can be detected which have a lower isoelectric point than the main Hb A. These are designated A_{Ia}, A_{Ib}, and A_{Ic}. On zone electrophoresis at alkaline pH, these components appear as a smear (sometimes designated as Hb A_3) running anodal to the main component. Hemoglobin A_{Ic} makes up about 5 per cent of the hemoglobin in normal adult red cells. Its structure differs from Hb A only at the N-terminal amino group of each β chain which is covalently linked to glucose by a Schiff base (Bookchin and Gallop, 1968; Bunn et al., 1975a). This glycoprotein is increased in patients with diabetes mellitus (Rahbar, 1968; Trivelli et al., 1971). About 20 per cent of Hb F in the developing fetus has a similar structural modification: the N terminus of each γ chain is acetylated (Hb F_1) (Schroeder et al., 1962).

Primary and Secondary Structure

Alpha chains contain 141 amino acids in linear sequence, while β, δ, and γ chains have 146 residues. The amino acid sequence for each of these polypeptide chains has been established by chemical methods, including enzymatic digestion followed by amino acid analysis of the resultant peptides. More recently, Edman degradation has also proved useful for determining primary amino acid sequence. Such techniques are used for the structural analysis of human hemoglobin variants. Furthermore, at this time the primary structure has

ALPHA CHAIN

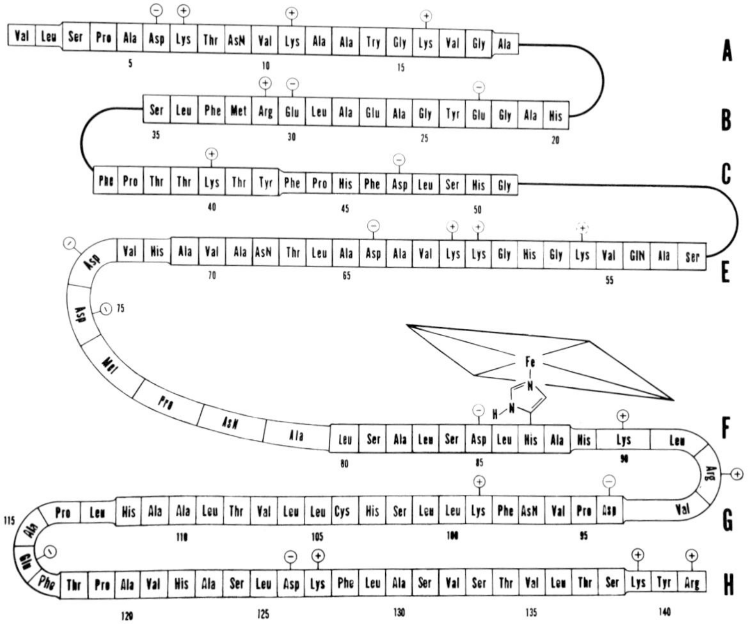

BETA CHAIN

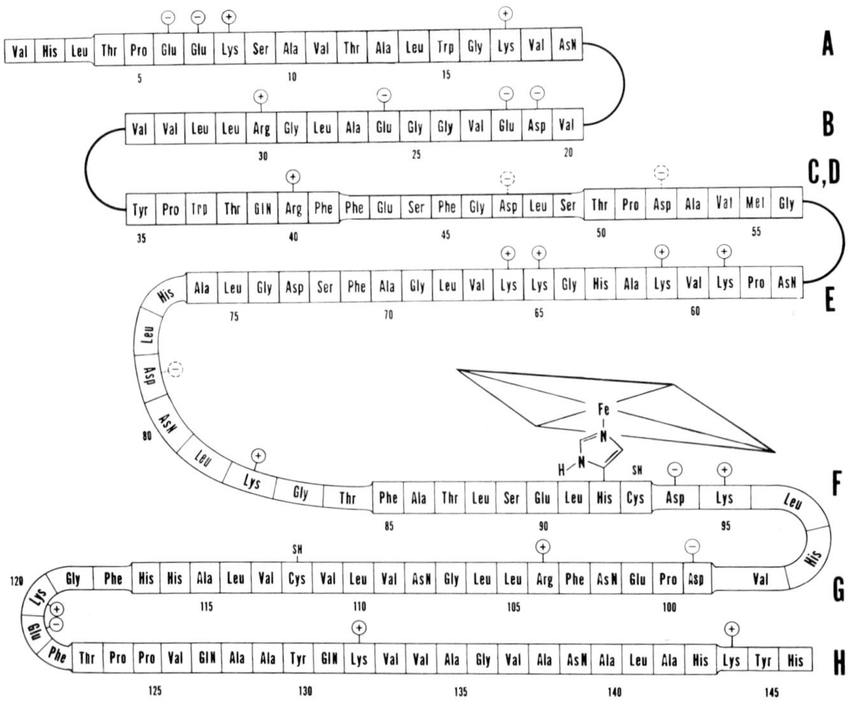

Figure 1–1. See legend on opposite page.

been worked out for some 26 mammalian hemoglobins and for a few avian and amphibian hemoglobins. This information has been useful in analyzing structural homology among the α chains and β chains of various species. Certain segments of these proteins have specific amino acids in common. Such invariant residues have been shown to be crucial to the molecule's function.

Approximately 80 per cent of hemoglobin in its native state is in the form of an α helix. X-ray analysis has shown that each chain consists of eight helical segments (labeled A through H in Figure 1–1). Figure 1–1 shows the amino acid residues of the α and β chains of human hemoglobin that are oriented in an α helix. Thus, individual residues can be assigned to a specific helix. This has been very useful in establishing homology between globin subunits. Thus, the heme iron is linked covalently to histidines at F8, the eighth residue of the F helix. This is residue number 87 of the α chain and 92 of the β chain (Fig. 1–1). All hemoglobins whose primary structures are known have a histidine residue at F8.* Residues which have charged side groups, such as lysine, arginine, and glutamic acid, lie on the surface of the molecule in contact with the surrounding water solvent. Uncharged residues are commonly oriented toward the hydrophobic interior of the molecule.

TERTIARY AND QUATERNARY STRUCTURE

From x-ray analyses of crystals of horse and human hemoglobins, Perutz and his associates in Cambridge, England, have determined the conformation of human hemoglobin in three-dimensional space. This remarkable achievement has allowed considerable progress in relating structure to function (Perutz, 1970). The hemoglobin tetramer was shown to be a spheroid with a diameter of about 55 Å and a single (dyad) axis of symmetry. The polypeptide chains are themselves folded in such a way that the four heme groups lie in clefts on the surface of the molecule equidistant from one another. The x-ray analysis is of sufficiently high resolution that the coordinates of all atoms in the molecule are known to within 2.5 Å. As shown in Figure 1–2, the

*Two of the variant M hemoglobins are exceptions. These will be discussed in detail in Chapter 7.

Figure 1–1. The primary structure of the α chain (*A*) and β chain (*B*) of human hemoglobin A. Those residues which are oriented in the form of an α helix are depicted by squares and nonhelical residues by rectangles. The site for heme attachment is shown. (From Muramaya, M.: In *Molecular Aspects of Sickle Cell Hemoglobin.* Nalbandian, R. M. (ed.), 1971. Courtesy of Charles C Thomas, Publisher, Springfield, Illinois.)

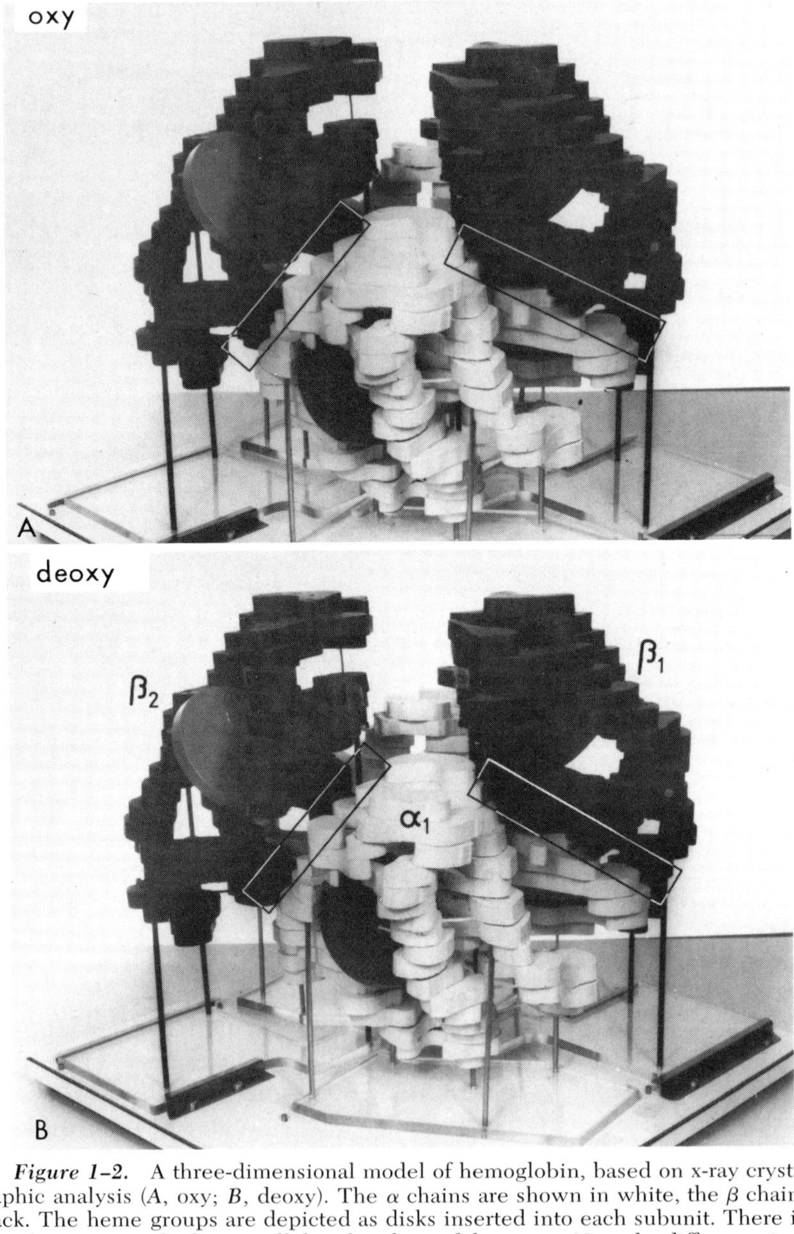

Figure 1–2. A three-dimensional model of hemoglobin, based on x-ray crystallographic analysis (*A*, oxy; *B*, deoxy). The α chains are shown in white, the β chains in black. The heme groups are depicted as disks inserted into each subunit. There is an axis of symmetry which is parallel to the plane of the paper. Note the difference in conformation between oxy- and deoxyhemoglobin. (From Muirhead, H., Cox, J. M., et al.: J. Mol. Biol. *28*:117, 1967.)

molecule undergoes a marked change in quaternary conformation upon deoxygenation. The β chains rotate apart by about 7 Å. In contrast, liganded forms, including oxyhemoglobin, carboxyhemoglobin, and cyanmethemoglobin, all appear to be isomorphous. This con-

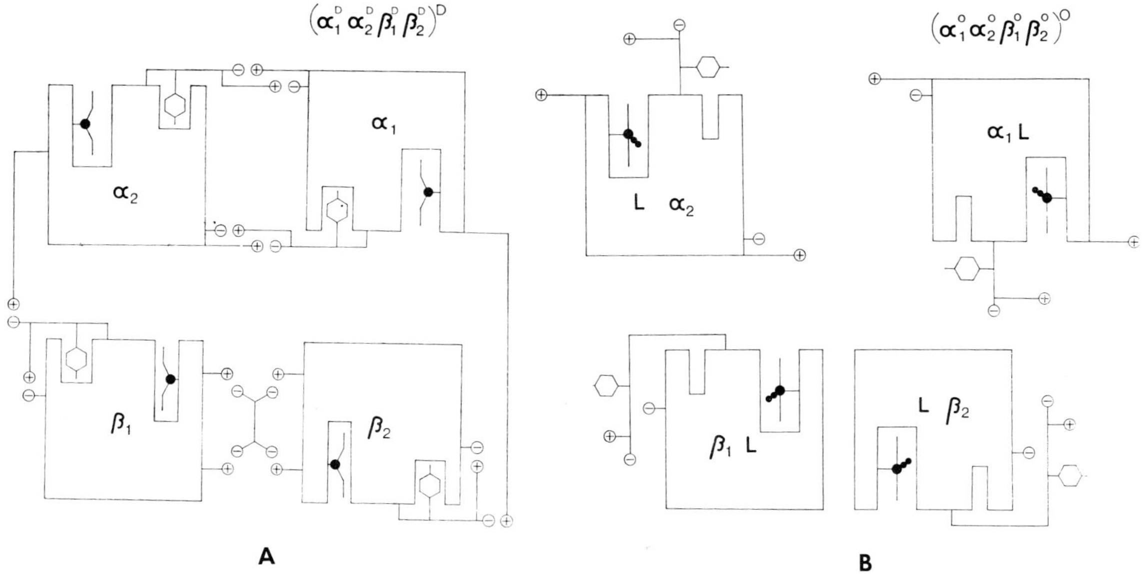

Figure 1–3. Diagrammatic representation of the quaternary configurations of deoxy-(*A*) and oxyhemoglobin (*B*). The salt bonds which stabilize the deoxy conformation are broken when the molecule is oxygenated. (From Perutz, M. F.: Nature [Lond.] 228:726, 1970.)

formational change which occurs upon removal and addition of ligand accounts for the many known differences in physical and chemical properties of oxy- and deoxyhemoglobins. Perutz has shown that deoxyhemoglobin is stabilized in a constrained or taut (T) configuration by the presence of inter- and intra-subunit salt bonds (Fig. 1–3) (Perutz, 1970). These include residues responsible for the Bohr effect and for the binding of 2,3-diphosphoglycerate (see below). Upon the addition of ligand, such as oxygen, these salt bonds are sequentially broken. The fully liganded hemoglobin is in the so-called relaxed (R) configuration. In this state, there is considerably less bonding energy between subunits, and the liganded molecule is able to dissociate reversibly according to the following reaction: $\alpha_2\beta_2 \rightleftharpoons 2\ \alpha\beta$. The formation of $\alpha\beta$ dimers is apparently required for hemoglobin to bind to haptoglobin (Bunn, 1967; Nagel and Gibson, 1967) and to traverse renal glomeruli (Bunn et al., 1969a). As shown in Figure 1–2, each subunit in the tetramer is oriented toward the two unlike subunits in different ways (i.e., α_1–β_1 and α_1–β_2). The dissociation of the liganded tetramer into dimers occurs at the $\alpha_1\beta_2$ interface. Thus, there is stronger binding energy between α_1 and β_1 subunits than between α_1 and β_2 subunits. Furthermore, during oxygenation and deoxygenation ($T \rightleftharpoons R$), there is considerable movement along the $\alpha_1\beta_2$ interface. As we shall discuss in Chapter 6, hemoglobin variants having an amino acid substitution in this region may have markedly abnormal functional properties.

HEMOGLOBIN FUNCTION

The oxygenation of hemoglobin, as depicted by the classic sigmoid oxyhemoglobin dissociation curve shown in Figure 1–4, can be characterized by two important properties: oxygen affinity and heme-heme interaction.* A convenient index of oxygen affinity is P_{50}, or partial pressure of oxygen at which hemoglobin is half saturated. If the oxyhemoglobin dissociation curve is shifted to the right, P_{50} is increased and oxygen affinity is decreased. Thus, P_{50} varies inversely with oxygen affinity. As discussed in detail in this section, P_{50} is dependent on temperature, pH, organic phosphates, and PCO_2. Under

*Data obtained from measurement of oxygen equilibria can be satisfactorily fitted by the empirical Hill equation: $\left(\frac{Y}{1-Y}\right) = \left(\frac{PO_2}{P_{50}}\right)^n$, where Y is the fractional saturation of hemoglobin with oxygen and n is an index of heme-heme interaction. If such interaction were absent, n would be 1.0. (This is true for myoglobin and isolated hemoglobin subunits.) If heme-heme interaction were maximal, n would be 4.0. In pure solutions of phosphate-free hemoglobin A, n is about 3.0, while in whole blood n is somewhat less (2.6 to 2.8). At the extremes of oxygen saturation ($Y < 0.1$, > 0.9), the experimentally derived points deviate from the Hill equation.

physiologic conditions (37° C, pH 7.40, 2,3-DPG = 5 mM, PCO_2 = 40 mm Hg), the P_{50} of normal adult blood is 26 mm Hg.

Heme-heme Interaction (Subunit Cooperativity)

When hemoglobin is partially saturated with oxygen, the affinity of the remaining hemes on the tetramer for oxygen increases markedly. This phenomenon can be considered in terms of the two hemoglobin conformations: deoxy (or T) and oxy (or R). The T form has a lower affinity for ligands such as O_2 or CO than has the R form. At some point during the sequential addition of oxygen to the four hemes of the molecule, a transition from the T to R configuration occurs. At this point the oxygen affinity of the partially liganded molecule increases markedly. In this way, hemoglobin can be considered a prototype of a more general class of allosteric enzymes, in which the interaction of protein and ligand alters binding affinity for another ligand at a different site on the same macromolecule.

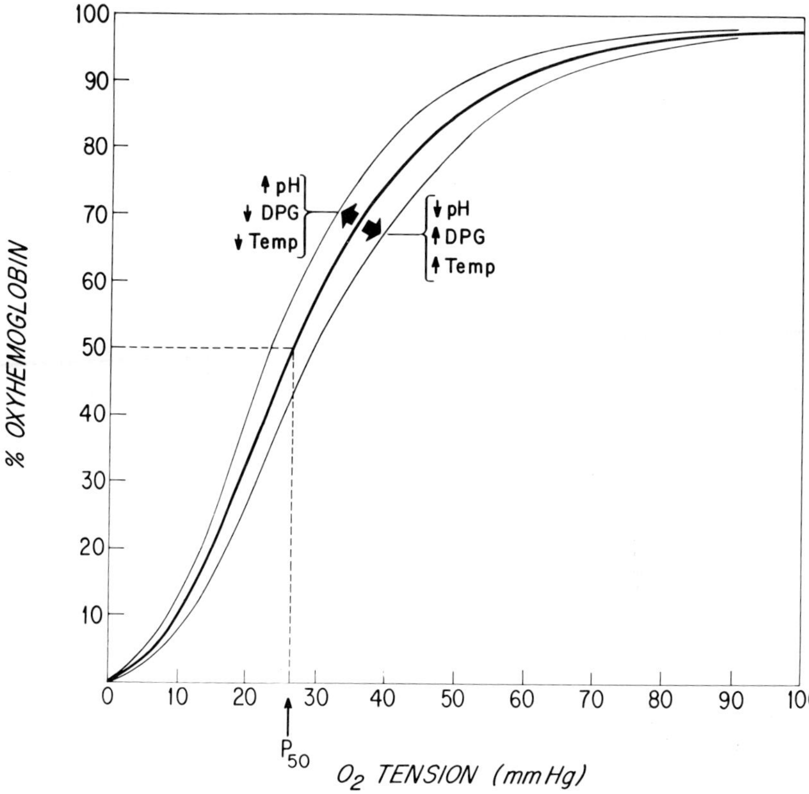

Figure 1–4. The principal factors which influence the position of the oxyhemoglobin dissociation curve.

How can the oxygenation of one heme cause sufficient alteration in the environment of other heme groups to affect their oxygen affinity? In deoxyhemoglobin, the iron atoms lie outside the plane of the porphyrin ring by about 0.6 Å (Perutz, 1970). The trigger which effects this allosteric transition appears to be the decrease in the atomic radius of heme iron upon the addition of ligand. The smaller iron atom is now able to snap into the plane of the porphyrin ring. The resulting alteration in heme configuration is amplified by a series of intra- and inter-subunit interactions, so that the environments of other hemes within the molecule are perturbed, resulting in increased ligand affinity. From a comparison of the immediate environment around the α and β chain hemes, Perutz (1970) has suggested that the first molecule of oxygen is more likely to bind to an α chain. However, there is no information as to which of the remaining three hemes would be oxygenated next. In general, the structural conformation of partially liganded hemoglobin is not well understood.

Heme-heme interaction (or subunit cooperativity) has considerable physiologic importance. This phenomenon dictates the familiar sigmoid shape of the oxyhemoglobin dissociation curve (Fig. 1–4). The S-shaped curve allows a considerable amount of oxygen to be released over a relatively small drop in oxygen tension. In contrast, heme proteins, such as myoglobin and hemoglobins H and Bart's, which lack subunit cooperativity, have a hyperbolic curve, which allows much less oxygen unloading.

THE BOHR EFFECT

In 1904, Bohr, Hasselbalch, and Krogh found that the oxygen affinity of hemoglobin decreased with increasing CO_2 tension (Bohr et al., 1904). It was later shown that this phenomenon was largely pH-dependent. Thus, over a pH range of 6.0 to 8.5, oxygen affinity varies directly with pH (Fig. 1–4). A thermodynamic corollary of this statement is that oxyhemoglobin is a stronger acid than deoxyhemoglobin. Under physiologic conditions, a molecule of hemoglobin releases about 2.8 protons upon oxygenation:

$$Hb \cdot H + 4\ O_2 \rightleftharpoons Hb\ (O_2)_4 + 2.8\ H^+$$

The recent high-resolution x-ray data in conjunction with experiments of Kilmartin and Rossi-Bernardi (1969) on chemically modified hemoglobins have permitted the identification of specific acid groups on hemoglobin which yield Bohr protons. In deoxyhemoglobin, the

N terminus of each α chain is linked by a salt bridge to the C terminus of the other α chain. This can be shown schematically as follows:*

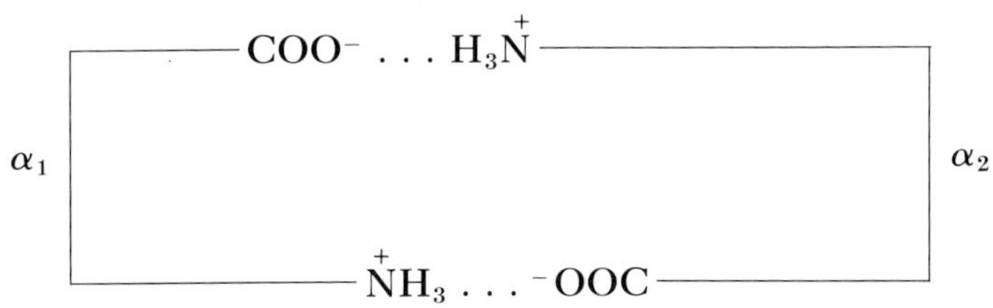

As part of the conformational isomerization that occurs upon oxygenation, these salt bonds are broken with the release of protons. These residues contribute about 25 per cent to the (physiologic or "alkaline") Bohr effect. About 50 per cent of the Bohr effect is due to intra-subunit salt bonds between the positively charged imidazole of β146-histidine and the negatively charged carboxyl of β94-aspartate. These salt bridges are among the important bonds which stabilize the deoxy conformation (see Figure 1–3).

The Bohr effect offers a physiologic advantage in facilitating oxygen unloading. At the tissue level, the drop in pH due to CO_2 influx lowers oxygen affinity, thereby enhancing oxygen release. In contrast, at the pulmonary level the increase in pH due to the efflux of CO_2 increases oxygen affinity and uptake. As further testimony to its adaptational advantage, the Bohr effect is present to a varying degree in virtually all mammalian species which have been tested and also in many types of lower animals.

Carbamino Formation

CO_2 affects hemoglobin function in two ways. It readily diffuses into red cells where, in the presence of a generous supply of carbonic anhydrase, carbonic acid is rapidly formed. The resulting decrease in pH lowers oxygen affinity (the Bohr effect). In addition, CO_2 can bind free amino groups on hemoglobin to form carbamino complexes according to the following reaction:

$$RNH_2 + CO_2 \rightleftharpoons RNHCOO^- + H^+$$

Only nonprotonated amino groups can react with CO_2. The only amino groups in globin whose pK's are low enough to be partially nonprotonated at physiologic pH are at the N termini. Hemoglobin having N-terminal amino groups blocked by cyanate is no longer able

*Also depicted diagrammatically in Figure 1–3.

to bind CO_2 (Kilmartin and Rossi-Bernardi, 1969). Deoxyhemoglobin forms carbamino complexes more readily than oxyhemoglobin. From this, it follows that, at a given pH, CO_2 lowers oxygen affinity. This effect becomes more marked as carbamino formation is favored at increasing pH. It is likely that, under physiologic conditions, the relatively low pH of the red cell precludes extensive carbamino formation. It is estimated that only about 10 per cent of the CO_2 produced by tissue metabolism is transported to the lungs in the form of carbamino hemoglobin (Rossi-Bernardi et al., 1972).

The Interaction of 2,3-Diphosphoglycerate with Hemoglobin

The red cell differs metabolically from other tissues in two important ways: (1) it derives its chemical energy almost solely through anaerobic glycolysis; and (2) it contains an unusually high concentration of 2,3-diphosphoglycerate (2,3-DPG). Normal human erythrocytes contain about 5 mM 2,3-DPG per liter (of packed cells), a concentration about fourfold that of the next most abundant organic phosphate, ATP. The *raison d'être* for such large amounts of 2,3-DPG in red cells remained elusive until the recent discovery that this compound is a potent modifier of hemoglobin function (Benesch and Benesch, 1967; Chanutin and Curnish, 1967). The addition of increasing amounts of 2,3-DPG to a solution of purified hemoglobin A results in a progressive lowering of oxygen affinity. This helps to explain the long-known fact that whole blood has a lower oxygen affinity than a solution of dialysed hemoglobin, studied under comparable conditions. The mechanism by which 2,3-DPG lowers oxygen affinity was

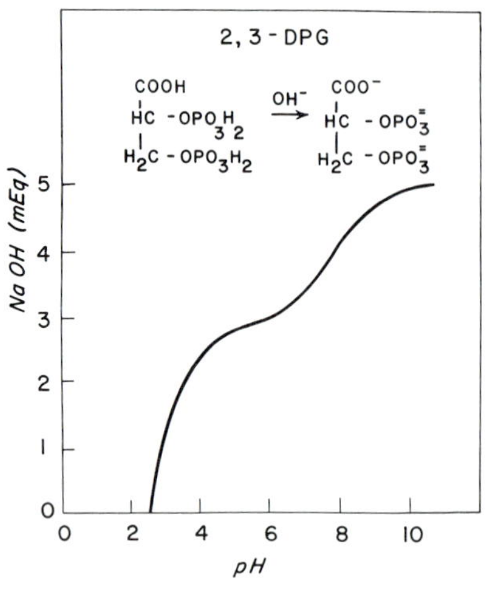

Figure 1–5. Structure of 2,3-DPG. From this titration curve it is apparent that, at physiologic pH, 2,3-DPG has about 3.5 negative charges per molecule.

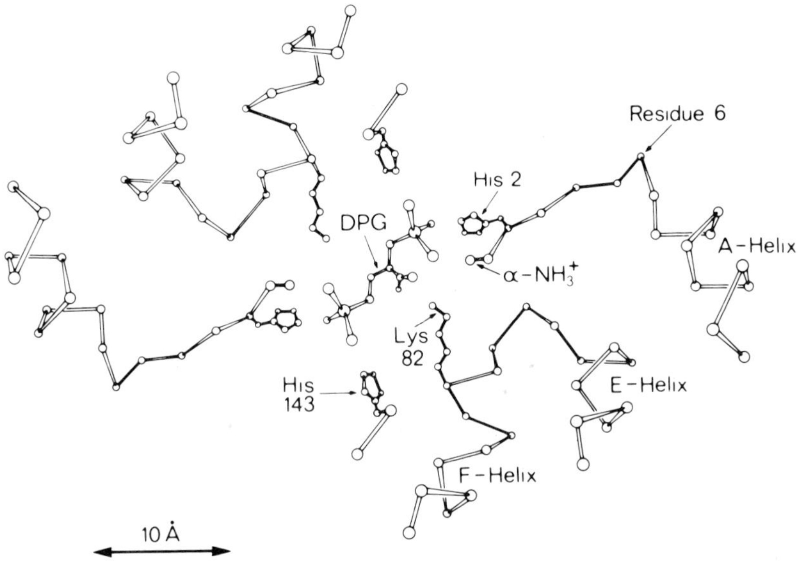

Figure 1–6. The site at which 2,3-DPG binds to the β chains of deoxyhemoglobin. This diagram shows a cross section of the molecule, the plane of which is perpendicular to the dyad axis of symmetry (compare with Figure 1–2). The diagram shows salt bonds between the phosphates of 2,3-DPG and positively charged groups at the β N terminus, β82 lysine and β143 histidine. (From Arnone, A.: Nature *237*:146, 1972.)

clarified when Benesch and his associates measured its binding to hemoglobin by a modified form of equilibrium dialysis (Benesch and Benesch, 1969). They showed that, at physiologic pH and ionic strength, 2,3-DPG bound to human deoxyhemoglobin rather avidly ($K = 2 \times 10^{-5}$ M) in a 1:1 molar ratio (1 molecule 2,3-DPG per hemoglobin tetramer). Furthermore, under these conditions, 2,3-DPG did not bind to liganded forms of hemoglobin such as oxy-, carboxy-, and cyanmethemoglobin. Furthermore, 2,3-DPG bound to hemoglobin H (β_4) but not to isolated α chains (Benesch and Benesch, 1969). As shown in Figure 1–5, 2,3-DPG is a strongly anionic compound. At physiologic pH, a molecule of 2,3-DPG has about three and one-half negative charges (Fig. 1–5). From their binding data, the Benesches concluded that 2,3-DPG binds electrostatically with the β chains of deoxyhemoglobin, probably in the central cavity along the dyad axis of symmetry.

A comparison of the reactivities of a number of human and animal hemoglobins of known structure with 2,3-DPG has suggested that the N-terminal amino groups of the β chains and the imidazoles of β143-histidine are specific residues responsible for 2,3-DPG binding (Bunn and Briehl, 1970). Model fitting and, more recently, x-ray diffraction measurements have confirmed these as the likely binding sites (Arnone, 1972; Perutz, 1970). Figure 1–6 shows a cross section of deoxyhemoglobin, with a plane perpendicular to that of Figure 1–2. The A E, and F helices of the β chains are shown (compare with Figure 1–2). 2,3-DPG is situated in the central cavity between the two β chains. Its negative charges are neutralized by positively charged groups mentioned above. In addition, β82-lysine and β2-histidine are also thought to be involved in 2,3-DPG binding (Arnone, 1972). In light of this information on the binding of 2,3-DPG to hemoglobin, the following simple reaction can be written:

$$Hb \cdot DPG + 4\ O_2 \rightleftharpoons Hb\ (O_2)_4 + DPG$$

(Note the similarity of this equation and that for the Bohr effect [see above].) This equilibrium expresses both the preferential binding of 2,3-DPG for deoxyhemoglobin and the 1:1 stoichiometry. Furthermore, changing concentrations of 2,3-DPG shift the oxygen binding equilibrium in accord with the experimental results cited above.

Other red cell phosphates are also able to lower the oxygen affinity of hemoglobin. In their degree of interaction with hemoglobin, these compounds can be ranked as follows: 2,3-DPG > ATP > ADP > AMP > pyrophosphate > inorganic phosphate. Although there is almost one-third as much ATP as 2,3-DPG in normal red cells, ATP probably plays an insignificant role in mediating intracellular hemoglobin function. First, it binds to deoxyhemoglobin less avidly than does 2,3-DPG. Second, an appreciable portion of red cell ATP is bound to magnesium ion. This complex does not interact with hemoglobin (Bunn et al., 1971).

ALTERATIONS IN BLOOD O_2 AFFINITY

The position of the oxyhemoglobin dissociation curve may be influenced by a number of factors. As depicted in Figure 1–4, the three most important are temperature, pH, and red cell 2,3-DPG. Oxygen affinity varies inversely with temperature. This phenomenon is physiologically appropriate since, during a period of relative hyperthermia, oxygen requirement is likely to be increased. The decrease in oxygen affinity at elevated body temperature would facilitate unloading of oxygen to tissues. The effects of pH and 2,3-DPG on hemoglobin function have already been discussed. Conventionally, whole blood oxygen saturation curves are corrected to pH 7.40, 37° C. Thus, the main variable leading to fluctuation in the position of the standardized oxygen dissociation curve is red cell 2,3-DPG.

Other factors which can also contribute include red cell ATP, PCO_2, alteration in cell hemoglobin concentration (mean corpuscular hemoglobin concentration [MCHC]), and extracellular-intracellular pH gradient. Red cell ATP and PCO_2 are probably of limited importance for reasons mentioned above. Changes in MCHC can affect oxygen affinity in several ways (Bellingham et al., 1971). Whether the range of MCHC encountered clinically is sufficiently large to influence hemoglobin function is not yet clear. Finally, because of the Bohr effect, any factor which changes the pH of the red cell relative to the plasma will be reflected in altered oxygen affinity. For example, any increase within the cell of an impermeant anion, such as hemoglobin or 2,3-DPG, will lower intracellular pH as a manifestation of the Gibbs-Donnan equilibrium.

How does the oxygen affinity of the blood affect the delivery of oxygen to tissues? This subject is considered in detail in a number of recent reviews (Adamson and Finch, 1975; Klocke, 1972; McConn, 1975; Thomas et al., 1974). At a given blood flow and hemoglobin concentration, the amount of oxygen that is unloaded is dependent upon the position of the oxyhemoglobin dissociation curve. As shown in Figure 1–7, red cells that are right-shifted have enhanced O_2 release when going from a normal arterial PO_2 (95 mm Hg) to a normal mixed venous PO_2 (40 mm Hg). This is due to the fact that at this Δ PO_2, a steeper portion of the oxygen dissociation curve is encompassed. In contrast, if the oxyhemoglobin dissociation curve is shifted to the left, less oxygen is unloaded at this Δ PO_2. From another viewpoint, it is apparent that if the oxygen affinity of the blood is increased, a given amount of oxygen will be extracted at a lower oxygen tension. This phenomenon bears on several clinical states to be discussed in detail, including hemoglobin variants associated with polycythemia, and blood transfusion therapy.

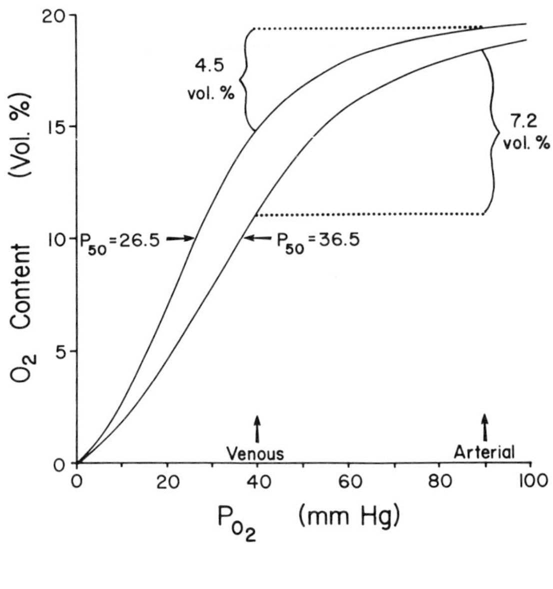

Figure 1–7. Enhancement of oxygen unloading due to a decrease in red cell oxygen affinity. Normal oxygen binding curve: P_{50} = 26.5 mm Hg; right-shifted curve: P_{50} = 36.5 mm Hg. (From Klocke, R. A.: Chest 62:795, 1972.)

Decreased Oxygen Affinity: Adaptation to Hypoxia

The uptake of oxygen (VO_2 [ml per min]) by a given tissue or the whole organism can be expressed in the following equation:

$$VO_2 = 1.39 \cdot Q \cdot Hb \cdot (S_aO_2 - S_{\bar{v}}O_2)$$

where 1.39 = the number of ml of O_2 which can bind to 1 g hemoglobin; Hb = the hemoglobin concentration of the blood (g per 100 ml); Q = blood flow (ml per min); and S_aO_2 and $S_{\bar{v}}O_2$ are the per cent saturation of arterial and venous blood, respectively (deVerdier, 1969). During hypoxic stress, VO_2 may be increased by alteration of one or more of these three variables:

1. Increase in blood flow ($\uparrow$ Q).
2. Increase in red cell mass ($\uparrow$ Hb).
3. Decrease in whole blood oxygen affinity ($\uparrow [S_aO_2 - S_{\bar{v}}O_2]$).

A shift to the right (decreased whole blood oxygen affinity) is encountered in various types of hypoxic states (Table 1–2). In each case, the decreased oxygen affinity can be explained by increased levels of red cell 2,3-DPG. In fact, several investigators have shown a close correlation between P_{50} (an index of oxygen affinity) and 2,3-DPG in a number of diverse disorders (Finch and Lenfant, 1972; Oski and Gottlieb, 1971) (Fig. 1–8). It is apparent from such data that

TABLE 1–2. Displacement of the Oxyhemoglobin Dissociation Curve in Various Clinical Disorders (Corrected to pH 7.4)

- I. Shift to the right
  - A. Increase in red cell 2,3-DPG
    1. High altitude adaptation
    2. Pulmonary hypoxemia
    3. Cardiac right to left shunt
    4. Severe anemia; decrease in red cell mass
    5. Congestive heart failure
    6. Decompensated hepatic cirrhosis
    7. Thyrotoxicosis
    8. Hyperphosphatemia (ATP also increased)
  - B. Functionally abnormal hemoglobin variants
- II. Shift to the left
  - A. Decrease in red cell 2,3-DPG
    1. Septic shock
    2. Severe acidosis
    3. Following transfusion of stored blood
    4. Hypophosphatemia
    5. Panhypopituitarism
    6. Neonatal respiratory distress syndrome
  - B. Functionally abnormal hemoglobin variants
  - C. Methemoglobinemia
  - D. Carbon monoxide intoxication

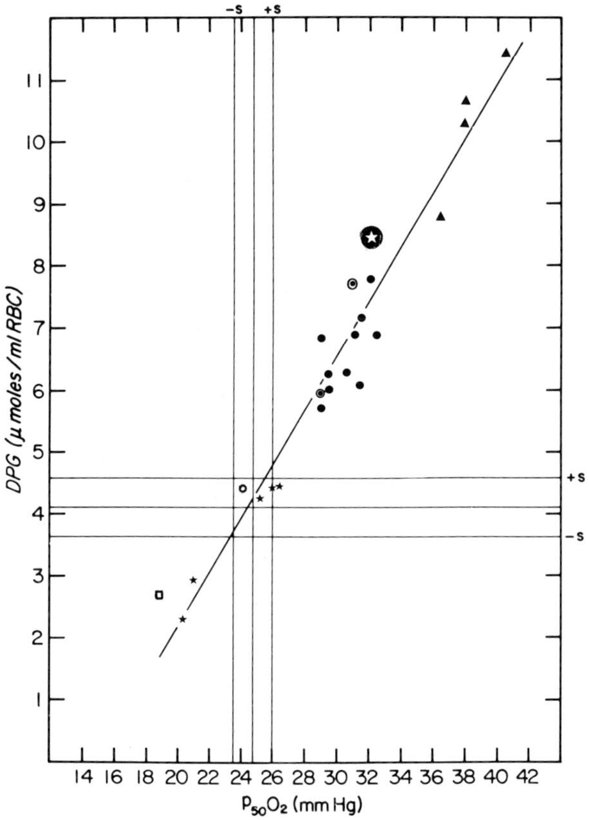

Figure 1–8. Correlation between alterations in red cell 2,3-DPG and P_{50} in a variety of clinical disorders: cyanotic congenital heart disease ●, pyruvate kinase deficiency ▲, hexokinase deficiency □, septic shock ★; postseptic shock ✪, thyrotoxicosis ◉, glucose-6-phosphate dehydrogenase deficiency ○. (From Oski, F. A., Gottlieb, A. J., et al.: Med. Clin. North Am. *54*:731, 1970.)

a decreased whole blood oxygen affinity, mediated through increased red cell 2,3-DPG, is a rather general phenomenon in a variety of hypoxic states.

2,3-DPG levels are quite variable in patients with chronic lung disease. It is difficult to assess the physiologic significance of the oxygen-binding curve in these individuals, since there may be concomitant respiratory acidosis (see below).

The regulation of the intracellular concentration of 2,3-DPG is poorly understood. (This subject is discussed in detail in Oski and Gottlieb, 1971 and in Rørth et al., 1972.) In particular, it is not clear how red cell 2,3-DPG can increase as much as twofold in various hypoxic states. One contributing factor may be an increase in intracellular pH. Patients with hypoxia of varying sorts commonly have respiratory alkalosis. Secondly, if there is an increase in the amount of oxygen extracted per red cell, intracellular pH will increase slightly because of the Bohr effect. Alkalosis not only stimulates glycolysis in

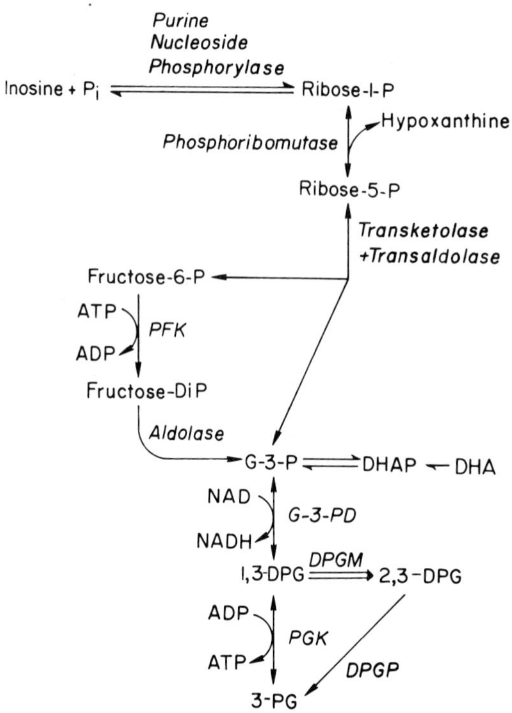

Figure 1–9. The pathway of red cell inosine metabolism to 2,3-DPG. Also shown in this figure is the Rapoport-Luebering cycle, wherein 1,3-DPG can be converted to 3-PG either directly or via 2,3-DPG. The conversion of dihydroxyacetone (DHA) to dihydroxyacetone phosphate (DHAP) is also shown. PFK, phosphofructokinase; G-3-PD, glyceraldehyde-3-phosphate dehydrogenase; PGK, phosphoglycerate kinase; DPGM, diphosphoglycerate mutase; DPGP, diphosphoglycerate phosphatase; P_i, inorganic phosphate; G-3-P, glyceraldehyde-3-phosphate; 3-PG, 3-phosphoglycerate. (From Oski, F. A., Travis, S. E., et al.: Blood 37:52, 1971, by permission of Grune & Stratton.)

general but may also affect the relative degree of 2,3-DPG formation and catabolism via the Rapoport-Luebering cycle (see Figure 1–9). A decreased oxygen saturation may also enhance red cell 2,3-DPG because of the specific binding of this organic phosphate to deoxyhemoglobin. The resulting fall in the intracellular concentration of free 2,3-DPG would relieve product inhibition of diphosphoglycerate mutase, thereby stimulating its own synthesis (Oski et al., 1970). There are two additional factors which may influence the level of 2,3-DPG within red cells:

1. 2,3-DPG falls during in-vivo cell aging (Bunn et al., 1969b). This may explain why patients with hypoplastic anemia and a relatively old population of red cells have somewhat lower 2,3-DPG than those with hemolysis and a comparable degree of anemia (Humpeler et al., 1974; Opalinski and Beutler, 1971).

2. Hormones may influence the absolute level of 2,3-DPG within the red cell. Increased red cell 2,3-DPG is encountered in patients with thyrotoxicosis (Oski and Gottlieb, 1971). Low levels are found in patients with panhypopituitarism (Rodriguez and Shahidi, 1971) but not in those with myxedema (unpublished observation). The administration of androgens to patients with chronic renal failure can cause a 60 per cent increase in red cell 2,3-DPG (Parker et al., 1972).

Although decreased oxygen affinity of blood containing normal hemoglobin is generally due to increased 2,3-DPG, some exceptions have been reported. A small shift to the right (1 to 3 mm Hg) has been observed in coronary sinus blood of patients with angina pectoris during atrial pacing (Shappell et al., 1970). This phenomenon could not be explained by any measurable increase in 2,3-DPG. Patients with hereditary spherocytosis who have undergone splenectomy have normal red cell 2,3-DPG but reduced whole blood oxygen affinity (shift to the right of 2.6 mm Hg) (Fernandez and Erslev, 1972).

The fact that decreased red cell oxygen affinity is so commonly found in hypoxic states does not constitute proof that the phenomenon is adaptive or beneficial to the organism. Is the position of the oxyhemoglobin dissociation curve an important determinant of tissue oxygenation? This question defies an easy answer. It is a technical challenge to monitor oxygen uptake at the cellular level. Clearly, there is a marked PO_2 gradient between the red cell and various intracellular organelles, such as mitochondria. Therefore, it is difficult to say what constitutes a critical PO_2 for various tissues. Recently, Oski and his associates (1971) have addressed themselves to this problem by comparing the hemodynamics of two teen-agers whose oxygen dissociation curves were abnormally fixed because of congenital red cell enzyme defects. Patient 1, with hexokinase deficiency, had a low red cell 2,3-DPG and consequently a left-shifted curve. In contrast, patient 2, with pyruvate kinase deficiency, had an elevated red cell 2,3-DPG and a right-shifted curve. Both individuals were equally anemic. However, patient 1 was a semi-invalid, while patient 2 had no appreciable limitations. During graded exercise, the patient with

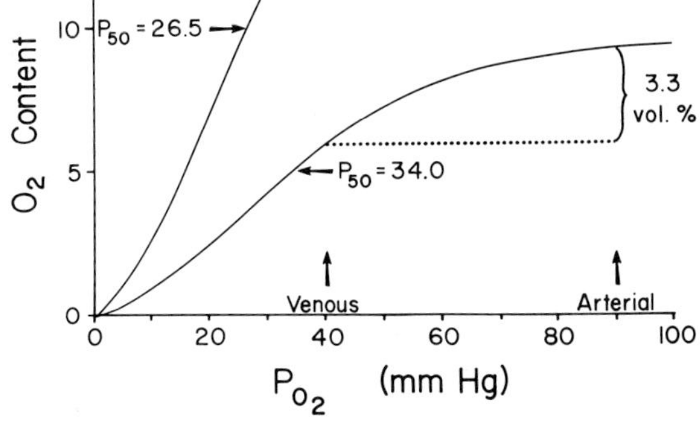

Figure 1–10. Enhancement of oxygen unloading by decreased red cell oxygen affinity in a patient with anemia. Anemic patient with a 50 per cent reduction in hemoglobin concentration has only a 27 per cent reduction in oxygen unloading. (From Klocke, R. A.: Chest *69*:795, 1972.)

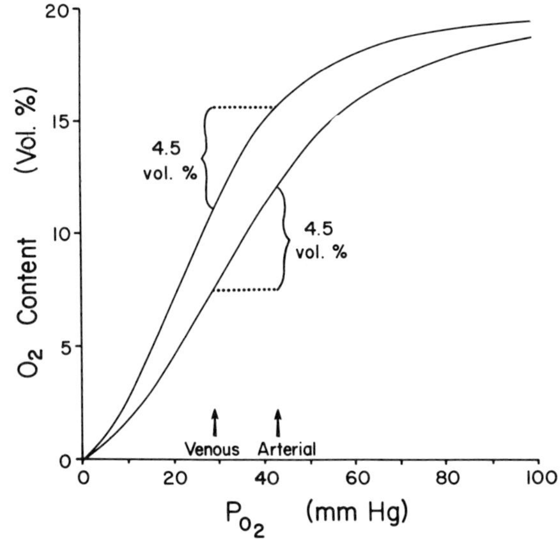

Figure 1–11. Failure of right-shifted oxygen binding curve to enhance oxygen unloading in patients with arterial hypoxemia. (From Klocke, R. A.: Chest 62:795, 1972.)

the left-shifted curve experienced a prompt fall in mixed venous PO_2 and a more marked increase in cardiac output.

As Figure 1–10 shows, the decreased oxygen affinity of blood from a patient with anemia provides a marked enhancement of oxygen delivery to tissues. This is not true, however, for individuals with arterial hypoxemia such as those adapted to high altitude or patients with severe chronic obstructive lung disease. As Figure 1–11 shows, when the arterial PO_2 is significantly decreased, the right-shifted curve provides no significant enhancement in oxygen unloading. Thus, not all types of patients with hypoxia derive benefit from having decreased oxygen affinity.

The position of the oxygen dissociation curve appears to be one important determinant of red cell mass, presumably via erythropoietin control. From a comparison of various hemolytic disorders, Bellingham and Huehns (1968) showed a strong correlation between hemoglobin level and oxygen affinity. The polycythemia secondary to high-affinity hemoglobin variants also attests to this relationship (see Chapter 6).

Increased Oxygen Affinity

From considerations developed here, it appears that increased whole blood oxygen affinity may lead to relative tissue hypoxia. In addition to the congenital disorders discussed above, a "shift to the left" may be encountered in a number of acquired conditions (Table 1–2). As previously noted, the concentration of 2,3-DPG in the red cell is markedly pH-dependent. Accordingly, patients with severe acidosis generally have low 2,3-DPG. The pH "corrected" oxygen dissociation curves of patients with acidosis are left-shifted. However, their in-vivo curve may be normally placed because the Bohr effect counterbalances the reduction in red cell 2,3-DPG. If metabolic acidosis is rapidly corrected by the infusion of bicarbonate, the prompt rise in blood pH is reflected in a proportional increase in oxygen affinity (the Bohr effect). However, there is a lag of several hours before the red cell 2,3-DPG increases to normal (Bellingham et al., 1970). During this time there is a "shift to the left" in both the in-vivo and the in-vitro oxygen dissociation curves. This phenomenon may compromise tissue oxygenation in patients who have diminished cardiovascular reserves. Low red cell 2,3-DPG has been documented in patients with septic shock (Chillar, 1971; Oski and Gottlieb, 1971). This may be in part because of concomitant metabolic acidosis. The resulting left shift in the oxyhemoglobin dissociation curve probably accounts for the increased mixed venous oxygen content often encountered in this condition. Again, an increase in blood oxygen affinity may have untoward effects in patients who already have severe circulatory dysfunction. Low red cell 2,3-DPG may be a grave prognostic sign in patients with sepsis.

In addition to metabolic acidosis, acquired deficiency of red cell 2,3-DPG (and ATP) may also be encountered in patients who have hypophosphatemia, due either to diarrhea (Jacob and Amsden, 1971; Lichtman et al., 1971) or to inadequate phosphate supplements during hyperalimentation (Travis et al., 1971). In both instances, the expected shift to the left has been observed.* In addition hemolysis may occur in association with rigid red cells (Jacob and Amsden, 1971). Finally, as mentioned above, low red cell 2,3-DPG has been found in patients with pituitary insufficiency (Rodriguez and Shahidi, 1971).

During the first week of storage of blood in acid-citrate-dextrose (ACD), red cells become depleted of 2,3-DPG and, as a result, have increased oxygen affinity (Akerblom et al., 1968; Bunn et al., 1969b; Valtis and Kennedy, 1954). Thus, patients who are transfused with large amounts of such blood will have a "left-shifted" oxyhemoglobin dissociation curve (Valtis and Kennedy, 1954). The clinical significance of this phenomenon has not been established. At the least, it is safe to say that the recipient does not derive the full physiologic benefit from blood depleted in 2,3-DPG. Following infusion of such donor cells into normal volunteers, their content of 2,3-DPG returns to normal within 6 to 24 hours (Beutler and Wood, 1969; Valeri and Hirsch, 1969). Considerable attention is now being focused on ways of

---

*In contrast, the slight but significant shift to the right encountered in normal children may be due to physiologically increased levels of plasma phosphate, resulting in a marked increase in red cell ATP and a modest increase in red cell 2,3-DPG (Card and Brain, 1973).

modifying storage media in order to preserve red cell 2,3-DPG and normal hemoglobin function. 2,3-DPG and P_{50} are better maintained in citrate-phosphate-dextrose (CPD), because of the higher pH of this medium (Huisman et al., 1969). The addition of inosine to the storage medium provides ribose-1-phosphate, a substrate which feeds directly into the glycolytic pathway (Fig. 1–9). The resulting increase in 2,3-DPG is potentiated by the addition of pyruvate or methylene blue, both of which oxidize NADH to NAD, thereby providing cofactor for the glyceraldehyde-3-phosphate dehydrogenase reaction (Oski et al., 1971). The transfusion of large amounts of blood stored in inosine may be limited by hyperuricemia resulting from the catabolism of this purine. More recently, dihydroxyacetone has been shown to be an effective additive, enabling the maintenance of 2,3-DPG and ATP during storage (Wood and Beutler, 1974) (Figure 1–9).

The oxygen affinity of fetal blood is substantially higher than that of maternal blood ($P_{50} = 19$ mm Hg compared with 26 mm Hg for normal maternal blood). This difference may be of physiologic importance in facilitating the transport of oxygen across the placenta. The content of 2,3-DPG in the red cells of the newborn is at least as high as that of maternal red cells. Furthermore, phosphate-free hemoglobins A and F have nearly the same oxyhemoglobin dissociation curves. The higher oxygen affinity of fetal blood is due to the fact that 2,3-DPG interacts less strongly with Hb F than with Hb A (Bauer et al., 1968). This can be explained by a comparison of the primary structure of the β and γ chains. β143-Histidine of Hb A has been shown to be an important binding site for 2,3-DPG (see above). In Hb F, γ143 is serine. This uncharged residue would not participate in electrostatic binding with 2,3-DPG.

ACQUIRED ABNORMALITIES OF HEMOGLOBIN STRUCTURE AND FUNCTION

Hemoglobinopathies are generally classified among the "inborn errors of metabolism." Indeed, the genetic bases for these disorders are well understood, and these disorders will be discussed in subsequent chapters. However, a number of acquired abnormalities of hemoglobin structure and function also deserve consideration. Some, such as methemoglobinemia and carbon monoxide poisoning, involve specific alterations of heme, the prosthetic group of the molecule. In contrast, acquired hemoglobin abnormalities may accompany such diverse entities as myeloproliferative disorders, diabetes mellitus, and lead poisoning.

METHEMOGLOBINEMIA

Congenital methemoglobinemia is due to a deficiency of NADH-dependent methemoglobin reductase (diaphorase I). Acquired methemoglobinemia is generally due to exposure to an agent capable of oxidizing heme iron to the ferric state. It has been demonstrated recently that individuals heterozygous for diaphorase I deficiency are much more likely than normals to develop clinically apparent methemoglobinemia following exposure to an oxidant stress (Cohen et al., 1968).

The extent of methemoglobinemia depends not only on the dose of the toxic agent but also on the susceptibility of the exposed individual. If methemoglobin exceeds 1.5 g per 100 ml (10 per cent of the total hemoglobin), cyanosis is readily apparent. At a methemoglobin level of about 35 per cent, the affected individual becomes symptomatic, experiencing headache, weakness, and breathlessness. Levels in excess of 70 per cent are incompatible with life.

The toxicity of methemoglobinemia can be readily explained in terms of our current understanding of hemoglobin function, as outlined in the beginning of this chapter. The fact that a certain proportion of hemes is no longer able to bind oxygen is not a serious physiologic handicap per se. Thirty per cent methemoglobinemia is much more deleterious than a 30 per cent decrement in red cell mass, because the oxidized hemes have a profound effect on the remaining functional hemes in the hemoglobin tetramer. The conformation of methemoglobin (as well as that of carboxyhemoglobin and of cyanmethemoglobin) is very close to that of oxyhemoglobin. Thus, a partially oxidized hemoglobin tetramer has the same tertiary and quaternary structure as a molecule which is comparably oxygenated. In each case, the affinity of the remaining hemes for oxygen is increased. For this reason, methemoglobinemia (as well as carbon monoxide [see below and Table 1–2]) causes a "shift to the left" of the oxyhemoglobin dissociation curve and, consequently, impairs unloading of oxygen to tissues. Recent high-resolution electrophoretic analysis has indicated that in hereditary methemoglobinemia both the α- and β-chain hemes are oxidized to an approximately equal extent (Bunn, 1973). However, there appears to be a heterogeneous distribution of methemoglobin among red cells in individuals with this disorder, the older red cells containing more methemoglobin (Feig et al., 1972; Keitt et al., 1966; Schwartz et al., 1972). Both congenital and acquired (toxic) methemoglobinemia can be readily reversed by the administration of methylene blue.

Carbon Monoxide Intoxication

Carbon monoxide (CO) has received belated recognition as an important and widespread industrial pollutant and toxin. This gas may be engendered from the combustion of any organic material but, in particular, that of hydrocarbons such as petroleum and tobacco tar.

In addition, one mole of CO is formed endogenously in the breakdown of heme into bile pigment. Accordingly, individuals with significant hemolysis or ineffective erythropoiesis have a measurably increased amount of circulating carboxyhemoglobin.

Like oxygen, CO is a ligand which binds reversibly to hemoglobin when heme iron is in the reduced (ferrous) state. The toxicity of CO is due to its very high affinity for heme, approximately 210 times that of oxygen. Following an acute exposure, CO remains so tightly bound to hemoglobin that about four hours are required for an individual with normal ventilation to expel half of it. Because of its slow disappearance time, a toxic level of carboxyhemoglobin may accumulate from continued exposure to a relatively low dose of CO. CO also binds to other heme proteins, such as cytochrome P-450. Whether this contributes significantly to the toxicity of CO is not yet known.

As expected, the clinical manifestations of CO intoxication are directly related to the duration and extent of exposure. Impaired visual and time discrimination have been documented in individuals with carboxyhemoglobin levels of 5 per cent (Coburn, 1970). Above approximately 20 per cent carboxyhemoglobin, more overt and subjective symptoms develop, such as headache, weakness, and so forth (Coburn, 1970). At levels of 40 to 60 per cent, unconsciousness is followed by death. Like methemoglobinemia, the toxic effect of CO is primarily due to increased oxygen affinity of the blood.

The mechanism by which CO shifts the oxyhemoglobin dissociation curve to the left is identical to that of methemoglobin (see above). However, a given per cent carboxyhemoglobin appears to be more deleterious than a comparable level of methemoglobin. This may be because of a more even distribution of CO among red cells of all ages.

The treatment of carbon monoxide intoxication is directed primarily at removing the source of toxic exposure and facilitating the expulsion of the gas by the lungs. Thus, it is very important to maintain adequate ventilation. If the patient is transferred from room air to 100 per cent oxygen, the disappearance half-time for CO is reduced from four hours to one hour. Other therapeutic approaches, such as hyperbaric oxygen or exchange transfusion, may have theoretical merit but are not readily available.

Acquired Alterations of Globin Structure

Minor hemoglobin components may increase in certain hematologic disorders. As mentioned previously, Hb A_2 may be elevated in megaloblastic anemia. Hemoglobin F may reach levels of about 5 per cent in such diverse diseases as aplastic anemia and pernicious anemia. Much higher levels of hemoglobin F have been encountered in children with chronic myelogenous leukemia. Finally, there are now several case reports of myeloproliferative disease, in which up to 10 per cent Hb H (β_4) has been documented (Hamilton et al., 1971).

Hemoglobin A_{Ic}, the "main" minor component of normal adults, is significantly increased in diabetics (Rahbar, 1968; Trivelli et al., 1971). This association is of considerable interest, since this hemoglobin is a glycoprotein having a glucose molecule covalently linked to the N terminus of the β chain.

In some children with plumbism, an abnormal hemoglobin of rapid (anodal) electrophoretic mobility has been documented (Charache and Weatherall, 1966). This component was more frequently observed in those children with hypochromic red cells. The hemoglobin did not contain any measurable lead. It is possible that the lead exposure in some way mediated oxidation of globin sulfhydryl groups. However, the abnormal component differed electrophoretically from the mixed disulfide which can be formed in vitro from hemoglobin and glutathione (Charache and Weatherall, 1966). Thus, the structure of this acquired hemoglobinopathy is not yet known. The abnormal hemoglobin may contain iron-free protoporphyrin groups in place of heme.

Chapter 2

THE THALASSEMIAS AND THE MOLECULAR GENETICS OF HUMAN HEMOGLOBIN SYNTHESIS

MOLECULAR GENETICS OF HUMAN HEMOGLOBIN SYNTHESIS

NORMAL HUMAN HEMOGLOBINS AND THEIR GENES

The protein portion of the various normal human hemoglobin molecules (Table 1–1) is made up of two α (or α-like) and two non-α polypeptide chains which are the products of separate and distinct genes or genetic loci.

Two embryonic hemoglobins, Gower-1 (? ϵ_4 or $\zeta_2\epsilon_2$) and Gower-2 ($\alpha_2\epsilon_2$), contain epsilon chains and are found only during the first 10 to 12 weeks of fetal development (Huehns et al., 1961, 1964; Hecht et al., 1966; Lorkin, 1973). They are presumably synthesized by erythroid cells derived from the yolk sac (Yoffey, 1971; Weatherall et al., 1974). Oxygen dissociation studies (Huehns and Farooqui, 1975) suggest that Hb Gower-1 may consist of two zeta chains and two epsilon chains rather than four epsilon chains, as initially proposed. In embryo and in normal cord blood (in trace amounts) one can detect another embryonic hemoglobin, Hb Portland-1 (Capp et al., 1967, 1970; Hecht et al., 1967), which is composed of two α-like chains (zeta chains) and two γ chains ($\zeta_2\gamma_2$). Increased levels of Hb Portland-1 are found in cord blood of infants with α thalassemia:Hb Barts-hydrops syndrome (Weatherall et al., 1970; Todd et al., 1970). The structure of zeta chains has been studied in a number of animal

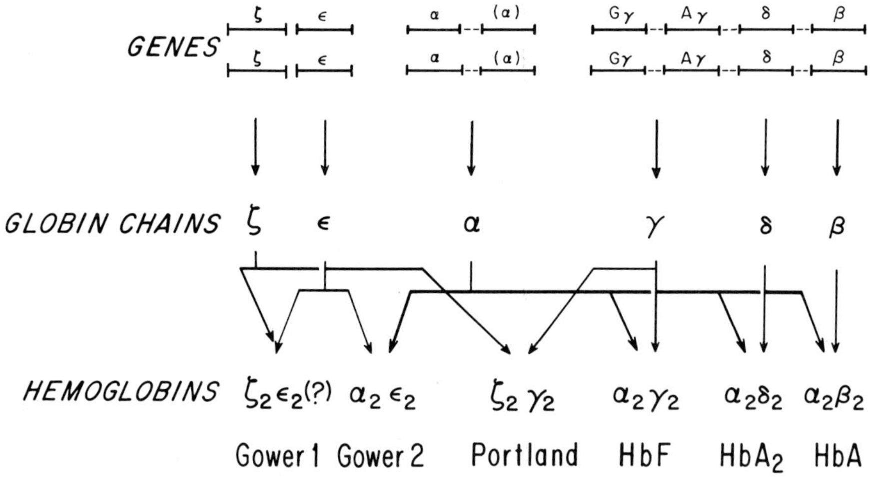

Figure 2–1. Schematic representation of the genes for the different human globin chains and their gene products.

species: it is similar in structure in different species and shares a great deal of homology with the sequence of α globin chains (Melderis et al., 1974). The similarity in structure of human α and ζ chains has led to the conclusion that ζ chains probably constitute an α-like embryonic chain (Kamuzora et al., 1974; Kamuzora and Lehmann, 1975).

Fetal hemoglobin, Hb F, consists of two α and two γ chains, and its appearance coincides with the shift in the site of erythropoiesis from the yolk sac to the liver and spleen. The adult hemoglobins, Hb A ($\alpha_2\beta_2$) and Hb A_2 ($\alpha_2\delta_2$), are normally the predominant hemoglobins present after the first year of life and are synthesized by erythroid precursor cells in the bone marrow. The synthesis of Hb A or Hb F is, however, not strictly limited to cells of marrow vs. liver or spleen origin. There exists at least one pair of allelic genes for each of these globin chains, as illustrated in Figure 2–1, and in the case of the α and γ globin chains there is evidence of gene duplication.

Alpha-chain Genes

Duplication of the α-chain locus has been demonstrated in many animal species, but there is still some controversy over the existence (or the incidence) of duplication of the human α-chain structural gene (Wasi, 1973). The most convincing evidence in favor of α-chain gene duplication consists of reports of families in which individuals have two different α-chain variants in addition to Hb A: (1) in a Hungarian family, three siblings were found to be heterozygous for two different α-chain variants (Hb J-Buda and Hb G-Pest) and still had approximately 50 per cent Hb A (Hollan et al., 1972); (2) in a number of individuals from a tribe in India two different α-chain variants (Hb Rampa and Hb Koya Dora) were found in addition to normal Hb A (DeJong et al., 1975); (3) red cells of an individual of black ancestry who was doubly heterozygous for the α-chain variants Hb G-Philadelphia and Hb-Seal Rock also contained Hb A (Bradley et al., 1975); (4) a presumed homozygote for the α-chain variant Hb Constant Spring also had substantial amounts of Hb A (Lie-Injo, 1974). The finding of two abnormal α chains in addition to normal α chains in heterozygotes for the α-chain variant Hopkins-2 has been used as further evidence of duplication of the human α gene (Ostertag et al., 1972b). The genetics of the α-thalassemia syndromes, especially Hb H disease (Lehmann and Carrell, 1968; Kattamis and Lehmann, 1970; Lehmann, 1970) in association with Hb Constant Spring (Wasi, 1973), also strongly support the concept of α-chain duplication without providing conclusive evidence for it. Finally, α-chain duplication is suggested by the fact that heterozygotes for most (but not all) α-chain variants have a lower percentage of the abnormal hemoglobin than do heterozygotes for β-chain structural variants (Lehmann and Carrell, 1968, 1969; White, 1972) (see Figure 3–4).

The evidence against α-chain gene duplication is the finding, in a Melanesian family, of the absence of Hb A in two homozygotes for the α-chain variant Hb J-Tongariki (Abramson et al., 1970). Three other individuals homozygous for Hb J-Tongariki have been found in New Guinea and they all lack Hb A (Beaver et al., 1972). Absence of Hb A in a patient homozygous for Hb G-Philadelphia, in Hb Q/α thalassemia (reviewed by Wasi, 1973) and in one case of Hb G/α thalassemia (Rieder et al., 1976) also favors the theory of a single α-chain locus, unless one postulates the existence of an α-thalassemia gene in cis with the α-chain variant (Wasi, 1973).

On the basis of all this evidence, one must conclude that α-chain gene duplication almost certainly occurs in some, but not necessarily all, human populations. Variations in the levels of the variant Hb present in black patients heterozygous for Hb G-Philadelphia (Baine et al., 1976) and in Algerian patients with Hb J-Mexico (Trabuchet et al., 1976) suggest, in fact, that even in individuals of the same race, there may be heterogeneity in the number of α-chain loci (see later section in this chapter).

Gamma-chain Genes

The presence of at least two structural genes for the gamma chain has been established by the finding, in individuals of a number of different populations, of two types of γ chains which have either glycine or alanine in position 136 of their amino acid sequence (Schroeder et al., 1968, 1972); these two different γ chains are referred to as the $^{G}\gamma$ and $^{A}\gamma$ chains, respectively. The $^{G}\gamma$ and $^{A}\gamma$ chains are the products of different genes and not due to a post-transcriptional process, because γ-chain variants are of either the $^{G}\gamma$ or the $^{A}\gamma$ type, but not both. The ratio of $^{G}\gamma$ to $^{A}\gamma$ chains in the Hb F of cord blood of neonates is 3:1, whereas in the Hb F of adult blood it is 2:3. When increased fetal hemoglobin is present in the course of various hematological conditions in the adult, either the 3:1 or the 2:3 ratio may be found. The reason for this variable ratio is not known; it may be related to the presence of more than one copy of either or both of the γ genes or may be due to other unknown regulatory mechanisms.

Huisman, Schroeder, and their colleagues (1972) have proposed an interesting model for the number of γ-chain genes, based on the study of the type ($^{A}\gamma$ vs. $^{G}\gamma$) and the relative proportions (% of total Hb F) of the various fetal hemoglobin structural variants (Huisman et al., 1972a; Schroeder et al., 1973). According to this model there would be four nonallelic structural genes for the γ chain: two $^{A}\gamma$ and two $^{G}\gamma$ genes, each with a different quantitative output of a gene product. These genes have been labeled $^{G}{}_{m}\gamma$, $^{G}{}_{l}\gamma$, $^{A}{}_{m}\gamma$, $^{A}{}_{l}\gamma$ (where m and l indicate *m*ore and *l*ess) or $^{G}\gamma$, $^{g}\gamma$, $^{A}\gamma$, $^{a}\gamma$ (where the capital and lower case letters indicate genes with a relatively high or low output of gene product, respectively). These genes would be arranged in the following order on the chromosome (going from N-terminal to C-terminal coding sequences of the genes, or from left to right as in Figure 2–1): $^{G}\gamma$, $^{g}\gamma$, $^{A}\gamma$, $^{a}\gamma$. If the production rate by $^{a}\gamma$ (the lowest output of the four genes) is arbitrarily given a value of one, the proportion of $^{G}\gamma$ and $^{A}\gamma$ in fetal and adult red cells may be explained by the following scheme:

	GENE			
	$^{G}{}_{m}\gamma$	$^{G}{}_{l}\gamma$	$^{A}{}_{m}\gamma$	$^{A}{}_{l}\gamma$
or	$^{G}\gamma$	$^{g}\gamma$	$^{A}\gamma$	$^{a}\gamma$
Production in fetal cells	4	2	2	1
Production in adult cells	0	2	2	1

This model is totally arbitrary and is based on the probably erroneous assumption that the cellular content of an abnormal gene product is directly proportional to the number of genes coding for that protein. The model does, however, provide a plausible explanation for the fact that fetal red cells have a $^{G}\gamma$:$^{A}\gamma$ ratio of approximately 3:1 (70:30), whereas adult red cells have a ratio of 2:3. If it is correct, the model may prove quite useful in furthering our understanding of the fetal to adult hemoglobin "switch" and the distribution of fetal hemoglobin subtypes in hereditary persistence of fetal hemoglobin (HPFH) and thalassemia.

Chromosomal Arrangement of Human Globin Genes

The precise location of the globin-chain genes on human chromosomes is not known. There is a report of presumptive identification of the chromosomes bearing the human globin genes by means of in situ hybridization of radioactive rabbit globin mRNA to metaphase chromosomes of human lymphocytes (Price et al., 1972). However, there are serious criticisms of the work (Bishop and Jones, 1972; Prensky and Holmquist, 1973). There is slight evidence favoring linkage of the beta (and delta) locus with the Duffy blood group locus (Nance et al., 1970), and it is known that the Duffy locus is located on chromosome No. 1 (Donahue et al., 1968). Although there is increased fetal hemoglobin associated with the D1 trisomy (trisomy 13), this is thought to result from a defect in normal fetal maturation rather than being an indication of localization of the gamma genes on chromosome 13 (Wilson et al., 1967; Bard, 1972).

Linkage studies show clearly that the α and β genes are not closely linked to each other and may even be on different chromosomes (Smith and Torbert, 1958; Wong and Huisman, 1972). Localization of α and β genes on different chromosomes has recently been confirmed by analysis of somatic cell hybrids (Deisseroth et al., 1976). However, the beta and delta genes are closely linked to one another as evidenced by the study of a number of families in which both a delta- and a beta-chain variant occur: there was no recombination, in 41 opportunities, between the two loci (Boyer et al., 1963). The occurrence of a delta-beta hybrid globin chain in Hb Lepore (Gerald and Diamond, 1958), presumably the result of a nonhomologous crossover between δ- and β-structural genes (Baglioni, 1962), also supports the close proximity of these two genes. The Lepore globin chain has the N-terminal sequence of the δ chain and the C-terminal sequence of the β chain, and in homozygotes for Hb Lepore, there is total absence of normal Hb A and Hb A_2. These findings definitively situate the δ-chain gene to the N-terminal coding side of the β-chain gene. The origin of the Lepore $\delta\beta$ chain is illustrated diagrammatically in Figure 2–2A and is discussed in detail in Chapter 3; the clinical and biochemical features of this condition are discussed later in this chapter.

The precise location of the γ genes is not certain but there is evidence to indicate close proximity of the γ genes to the β and δ genes:

(1) In families where a β-chain structural variant (or β thalassemia) occurs in association with hereditary persistence of fetal hemoglobin (HPFH), β-chain and HPFH genes behave as alleles, in-

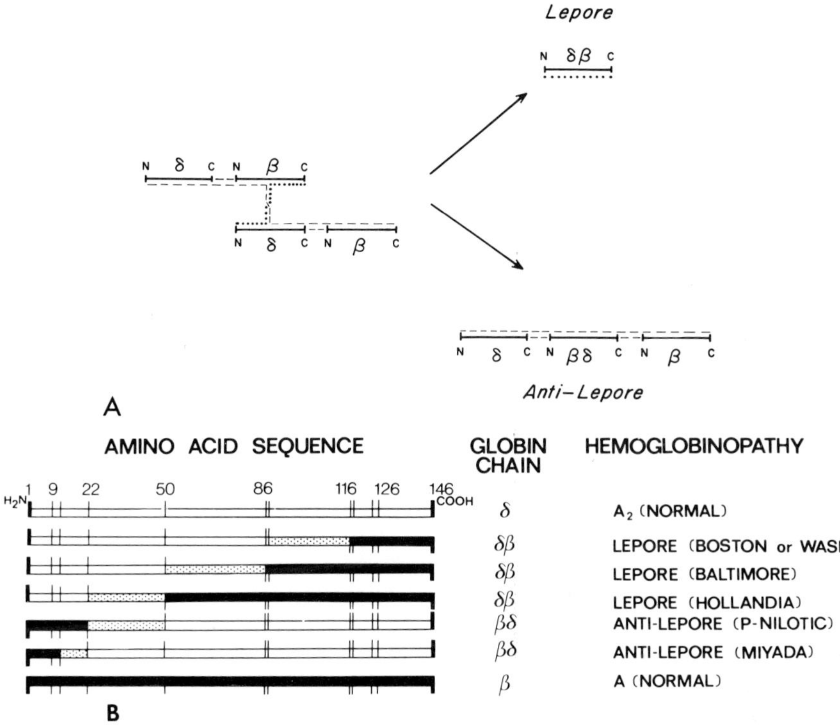

Figure 2–2. A, Origin of the Lepore and anti-Lepore globin chains by nonhomologous crossing over between δ- and β- globin genes. N and C refer to the extremities of the gene coding for the amino-terminal (N) and carboxy-terminal (C) ends of the globin chains. *B*, Different types of Lepore and anti-Lepore globin chains. The numbers refer to the position of amino acid residues in the globin chain: the 10 positions where δ and β sequences differ are indicated by the lighter vertical lines. The dotted area represents the region in which the δβ crossover occurred. (From Benz, E. J., and Forget, B. G.: *In* Brown, E. B. (ed.): Progress in Hematology. Vol. IX, New York, Grune & Stratton, 1975, p. 107. By permission of Grune & Stratton.)

dicating close linkage between the two loci (Weatherall and Clegg, 1972).

(2) In individuals homozygous for HPFH or doubly heterozygous for HPFH and a β- or δ-chain structural variant, there is no synthesis of normal β or δ chain associated with the HPFH gene (Weatherall and Clegg, 1972). This is the so-called "cis-effect," i.e., the β- and δ-chain genes in the cis position of the HPFH gene are usually totally inactive.

(3) Finally, there exists Hb Kenya, a fused γβ globin chain (Huisman et al., 1972b) which has the N-terminal sequence of the γ chain and the C-terminal sequence of the β chain. The Kenya γβ chain presumably resulted from nonhomologous crossing over of the γ- and β-structural genes in a manner analogous to the δβ crossover of Hb Lepore (see Figure 2–3 and Chapter 3). Individuals heterozygous for Hb Kenya (or doubly heterozygous for Hb Kenya and Hb S) synthesize Hb F only of the $^{G}\gamma$ type, presumably from the remain-

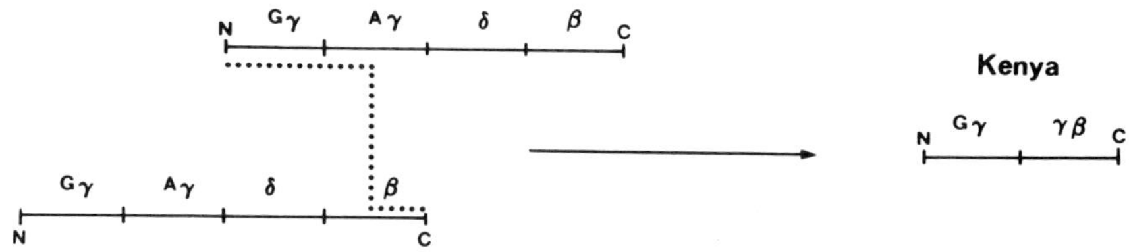

Figure 2–3. Origin of Kenya globin chain by nonhomologous crossing over between γ- and β-globin genes. N and C have the same designation as in Figure 2–2A.

ing intact γ-chain genes in cis to the fused Kenya γβ-chain gene. These findings indicate that the $^{A}\gamma$ gene(s) is involved (or deleted) in the crossover event and is therefore localized (perhaps, but not necessarily, with the $^{G}\gamma$ gene[s] as well) to the N-terminal coding side of the δ- and β-chain genes (Fig. 2–1). The clinical features of the Hb Kenya syndromes are discussed later in this chapter.

The close proximity of the γ-, δ-, and β-chain genes on the same chromosome and the similarities in the amino acid sequences of these globin chains (10 amino acids different out of 146 between δ and β chains and 39 differences between γ and β) support the theory that the δ- and γ-chain genes may have evolved as a result of reduplication of the β-chain gene.

The location and relationship of the epsilon- and zeta-chain genes to one another and to other globin-chain genes are not known.

Changes in Hemoglobin During Development

The time of appearance and relative proportions of the various globin chains present during fetal and neonatal development are schematically represented in Figure 2–4. Alpha chains appear early and persist throughout development. Epsilon chains can be detected in the fetus from an early age but they disappear by the 10th to 12th week of gestation (Huehns et al., 1964; Lorkin, 1973) when γ chains begin to appear in large quantity. The time of onset and pattern of zeta-chain synthesis has not yet been determined in humans; its synthesis probably parallels that of ε chains, but it must persist at a low level in the later stages of fetal development because of the finding of trace amounts of Hb Portland-1 in normal cord blood. Alpha- and γ-chain synthesis predominates after the first 10 to 12 weeks of fetal development. A small amount of β-chain synthesis can be detected in fetuses as early as 6 to 8 weeks of gestation (Hollenberg et al., 1971; Basch, 1972; Kan et al., 1972a; Pataryas and Stamatoyannopoulos, 1972; Kazazian and Woodhead, 1973; Wood and Weatherall, 1973; Cividalli et al., 1974a). However, β chains appear in substantial

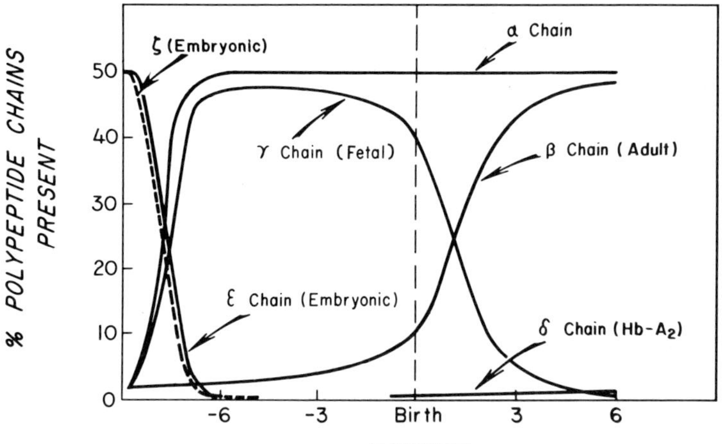

Figure 2–4. Diagrammatic representation of the changes in human globin synthesis during prenatal and neonatal development. (Modified from Beck, W. S. (ed.): Hematology. 2nd ed. Boston, MIT Press, 1976.)

amounts only near term. Studies of globin synthesis in cord blood (Bard et al., 1970; Kan et al., 1972b; Bard, 1975) show that there is approximately one-third to one-half as much β- as γ-chain synthesis at term. During the first 3 months of life, β-chain synthesis rapidly increases as γ-chain synthesis ceases. By 6 months of age β-chain synthesis has usually achieved its maximal adult rate, and γ-chain synthesis is normally reduced to 1 per cent or less of the total hemoglobin. This phenomenon is variable, however (Colombo et al., 1976), and in some normal children higher levels of Hb F (2 to 5 per cent) persist for 12 to 24 months (Chernoff and Singer, 1952). Delta-chain synthesis probably starts only late in the third trimester of intrauterine life, and cord blood contains only trace amounts of Hb A_2. Its synthesis increases gradually during the first 6 to 12 months of life until it reaches the normal adult level (approximately 2.5 per cent of the total hemoglobin). The reason for this low level of δ-gene expression is unknown. As will be discussed later in this chapter in relation to Hb Lepore, the synthesis of δ chains is active only in nucleated erythroid precursor cells and is virtually absent in reticulocytes; the cause of this phenomenon is also unexplained.

The sequence of appearance of the various globin chains is important for the understanding of the development of clinical manifestations in the thalassemia syndromes and other hemoglobinopathies. A deficiency in α-chain or γ-chain synthesis should be obvious at birth, whereas β-chain deficiency will not become clinically manifest until several months of age. Similarly, β-chain structural variants such as Hb S will not accumulate in sufficient quantities to cause clinical symptoms until the latter half of the first year of life. On the other hand, the low but measurable levels of β-chain synthesis in normal fetuses make possible the prenatal diagnosis of β-chain hemoglobinopathies before the 20th week of gestation (see later section in chapter).

There is definite physiological advantage for the developing fetus to have Hb F rather than Hb A. Hemoglobin F, because of its structure and its decreased ability to bind 2,3-DPG, has a relatively high oxygen affinity. Therefore, in the low oxygen tension environment of the placenta, Hb F can effectively compete with Hb A for its oxygen. The high O_2 affinity of fetal red cells, however, does not appear to prevent adequate oxygenation of fetal tissues because the PO_2 of fetal tissues is very low (as low as 15 mm Hg), and this allows approximately 50 per cent extraction of oxygen. The presence of fetal red cells, however, is not totally essential for fetal viability and oxygenation: complete intrauterine exchange with adult red cells still allows the fetus to go to term.

The possible biological or physiological significance of Hb A_2 and the embryonic hemoglobins is unknown.

The Switchover from Fetal to Adult Hemoglobin Synthesis

The mechanism of the "switch" from γ- to β-chain synthesis is unknown. The switch seems to be regulated more by gestational age than by the extrauterine environment, since prematurity seems to have little effect on the process (Bard, 1971, 1973). However, various forms of anoxia (Cooper and Hoagland, 1972), intrauterine growth retardation (Bard, 1970), maternal anoxia (Bromberg et al., 1956), and the D1 trisomy syndrome (Wilson et al., 1967; Bard, 1972) seem to delay the switch. The cord blood of infants with erythroblastosis fetalis contains increased amounts of Hb A compared to normal cord blood (Cooper and Hoagland, 1972; Fraser, 1972). However, this finding is not universal (Bhoyroo and Storrs, 1971), and it is not related to the actual levels of synthesis of γ and β chains by the reticulocytes of the infants: the relative amounts of Hb A and Hb F synthesized are not different from those of normal neonates of the same gestational age (Bard et al., 1971; Kan et al., 1972b). The preponderance of Hb A probably results from the destruction of the older Hb F-containing cells. Previous intrauterine transfusion (Bard et al., 1970) or exchange transfusion at birth (Fraser, 1972) does not seem to affect the relative synthesis of Hb A and Hb F at birth or during neonatal development. In normal cord blood, small amounts of Hb Bart's (γ_4) can be detected; this finding suggests that in the γ to β switching process there is some imbalance between α and $\beta + \gamma$ synthesis, with a small relative excess of γ chains produced (Weatherall, 1963). An even greater excess of γ- to α-chain synthesis has been observed during the course of fetal development in sheep (Kazazian et al., 1976).

Once the switch has occurred it is not usually reversible, although in certain medical conditions (Cooper and Hoagland, 1972; Lorkin, 1973) usually associated with some hematological stress, an increase in fetal hemoglobin is observed (see Chapter 1). In such instances the Hb F is heterogeneously distributed among the red cells and usually only a small proportion of the red cells contains significant amounts of Hb F. In the neonatal "switch" there is true reciprocal relationship between Hb A and Hb F production. However, in cases of persistence or reactivation of Hb F synthesis associated with other medical conditions, the synthesis of Hb A does not decrease proportionally, and the Hb F is accumulated as an "extra package" which increases the Hb content of the cell (Weatherall et al., 1974). In certain conditions, however, such as juvenile chronic myeloid leukemia and rare cases of erythroleukemia (Weatherall et al., 1968; Maurer et al., 1972; Weatherall et al., 1975b), there is near total reversion to a state of fetal red cell protein synthesis, with a decrease in Hb A and Hb A_2, a decrease in carbonic anhydrase and I-antigen titer, and an increase in i-antigen titer.

Changes in the types of hemoglobin synthesized during fetal development are associated with changes in the site of erythropoiesis. Embryonic hemoglobins are presumably synthesized in cells of yolk sac origin; fetal hemoglobin is synthesized when erythropoiesis is maximal in liver and spleen but adult hemoglobin synthesis increases when erythropoiesis shifts from liver and spleen to bone marrow. However, there is no evidence that the type of hemoglobin synthesized by an erythroid cell is strictly determined by the site or organ of its origin. In fact, fetal and adult hemoglobins are both present in many neonatal red cells (Shepard et al., 1962; Tomada, 1964). Furthermore, the ratio of Hb F to Hb A synthesis is the same in fetal erythroid cells derived from marrow, liver, and spleen at all stages of development (Wood and Weatherall, 1973). When extramedullary hematopoiesis develops in the adult there is rarely a significant amount of fetal hemoglobin synthesis. Furthermore, when increased fetal hemoglobin synthesis occurs in the course of various hematological disorders, there is rarely any associated extramedullary hematopoiesis. Another striking example of the lack of site specificity of fetal hemoglobin synthesis is the finding that in leukemic patients recovering from chemotherapy and in patients receiving homologous adult bone marrow transplants, there is an initial burst of fetal hemoglobin synthesis by the regenerating or engrafted marrow cells which then switches to Hb A synthesis (Alter et al., 1975; Weatherall et al., 1975b).

The finding of increased maternal synthesis of fetal hemoglobin during pregnancy (Pembrey et al., 1973) suggests the possible role of a humoral factor in the control and maintenance of fetal hemoglobin synthesis. There is, however, no definitive information on the possible nature of this putative humoral factor or its origin from either fetus, mother, or placenta. The maternal synthesis of Hb F occurs as a short burst for a few weeks in the first trimester and accounts for approximately 5 per cent of total Hb synthesis during that time; it coincides with the time of peak excretion of human chorionic gonadotropin (Pembrey et al., 1973).

The role of erythropoietin in the control of fetal erythropoiesis and the Hb A→Hb F switch remains controversial. No definite role has been demonstrated for erythropoietin in the activation of neonatal Hb A synthesis. It is generally agreed that yolk sac erythroid cells are insensitive to erythropoietin. However, fetal liver erythroid cells are responsive to the hormone. In humans, fetal liver erythroid cells do show sensitivity to erythropoietin in short-term culture systems (Basch, 1972; Shchory and Weatherall, 1975). The degree of responsiveness varies with the fetal age, but no change in the ratio of Hb A to Hb F synthesis in vitro was observed as a result of the erythropoietin stimulation (Basch, 1972). Nevertheless, erythropoietin can be detected in vivo in blood, urine, and amniotic fluid of human fetuses in the third trimester, and these levels are increased in hypoxic and hemolytic states (Finne and Halvorsen, 1972). These findings suggest that erythropoietin may play a role in the regulation of erythropoiesis in the third trimester of intrauterine life, although its role in the Hb F to Hb A switch remains to be demonstrated.

In sheep and goats, the induction of fetal anemia will result in an increase in erythropoietin levels in the fetuses, probably from an extrarenal source (Zanjani et al., 1974a). Furthermore, the administration of antierythropoietin serum results in suppression of erythropoiesis in fetal sheep (Zanjani et al., 1974b). Bleeding of fetal sheep can actually cause premature activation of the fetal to adult switch (Kazazian et al., 1976) but it is not known if this effect is directly mediated by erythropoietin.

A different type of hemoglobin switching phenomenon in goats and sheep is, however, directly mediated by erythropoietin: the Hb A to Hb C switch which occurs in certain types of sheep and goats when they are made anemic (Blunt and Evans, 1963; Van Vliet and Huisman, 1964). The change of Hb type under the stress of anemia is associated with suppression of the synthesis of β^A chains of Hb A and activation of synthesis of another globin chain, the β^C chain of Hb C, which is different from the non-α chain of ovine fetal Hb (Boyer et al., 1967; Wilson et al., 1966). This phenomenon has been conclusively shown to be mediated by erythropoietin (Thurmon et al., 1970; Adamson and Stamatoyannopoulos, 1973). The switch operates at the level of individual cells and not at a clonal level, since both Hb A and Hb C can be detected in the same red cells (Garrick et al., 1973; Nienhuis and Bunn, 1974). This phenomenon does not represent a true fetal to adult (or adult to fetal) switch but it does provide an experimental system for the study of molecular mechanisms involved in the process of differential globin gene expression.

Another consideration in the control of switching from γ- to β-chain synthesis is whether the γ- and β-chain genes on the same chromosome are active at the same time. Even though neonatal cells individually contain both Hb F and Hb A, it is not known with certainty if all the cells' γ- and β-chain genes are active simultaneously or whether γ-chain synthesis and β-chain synthesis are each specified by a different chromosome. This problem was studied by Kabat (1974) in red cells from neonates heterozygous for Hb S ($\alpha_2\beta_2{}^S$). He found that individual red cells of these infants probably contain either Hb A + Hb S, Hb A + Hb F, or Hb S + Hb F, but not all three hemoglobins simultaneously. He concluded that it is unlikely that γ- and β-chain genes on the same chromosome are simultaneously active in the neonatal period. One can, however, question the sensitivity of the cytological methods used to detect the various hemoglobins. It is possible that very small quantities of a given type of hemoglobin could be present in a given cell but go undetected by purely cytological techniques. Even if this were the case, however, the results still indicate that the majority of the red cells in AS neonates do not contain substantial amounts of all three possible hemoglobins (A, S, and F).

Yet another issue in the fetal to adult hemoglobin switch is the nature of the low level (1 per cent) of Hb F synthesis observed in normal adults. Do most red cells synthesize very low levels of Hb F, or do small numbers of red cells synthesize the bulk of Hb F? Boyer et al. (1975) and Wood et al. (1975) have studied this phenomenon using sensitive immunochemical techniques. The results indicate that normal adults contain small numbers of cells which show substantial immunofluorescence using anti-Hb F antibodies, whereas most cells show no fluorescence. These findings suggest that adult synthesis of Hb F is limited to a small clone of cells. Such fetal clones could expand in response to various hematological stresses.

In hereditary persistence of fetal hemoglobin (HPFH) the fetal to adult hemoglobin switchover does not occur. The red cells of adult black patients homozygous for this disorder contain 100 per cent Hb F. The complete absence of Hb A (and Hb A_2) in such homozygotes indicates that the defect is not simply a failure of switching over from the low levels (10 per cent) of Hb A synthesis in utero to the adult levels; there is a total lack of expression of the affected β (and δ) globin gene. In fact, this condition has been shown, in black homozygotes, to be associated with a β-globin gene deletion

(Kan et al., 1975d; Forget et al., 1976b). HPFH is, however, genetically and biochemically heterogeneous: in some cases, β-chain synthesis in cis to the HPFH gene has been observed. Although most cases of HPFH synthesize both $^{A}\gamma$ and $^{G}\gamma$ chains in the usual *adult* ratio, cases have been described in which only $^{G}\gamma$ or $^{A}\gamma$ chains are synthesized. The genetic, clinical, and biochemical findings observed in HPFH will be discussed in more detail later in this chapter.

In conclusion, we know very little about the precise molecular mechanisms which are involved in the fetal to adult hemoglobin switch in humans. Better knowledge of these mechanisms is of great practical as well as theoretical interest, because the ability to manipulate and preserve γ-chain synthesis into adult life might provide an effective future means of treatment of β thalassemia and other β-chain hemoglobinopathies such as sickle cell anemia.

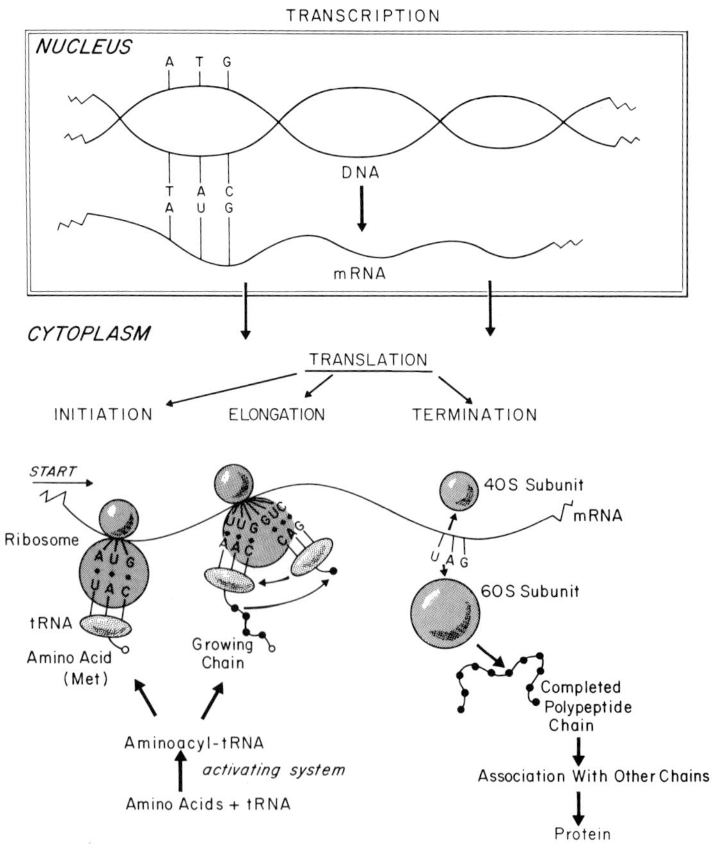

Figure 2–5. Schematic representation of the mechanism of polypeptide-chain synthesis.

MECHANISM OF POLYPEPTIDE-CHAIN SYNTHESIS

The major steps involved in protein synthesis are illustrated schematically in Figure 2–5 and pertain to the synthesis of globin as well as of any other polypeptide chain. The genetic information for the structure of a given protein is encoded in the nucleotide sequence of the DNA, which makes up a gene located on a chromosome within the cell nucleus. Each amino acid is specified by a sequence of three nucleotide bases, called a codon (Table 2–1). A given amino acid can be specified by many different codons, but each codon is specific for only one amino acid and for a different specific transfer RNA (tRNA) molecule necessary for transporting that

TABLE 2–1. *The Messenger RNA Codons for the Various Amino Acids**

Alanine	*Arginine*	*Asparagine*	*Aspartic acid*	*Cysteine*
GCU	CGU	AAU	GAU	UGU
GCC	CGC	AAC	GAC	UGC
GCA	CGA			
GCG	CGG			
	AGA			
	AGG			
Glutamic acid	*Glutamine*	*Glycine*	*Histidine*	*Isoleucine*
GAA	CAA	GGU	CAU	AUU
GAG	CAG	GGC	CAC	AUC
		GGA		AUA
		GGG		
Leucine	*Lysine*	*Methionine*	*Phenylalanine*	*Proline*
UUA	AAA	AUG	UUU	CCU
UUG	AAG		UUC	CCC
CUU				CCA
CUC				CCG
CUA				
CUG				
Serine	*Threonine*	*Tryptophan*	*Tyrosine*	*Valine*
UCU	ACU	UGG	UAU	GUU
UCC	ACC		UAC	GUC
UCA	ACA			GUA
UCG	ACG			GUG
AGU				
AGC				

SPECIAL CODONS

Chain initiation	*Chain termination (nonsense codons)*
AUG	UAA
	UAG
	UGA

*Adapted from Watson, 1970. The first letter shown for each triplet codon represents the 5′ extremity of the mRNA codon. Note that AUG serves both as chain initiation codon and as methionine codon.

amino acid. The genetic information is relayed to the cytoplasm of the cell, where protein synthesis must occur, by the synthesis of a strand of RNA called messenger RNA, or mRNA. The mRNA is complementary to, or the mirror image of, the DNA according to Watson-Crick base pairing (C gives G, A gives U, G gives C, and T gives A). The synthesis of mRNA from DNA by the enzyme RNA polymerase is called the process of transcription.

The mRNA is then transported from the nucleus to the cytoplasm where it binds to ribosomes, which are the subcellular organelles on which protein synthesis occurs. The following process by which the mRNA directs the synthesis of a specific polypeptide chain is called translation, and it involves a number of different steps. The initial step of mRNA binding to ribosomes is called initiation: it is a complex enzymatic reaction which brings together the mRNA; the smaller (40S) ribosomal subunit; a special initiator tRNA, which carries the amino acid methionine; and the larger (60S) ribosomal subunit. The reaction requires a number of separate protein factors (initiation factors), GTP, and ATP. In mammalian systems, just as in bacterial systems, the first amino acid incorporated into a protein chain is methionine, but contrary to the bacterial systems this initial amino acid does not have a blocked (formylated) amino group and it is later cleaved from the nascent polypeptide chain during its elongation. The completed mammalian polypeptide chain, therefore, does not necessarily have an N-terminal methionine.

Once initiated, the synthesis of a protein chain continues by the process of elongation, which involves the sequential addition of amino acids to the initial amino acid by peptide bond formation, resulting in gradual lengthening of the polypeptide chain. Protein synthesis begins at the N-terminal amino acid residue and proceeds toward the C-terminal residue of the polypeptide chain. Each amino acid is brought to its specific position by a specific tRNA to which it is attached (the complex is called aminoacyl-tRNA). The aminoacyl-tRNA binds to the ribosome and the specific codon sequence of the mRNA by a complementary nucleotide sequence of its own, called the anticodon, which is located in a specific site of the tRNA. The nascent peptide chain which is attached to the previous tRNA is transferred to the new tRNA, and a peptide bond is formed with the new amino acid. This new peptidyl-tRNA complex then moves to the position of the previous tRNA, which is released as the ribosome moves along to the next codon. A new aminoacyl-tRNA binds to this new codon, and the process is repeated. This process involves a complex set of reactions which involve many enzyme factors and GTP. Chain elongation continues until the ribosome, traveling down the messenger RNA in "ticker-tape" fashion, reaches a specific nucleotide codon which signifies chain termination, at which time the polypeptide chain is released from the ribosome which dissociates into two subunits and separates from the mRNA. The polypeptide chain then assumes its secondary and tertiary structure and may bind to other polypeptide subunits and other cellular components to form a mature protein. The details of this complicated process of eukaryotic protein synthesis have recently been reviewed (Benz and Forget, 1974).

The synthesis of globin is accomplished by this same basic mechanism. In fact, much of the process of eukaryotic protein synthesis was elucidated by the study of globin-synthesizing cells and cell-free systems. Once synthesized, the globin chains bind heme and combine with one another to form appropriate tetramers of complete hemoglobin molecules.

THE THALASSEMIAS

Definition

The thalassemia syndromes are a group of hereditary disorders in which there is a defect in the synthesis of one or more of the normal polypeptide chains of hemoglobin. This defect causes absent or decreased synthesis of the affected chain. As a result, the erythrocytes have a low intracellular hemoglobin content (hypochromia) and are smaller than normal (microcytosis). In addition, the continued normal synthesis of the unaffected globin chain leads to the accumulation of unstable aggregates of these unmatched chains. These aggregates precipitate within the red blood cell, damage its membrane, and cause its premature destruction in the peripheral circulation or at an earlier stage in the bone marrow. In α thalassemia, synthesis of the α chain of normal adult hemoglobin (Hb A: $\alpha_2\beta_2$) is impaired, whereas in β thalassemia, it is the synthesis of β chains which is reduced or absent.

Incidence and Population Genetics

Thalassemia primarily affects people of Mediterranean, African, and Asian ancestry. However, sporadic cases have been reported in many varied ethnic groups. It is believed that malaria has exerted a selective pressure for the propagation of the thalassemia genes (Weatherall and Clegg, 1972), although the scientific basis for the proposed protection of the thalassemia heterozygote against malaria is unknown.

The actual incidence of thalassemia in various populations can be estimated only on the basis of limited surveys. In Southern

Italian, Sicilian, and Greek populations approximately 10 per cent of individuals are heterozygotes for β thalassemia. On certain Greek islands and in some villages of Sardinia the incidence can reach 20 to 30 per cent. In blacks, fewer than 5 per cent are affected with α or β thalassemia. In Thailand as many as 20 per cent of the population carry the trait for one or another type of thalassemia (Wasi et al., 1969). In Thailand α thalassemia is much more common than β thalassemia, but in other Oriental populations α and β thalassemia are probably equally prevalent.

Genetics of the Thalassemia Syndrome

Alpha and beta thalassemia are inherited as autosomal dominant traits. The location of the α and β thalassemia genes is not known with certainty, but there is good evidence that they are closely linked to the structural genes for the α and β globin chains, respectively. This conclusion is confirmed by the study of the interaction of α and β thalassemia with α and β globin chain structural variants: the genes for β-chain structural variants and β thalassemia behave as alleles, as do the genes for α-chain structural variants and α thalassemia (Weatherall and Clegg, 1972).

There has been no convincing evidence of crossing over between the β-thalassemia and β-structural genes. The study of families in which genes for both β thalassemia and a δ-chain variant coexist makes it possible to evaluate the proximity of these two genes: in four such families, providing 31 opportunities for crossing over between β-thalassemia and δ-structural genes, there is indeed evidence of two likely instances of such a crossover (Pearson et al., 1965; Thompson et al., 1965b). On the other hand, there has been no evidence of recombination, in 50 opportunities, between β-structural and δ-structural genes (Weatherall and Clegg, 1972). These findings suggest that the β-thalassemia gene is located farther away from the δ-structural gene than is the β-structural gene. Further family studies are necessary to confirm this conclusion.

There are only two families which provide genetic evidence for the linkage of the α-thalassemia and α-chain structural loci: in four offspring of two individuals doubly heterozygous for α thalassemia and an α-chain structural variant (Hb I or Hb G-Philadelphia) no crossing over occurred, indicating close linkage of the α-thalassemia to the α-chain structural gene(s) (Atwater et al., 1960; Rieder et al., 1976).

The genetics of α-thalassemia are otherwise quite confusing (reviewed in Weatherall and Clegg, 1972), and much of the confusion centers on whether or not the α-chain locus is duplicated in man and, if it is duplicated, whether the two genes are linked or independent. The evidence for and against α-chain locus duplication was reviewed earlier in this chapter. Study of various α-thalassemia syndromes and the interaction of α thalassemia with α globin chain structural variants has not definitively resolved the issue (see later section in this chapter). However, the genetics of α thalassemia, especially in association with Hb Constant Spring, can be most easily explained if one accepts the presence of duplicated α-chain loci, at least in the Asian population in which α thalassemia is most prevalent. The detailed evidence for this conclusion will be reviewed in the section of this chapter dealing with the various α-thalassemia syndromes.

Molecular Pathology of the Thalassemia Syndromes

As previously stated in this chapter, the thalassemia syndromes are all characterized by absent or decreased synthesis of one or more of the globin chains of human hemoglobin. In those cases where some of the affected globin chain is synthesized, the resulting globin chain is structurally normal (Guidotti, 1962; Baglioni, 1963; Jones and Schroeder, 1963). In this respect, the thalassemia syndromes differ from the other hemoglobinopathies, such as sickle cell anemia, in which a structurally abnormal globin chain is synthesized. The molecular basis of most structural hemoglobin variants is well understood and is discussed in Chapter 3. The precise molecular basis for the quantitative defect in globin-chain synthesis in thalassemia, on the other hand, has not been established in most cases. Nevertheless, a great deal of information has been obtained which clearly implicates certain molecular mechanisms in the pathogenesis of thalassemia. This information will now be reviewed.

STUDIES OF GLOBIN SYNTHESIS IN INTACT THALASSEMIC ERYTHROID CELLS

The thalassemic defect—the imbalance of globin-chain synthesis—was first directly demonstrated in thalassemic cells by three different laboratories between 1964 and 1966 (Heywood et al., 1964, 1965; Weatherall et al., 1965; Bank and Marks, 1966). The technique which was used consists of incubating peripheral blood reticulocytes for 1 to 2 hours in the presence of a radioactive amino acid precursor, usually leucine or valine. Globin is then prepared from the total cell lysate or from the Hb A purified from the lysate by column chromatography. The globin is fractionated by carboxymethyl-cellulose column chromatography in the presence of 8 molar urea, which separates the α, β, and γ globin chains. An example of a chromatogram obtained with globin isolated from normal nonthalassemic peripheral reticulocytes is shown in Figure 2–6*A*. It can be seen that roughly equal amounts of radioactive, newly synthesized α and β chains are found under the α and β globin chain optical density peaks. One can thus obtain a quantitative ratio of β to α globin-chain synthesis (β/α synthetic ratio), which, in a normal cell, will be equal to 1.0. When applied to the study of thalassemic reticulocytes, the initial studies

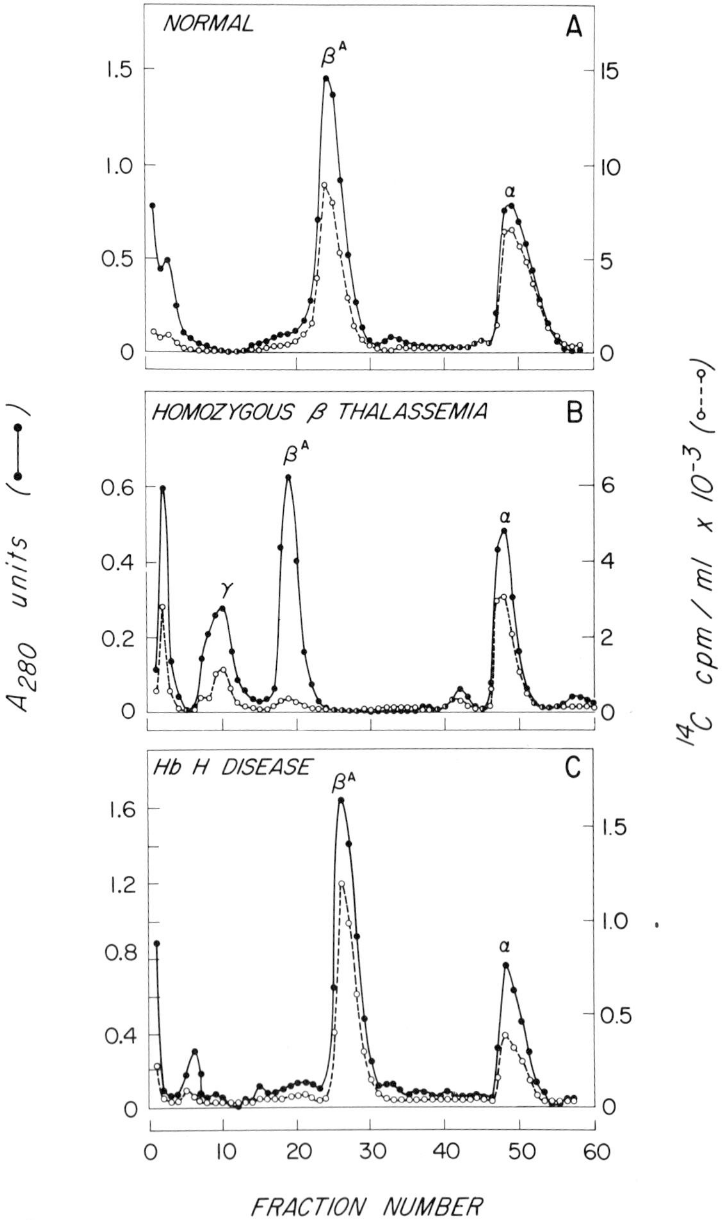

Figure 2–6. Globin synthesis in reticulocytes of patients with nonthalassemic hemolytic anemia, homozygous beta thalassemia, and Hb H disease. Peripheral blood was incubated with ^{14}C-leucine; globin then was prepared from the red cells and fractionated by carboxymethyl cellulose column chromatography. •——• represents optical density of globin chains. ○——○ represents radioactivity incorporated into newly synthesized globin chains.

all demonstrated a decrease in incorporation of radioactivity into the β chain of hemoglobin A in β-thalassemic reticulocytes. Similar studies have since been repeated in a number of laboratories and the results of these studies all indicate marked decrease of β-chain synthesis relative to α-chain synthesis in β thalassemia (Bargellesi et al., 1967; Modell et al., 1969; Weatherall et al., 1969; Conconi et al., 1970).

In the usual heterozygotes for β thalassemia, approximately half as much radioactivity is incorporated into β chains as into α chains, but in American blacks with β-thalassemia trait, the β/α ratio can be virtually normal (Friedman et al., 1972, 1973; Braverman et al., 1973). In homozygotes for β thalassemia, there is either total absence of β-chain radioactivity or a marked decrease in β-chain radioactivity with β/α ratios of 0.1 to 0.3 (Fig. 2–6*B*). It should be pointed out that this technique does not measure absolute rates of α- and β-chain synthesis but expresses only a ratio of one to another. An attempt has been made to express the data in terms of absolute rates (Bank et al., 1968), and the findings are consistent with a normal rate of α-chain synthesis in β thalassemia; therefore the low β/α ratio is due to decreased β-chain synthesis rather than to increased α-chain synthesis.

The same techniques have been applied to the study of α thalassemia (Weatherall et al., 1965; Clegg and Weatherall, 1967; Kan et al., 1968). In severe homozygous α thalassemia (hydrops fetalis with Hb Bart's) there is a total absence of α-chain synthesis (Weatherall et al., 1970). In Hb H disease, a less severe α-thalassemia syndrome, the globin synthesis profile reveals decreased incorporation of radioactivity into α chains compared to β chains (Fig. 2–6*C*), with an α/β ratio of 0.3 to 0.6 (Kan et al., 1968). When globin-chain synthesis is studied in α-thalassemia heterozygotes, a less striking imbalance in globin-chain synthesis is observed in comparison to the β-thalassemia heterozygotes (Kan et al., 1968). In the phenotypically obvious form of heterozygous α thalassemia (α-thal 1 trait), the α/β ratio is 0.70 to 0.80, whereas in the mild form of heterozygous α thalassemia (the "silent carrier" state or α-thal 2 trait), it is 0.80 to 0.95 (Kan et al., 1968). Alpha thalassemia in American blacks does not demonstrate as marked or as consistent an imbalance in globin-chain synthesis (Schwartz and Atwater, 1972).

The range of β/α ratios obtained in a large series of patients with various α- and β-thalassemia syndromes is shown in Figure 2–7.

When globin synthesis was studied in marrow of patients with β thalassemia, interesting observations were made. In homozygous β thalassemia, the β/α synthetic ratio was still abnormal but the value was closer to normal than in the peripheral blood of the same patient (Braverman and Bank, 1969; Friedman et al., 1972). Other workers

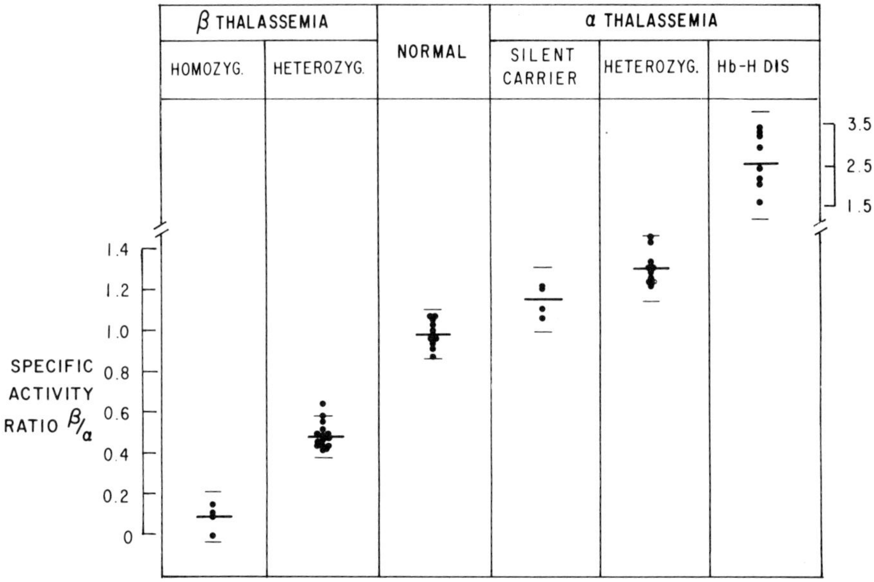

Figure 2–7. Range of values obtained for the ratio of β- to α-chain synthesis in nonthalassemic reticulocytes and in reticulocytes of patients with various α- and β-thalassemia syndromes. (From Nathan, D. G.: N. Engl. J. Med. *286*:586, 1972.)

have not been able to demonstrate such a striking difference between marrow and peripheral blood globin synthesis in β thalassemia (Bargellesi et al., 1967; Shchory and Ramot, 1972; Nienhuis et al., 1973). It is likely that some artifact in the technique is responsible for these discrepancies rather than some fundamental difference in the expression of the β-thalassemic defect between marrow and peripheral blood cells.

In heterozygous β thalassemia, an even more interesting observation has been made by Schwartz (1970). In the marrow of such persons, he found that the β/α synthetic ratio is very close to 1.0. This observation has been confirmed in a number of different laboratories (Clegg and Weatherall, 1972; Gill et al., 1972; Kan et al., 1972c; Shchory and Ramot, 1972; White et al., 1972; Natta et al., 1973; Nienhuis et al., 1973). The findings are difficult to interpret. It is unlikely that there is decreased β-chain synthesis only in reticulocytes and not in marrow, because over 90 per cent of globin-chain synthesis occurs in the marrow, and if decreased β-chain synthesis occurred only at the reticulocyte stage, then the β-thalassemic heterozygotes should not be anemic and their red cells should not be hypochromic and microcytic. Another possible explanation for hypochromia despite relatively equal amounts of α- and β-chain synthesis is that the α-chain synthesis as well as β-chain synthesis is decreased in the marrow cells of patients with heterozygous β thalassemia, whereas in the reticulocytes, the imbalance becomes manifest as α-chain synthesis returns to normal (Nathan, 1973).

There is as yet no experimental evidence to support this type of presumed feedback inhibition of synthesis of the nonaffected globin chain in thalassemia. Studies by Clegg and Weatherall (1972) on globin synthesis in heterozygous β-thalassemia marrow indicate that despite the β/α synthetic ratio of nearly 1.0, there is indeed imbalance between β and α globin chain synthesis in marrow, evidenced by the finding of a large pool of free α globin chains in such marrow cells. The authors postulate two explanations for the finding of β/α synthetic ratios close to 1.0: first, in marrow, nonglobin peptides may co-chromatograph with the β chain, thereby falsely increasing the radioactivity in the β-chain region; second, the authors also provide some evidence that, in vitro, α chains are more unstable in marrow as compared to those in peripheral blood and may undergo proteolysis in time, thereby falsely lowering the radioactivity found in the α-chain peak.

Studies by Wood and Stamatoyannopoulos (1975) failed to demonstrate a contaminating nonglobin peptide, but experiments using purified erythroid precursor cells did demonstrate increased free pools of α chains even in the most immature erythroid precursor cells in heterozygous β thalassemia. Their studies also provided convincing indirect evidence that turnover (? proteolysis) of α chains is the most likely explanation for the unexpected finding of a β/α synthetic ratio of 1.0 in heterozygous β-thalassemia marrow. A more recent report by Chalevelakis et al. (1975) has shown the presence of a minor nonglobin (? marrow granulocyte) protein contaminating the β-chain peak on CMC columns. More importantly, however, in short pulse-labeling experiments the authors demonstrated clearly that the β/α synthetic ratio in heterozygous β-thalassemia marrow changes with time, being abnormal (0.5) after short incubations and nearing unity after longer periods of incubation. Increased α-chain turnover is again implicated as the primary cause of the phenomenon. Assays of globin mRNA in purified nucleated marrow cells of patients with heterozygous β thalassemia have in fact demonstrated the expected deficiency of β mRNA (β/α mRNA content 0.4 to 0.6) (Pritchard et al., 1975).

Recently, cases of heterozygous β thalassemia of unusual severity have been reported in which the marrow β/α synthetic ratio ranges between 0.7 and 0.8 whereas the peripheral blood ratio remains at the usual level of 0.5 (Friedman et al., 1976a; Stamatoyannopoulos et al., 1974).

Molecular Basis of Thalassemia

The details of the normal process of protein and hemoglobin biosynthesis were reviewed earlier (see Figure 2–5). It is easy to see that, in the complex process of protein synthesis, a number of regulatory events could occur which would affect the rate of synthesis of a given protein and result in the presence of decreased amounts of an otherwise structurally normal protein in the cells. Various defects in the process of protein synthesis have been searched for to explain the decreased synthesis of structurally normal globin chains which occurs in thalassemia. This topic has been reviewed in detail elsewhere (Forget, 1974; Forget and Nathan, 1975; Benz and Forget, 1975) and will be summarized here.

If chain termination were defective (abnormally slow), less protein would accumulate in the cell. In thalassemia, however, there is no evidence for slow release of chains from ribosomes to cytoplasm (Clegg et al., 1968). At the level of chain elongation, decreased output of a structurally normal protein chain could result from a nucleotide sequence change (base substitution) in the messenger RNA, which results in its coding, not for a different amino acid, but for a different transfer RNA for the same amino acid; if the specific tRNA were in short supply in the cell, there would result an overall slowing of the rate of synthesis of the affected chain. This is the so-called modulation hypothesis to explain thalassemia (Ingram, 1964; Itano, 1965). However, there is good evidence that this phenomenon does not occur in thalassemia, since pulse-labeling experiments and peptide analysis (Dintzis' plots) of the nascent globin chains in β thalassemia have revealed normal rates of chain assembly and elongation of the β globin chain (Clegg et al., 1968; Rieder, 1972). At the level of initiation, decreased synthesis could occur if there is decreased initiation of the messenger RNA due to an abnormality in the messenger RNA, an abnormality of the ribosome, or abnormalities in the various initiation factors.

The following areas of study have revealed no abnormalities or differences in thalassemic cells compared to nonthalassemic cells: ribosome quantity and radioactive profile or polysomes (Burka and Marks, 1963); effect of added nonthalassemic ribosomal subunits to thalassemic ribosomes (Fuhr et al., 1969); translation by thalassemic ribosomes of synthetic mRNA (poly [U]) (Bank and Marks, 1966) and natural mRNA (rabbit globin mRNA) (Nienhuis et al., 1971); effect of added human and/or rabbit initiation factors to thalassemic ribosomes (Gilbert et al., 1970); the distribution of nascent α and β chains on thalassemic reticulocyte and marrow polysomes, as an index of specific chain initiation and elongation (Nathan et al., 1971; Cividalli et al., 1974b); and the specific mechanism of globin chain initiation (use of initiator tRNA) and initial dipeptide formation (Crystal et al., 1973).

All evidence therefore indicates the presence of a defect in the messenger RNA for the affected globin chain as the basis for the imbalanced globin-chain synthesis which occurs in the thalassemia syndromes. On the basis of the above evidence, the messenger RNA could be either quantitatively deficient or qualitatively (structurally) abnormal in its nontranslated portions. Such a structural defect of the mRNA might lead to more rapid degradation, and eventually concomitant quantitative deficiency of the mRNA, or it might lead to abnormal function of the mRNA such as absent or decreased binding to ribosomes without actual quantitative deficiency of the mRNA. The involvement of globin mRNA in the expression of the thalassemic defect has in fact been directly demonstrated in a number of laboratories (Benz and Forget, 1971; Nienhuis and Anderson, 1971; Benz et al., 1973; Dow et al., 1973; Grossbard et al., 1973; Natta et al., 1973a; Nienhuis et al., 1973)—messenger RNA isolated from thalassemic reticulocytes or marrow cells, when it is translated in a heterologous cell-free protein synthesizing system, will duplicate the imbalance of globin-chain synthesis, which is characteristic of the intact thalassemic reticulocyte. Although these observations demonstrate direct involvement of globin mRNA in the expression of the thalassemic defect, they still do not differentiate between overall quantitative or chemical deficiency of mRNA and simple deficiency of mRNA function. On the other hand, RNA-DNA hybridization studies (Housman et al., 1973; Kacian et al., 1973) and primary structure studies (Forget et al., 1974b; Marotta et al., 1974) of the messenger RNA isolated from thalassemic reticulocytes indicate that the messenger RNA for the affected (thalassemic) globin chain is indeed quantitatively deficient in these reticulocytes.

These latter observations were made possible by use of the RNA-dependent DNA polymerase (or reverse transcriptase) of RNA tumor viruses. This enzyme will synthesize, in vitro, a radioactive DNA copy (cDNA) of globin mRNA. The radioactive cDNAs of α and β mRNA can then be used as probes for the quantitation, in RNA-DNA hybridization experiments, of the relative chemical amounts of α and β mRNA in reticulocyte RNA of thalassemic patients. The cDNA can also be used as a template for RNA polymerase which will synthesize a highly radioactive ^{32}P-labeled RNA copy of the cDNA suitable for nucleotide sequence analysis by standard RNA sequencing techniques. Both of these general approaches were applied to the study of thalassemic mRNA, and both approaches demonstrated quantitative deficiency of β mRNA in β thalassemia and deficiency of α mRNA in α thalassemia (Housman et al., 1973, 1974; Kacian et al., 1973; Forget et al., 1974a, 1974b; Marotta et al., 1974). The results and interpretations of these studies have been reviewed in detail elsewhere (Forget, 1974; Forget and Nathan, 1975; Benz and Forget, 1975).

Subsequent studies have demonstrated even more directly quantitative deficiency of chain-specific globin mRNA in α and β thalassemia. It is possible to separate α from β globin mRNA by acrylamide-gel electrophoresis in the presence of formamide, a solvent which completely denatures nucleic acids. When nonthalassemic globin mRNA is fractionated by this technique, roughly equal amounts of α mRNA and β mRNA are revealed. On the other hand, when α- or β-thalassemic mRNAs are fractionated, marked deficiency of α and β mRNA, respectively, can be demonstrated (Forget et al., 1975a; Kazazian et al., 1975).

The demonstration of quantitative deficiency of globin mRNA in thalassemic reticulocytes and unfractionated marrow cells still leaves open the question of whether the messenger RNA is initially transcribed in abnormally low amounts from the DNA or whether it is transcribed initially in normal amounts but later becomes deficient owing to defects in mRNA processing or transport or to some structural defect which renders it unstable and susceptible to premature degradation. A defect at either the transcriptional or the post-transcriptional level could explain the deficiency of mRNA observed in thalassemia. Studies of globin-chain synthesis in purified β-thalassemic erythroid precursor cells before and after culture and differentiation in vitro indicate that the thalassemic imbalance of globin-chain synthesis is expressed at all stages of red cell maturation in homozygous β-thalassemia (Kim et al., 1976).

A different set of molecular mechanisms could be responsible for the cases of thalassemia in which there is totally absent synthesis of the affected globin chain (β^0 and α^0 thalassemia). A gene deletion and therefore total absence of mRNA could explain the findings, but other mechanisms must be ruled out. One such mechanism is a nonsense mutation in which there is a nucleotide base substitution in the mRNA which converts an amino acid codon into a chain termination codon. In such cases, only a short portion of the affected peptide chain is synthesized and then prematurely released. If this mechanism were responsible for β^0 or α^0 thalassemia, one should find within the cells α or β peptides corresponding to the incomplete chains, assuming there is no proteolytic destruction of the abnormally short chains (Baglioni et al., 1969). Such peptides have been sought but not found in both β^0 thalassemia of the Ferrara type (Dreyfus et al., 1972) and the α^0-thalassemia syndrome of hydrops fetalis with Hb Bart's (Weatherall et al., 1970).

In β^0 thalassemia of patients from Ferrara (Italy) there is evidence that β mRNA may be present in the cells, because β-chain synthesis can apparently be induced in a cell-free system by adding nonthalassemic (β^A or β^S) reticulocyte supernatant fraction to Ferrara-thalassemia ribosomes (Conconi et al., 1972; Rowley and Kosciolek, 1972). The results were interpreted as indicating the deficiency in these patients of a factor necessary for β mRNA translation (Conconi and Del Senno, 1974). These authors have also reported experiments in which the transfusion of blood to patients with β^0 thalassemia of the Ferrara type apparently resulted in the synthesis in these patients of some β chains 10 to 15 days after the transfusion

(Conconi and Del Senno, 1974; Conconi et al., 1975). More recently, RNA-cDNA hybridization assays have confirmed the presence of β-like mRNA in this disorder but in reduced amounts compared to α mRNA (Ramirez et al., 1976; Ottolenghi et al., Nature *266*:231, 1977).

Beta^0 thalassemia is probably genetically and biochemically heterogeneous. Studies of mRNA isolated from reticulocytes of various patients with β^0 thalassemia other than the Ferrara type have shown no evidence of β-chain mRNA activity when the mRNA was translated in various heterologous cell-free protein synthesizing systems (Dow et al., 1973; Nienhuis et al., 1973; Benz et al., 1975b; Kan et al., 1975e; Tolstoshev et al., 1976). On the other hand, RNA-cDNA hybridization studies have given variable results in β^0 thalassemia. In some cases, it is possible to demonstrate virtual absence of β mRNA in β^0 thalassemia (Forget et al., 1974c; Ottolenghi et al., 1975; Tolstoshev et al., 1976). However, in other cases, the hybridization assay does reveal the presence of a significant level of β or β-like mRNA in β^0 thalassemia (Kan et al., 1975e; Ramirez et al., 1976; Forget et al., 1976c). It is therefore unlikely that cases of β^0 thalassemia are due to gene deletions. Such cases may be due to defects in transcription or due to structurally and functionally abnormal β mRNA. In fact, studies of gene dosage by DNA-cDNA hybridization in a number of cases of homozygous β^0 thalassemia (some with absent β mRNA) have yielded results which are not consistent with the presence of β-globin gene deletions in these cases (Ottolenghi et al., 1975; Tolstoshev et al., 1976; Kan et al., 1975e; Ramirez et al., 1976; Forget et al., unpublished observations).

Gene quantitation has also been accomplished using DNA of cultured fibroblasts and lymphocytes from patients with homozygous hereditary persistence of fetal hemoglobin (HPFH) in which there is total absence of Hb A and Hb A_2 synthesis (see later section of this chapter). In contrast to the findings in homozygous β^0 thalassemia, these studies have demonstrated absence of β-chain genes (and presumably δ-chain genes) in the two cases studied (Kan et al., 1975d; Forget et al., 1976b). There was also total absence of β-chain mRNA in the one case in which it was measured (Forget et al., 1976b). It has also been shown that β- (and δ-) gene deletion exists in homozygous $\delta\beta$ thalassemia in which there is total absence of Hb A and Hb A_2 synthesis (Ottolenghi et al., 1976; Ramirez et al., 1976). Since both $\delta\beta$ thalassemia and HPFH appear to be associated with β-gene deletions, the difference in phenotypic expression between the two syndromes is not explained by this fact alone. It is possible that the extent of the chromosomal deletion, especially the involvement of intergene material between γ and δ genes, is different in both cases and that this material is involved in the differential expression of the γ genes in these two syndromes. This is pure speculation, however.

In the case of α^0 thalassemia, on the other hand, there is definitive evidence that the molecular basis of this disorder is deletion of the α globin chain loci. Incubation of α cDNA with liver DNA from hydropic infants with homozygous α thalassemia (Hb Bart's syndrome) reveals no significant hybridization, indicating deletion of the α globin chain genes (Ottolenghi et al., 1974; Taylor et al., 1974; Ramirez et al., 1975b). Subsequent hybridization studies utilizing DNA from the spleen of a patient with Hb H disease revealed deficiency of α globin genes to a level of approximately 25 per cent of normal (Kan et al., 1975a). These results are consistent with deletion of three of the α globin genes in Hb H disease and lend additional support to the presence of duplicated α-chain loci at least in the Asian population in which α thalassemia is prevalent: if the α-chain loci were not duplicated, the expected deficiency of α-chain genes would be 50 per cent (rather than 75 per cent) in Hb H disease (Kan et al., 1975a).

Thalassemia-like Disorders Associated with Structurally Abnormal Globin Chains

In the usual forms of thalassemia, the affected globin chain, which is synthesized in decreased amounts, is structurally normal, i.e., it shows no evidence of an amino acid substitution. There are two groups of thalassemia-like disorders, however, in which an abnormal globin chain is in fact synthesized: the Hb Lepore syndromes and the Hb Constant Spring syndromes.

The Hemoglobin Lepore Syndromes. Hb Lepore is a structurally abnormal hemoglobin in which the abnormal globin chain is a hybrid or fused globin chain, having the N-terminal amino acid sequence of the normal δ chain and the C-terminal amino acid sequence of the normal β chain (Baglioni, 1962). The Lepore defect appears to have resulted from mispairing of δ and β loci during meiosis and subsequent nonhomologous crossing over of the chromosomes in the area of the mispaired δ and β loci (Baglioni, 1962). As illustrated in Figure 2–2*A*, such a crossover event would yield, on one chromosome, a fused $\delta\beta$ locus (without adjacent intact δ or β loci) and, on the other chromosome, a locus for a hybrid or fused globin chain having the N-terminal amino acid sequence of the β chain and the C-terminal sequence of the δ chain (an "anti-Lepore" chain) situated between a normal δ-chain locus and a normal β-chain locus. The Hb Lepore gene behaves as a β-thalassemic gene because there is only a low level of synthesis of its gene product (the $\delta\beta$ chain) and presumably absence of a normal β-chain locus on the affected chromosome. This latter assumption is confirmed by the findings in patients homozygous for Hb Lepore, in which there is total absence of normal Hb A and Hb A_2 (Weatherall and Clegg, 1972). Three different types of Lepore chains have been described in which the transition from δ to β amino acid sequence occurs in different areas of the sequence (see Figure 2–2*B* and Table 3–2).

The reasons for the low level of synthesis of Hb Lepore are not known. There may be decreased synthesis because of relative instability of the mRNA for the Lepore chain: globin synthetic studies reveal that synthesis of the Lepore $\delta\beta$ chain, like that of the δ chain of the Hb A_2, occurs primarily in marrow cells and is virtually absent in peripheral blood reticulocytes (Rieder and Weatherall, 1965; Gill et al., 1972; Roberts et al., 1972; White et al., 1972a). Alternatively, transcription of the Lepore $\delta\beta$ gene may be reduced because of adjacent control genes which are responsible for the normally low level of expression of the δ gene. In either case, it is difficult to explain why Hb Lepore accumulates to a level of 10 to 15 per cent of the total Hb, whereas Hb A_2 is rarely increased to levels much greater than 5 per cent of the total Hb. The 5′-terminal sequences adjacent to the δ-chain gene cannot be the only factors regulating the expression of the Lepore $\delta\beta$ gene, otherwise Hb Lepore would accumulate only at a level similar to that of Hb A_2. The relative contributions of transcriptional versus post-transcriptional control in these phenomena are not known. Despite absence of Lepore-chain synthesis in peripheral blood cells, substantial amounts of mRNA for the Lepore chain can still be detected in these cells by molecular hybridization assays (Benz et al., 1975a).

The condition in which the δ, $\beta\delta$, and β loci all occur on one chromosome is called the anti-Lepore syndrome, and its demonstration is important in confirming the nonhomologous crossover hypothesis for the origin of the Lepore $\delta\beta$ chain (Fig. 2–2*A*). Two instances of such an abnormal hybrid (N)$\beta\delta$(C) chain have recently been demonstrated, in Hb P-Congo (Hb P-Nilotic) (Lehmann and Charlesworth, 1970; Badr et al., 1973) and Hb Miyada (Ohta et al., 1971) (Fig. 2–2*B*). The anti-Lepore syndromes do not resemble β thalassemia because the affected chromosome carries, in addition to the mutant gene, normal β and δ genes with normal output. There is therefore no overall deficit (or imbalance) in globin-chain synthesis and, consequently, no thalassemic phenotype.

The anti-Lepore hemoglobins accumulate in the red cell to approximately the same levels as do the Lepore hemoglobins. The synthesis of Hb Miyada is virtually limited to the bone marrow as is that of the Lepore hemoglobins (Roberts et al., 1973). This phenomenon has been interpreted as evidence of instability of the anti-Lepore globin mRNA and evidence that both the 5′- and 3′-terminal sequences of globin mRNA are important in maintaining its stability (Roberts et al., 1973; Clegg et al., 1974b). There could, however, also be effects of these mutations on the globin gene transcription process. The fact that the anti-Lepore hemoglobins are present at much lower levels than Hb A and at approximately the same levels as the Lepore hemoglobins indicates that the putative control genes at the 5′ extremity of the δ and β genes are not the sole factors regulating the expression of mutant fused $\delta\beta$ and $\beta\delta$ genes.

The Hemoglobin Constant Spring Syndromes. The second group of thalassemia-like conditions in which a structurally abnormal globin chain is synthesized are the hemoglobin Constant Spring syndromes (Clegg et al., 1971b; Milner et al., 1971). In Hb Constant Spring, an abnormally long α globin chain is synthesized, which is elongated at its C-terminal end by an additional 31 amino acids. This globin chain is produced in only small amounts and therefore the gene resembles an alpha-thalassemic gene. Red cells of patients heterozygous for Hb Constant Spring alone contain only 1 to 2 per cent of the mutant hemoglobin.

Three other similar hemoglobin variants have been described which have elongated α chains: Hb Icaria (Clegg et al., 1974a), Hb Koya Dora (DeJong et al., 1975), and Hb Seal Rock (Bradley et al., 1975). The three variants, like Hb Constant Spring, are also synthesized at very low levels. All four variants have different amino acids at portion 142 of their α chain (the first residue following the normal α-chain C-terminal residue at position 141). The following 30 amino acid residues, however, are the same in all four variants. These mutant hemoglobins probably arose by chain termination mutation (see Chapter 3).

The traits for Hb Constant Spring and Hb Icaria interact with heterozygous α thalassemia to give the more severe α-thalassemia syndrome, Hb H disease (see below). It is unclear how the chain termination mutation leads to the very low level of production of the elongated mutant globin chain. The synthesis of Hb CS, like that of Hb A_2, Hb Lepore, and Hb Miyada, is virtually limited to bone marrow cells and essentially absent in peripheral blood cells (Kan et al., 1974c). These findings suggest instability of the Hb Constant Spring mRNA but it is difficult to conceive how a single base substitution in the termination codon could lead in itself to instability of the mRNA. Other phenomena may be operative, such as decreased transcription and/or degradation of the mRNA during the "read-through" process. Hb CS was not initially considered to be an unstable hemoglobin (Clegg et al., 1971b), but recent results suggest that the elongated chain is quickly degraded to shorter forms (Pootrakul et al., 1976).

Pathophysiology of the Anemia

There are many primary and secondary causes for the anemia observed in thalassemia. It is easy to understand how reduced synthesis of one or another of the globin chains of hemoglobin A will result in an overall deficit of hemoglobin A synthesis and cause a hypochromic, microcytic anemia with a low mean corpuscular hemoglobin level of the red cells. This is true in both the heterozygous and homozygous states. In the homozygous state, however, another pathophysiological process worsens the anemia and is responsible for the major clinical manifestations of Cooley's anemia. The continued synthesis in normal amounts of the nonaffected globin chain results in the accumulation, within the red cells, of excessive amounts of these normal chains. Not finding complementary globin chains with which to bind, these chains form aggregates, precipitate within the cell, and become attached to the cell membrane (Bargellesi et al., 1968; Weatherall et al., 1969). These precipitates then lead to membrane damage (Gunn et al., 1972) and premature destruction of the red cell (Nathan and Gunn, 1966; Nathan et al., 1969). In β thalassemia, the resulting α-chain aggregates are called inclusion bodies or, perhaps improperly, Heinz bodies. In contrast to true Heinz bodies which are made up of total precipitated hemoglobin ($\alpha_2\beta_2$), these inclusion bodies have been shown, convincingly, to consist of only α globin chains (Fessas et al., 1966), which do have some attached heme, perhaps in the form of hemichromes (Rachmilewitz and Thorell, 1972). In α thalassemia, the resulting β_4 tetramers constitute Hb H, which is less insoluble than α-chain aggregates. In the neonatal and fetal periods, γ_4 tetramers occur in α thalassemia and constitute Hb Bart's. (Hemoglobin Bart's is seen in occasional adults with Hb H disease, particularly those with Hb Constant Spring.) The process of inclusion-body formation occurs in the erythroid precursors as well as in the mature red cells. It is responsible for the marked ineffective erythropoiesis and the hemolytic component seen in both the α- and β-thalassemia syndromes.

In β thalassemia, the role of thalassemic inclusions in the pathophysiology of the hemolytic anemia is manifested in the heterogeneous red cell population which is present in this disorder. Fetal hemoglobin is very heterogeneously distributed in the β-thalassemic red cells. Those cells which have the most fetal Hb are those which will have the least relative excess of α chains, since the γ chains combine with α chains to form Hb F. It has been demonstrated in β thalassemia that Hb A has a more rapid turnover (shorter half life) than Hb F (Gabuzda et al., 1963). This finding is consistent with the presence of different populations of red cells: those containing mainly Hb A are short lived and those containing much more Hb F have longer survival (Gabuzda et al., 1963). Indeed, differential centrifugation of red cells in β thalassemia reveals that the older, more rapidly sedimenting red cells contain much Hb F and have relatively few α-chain inclusions, whereas the younger, more slowly sedimenting cells are relatively deficient in Hb F and contain many α-chain inclusions (Loukopoulos and Fessas, 1965; Nathan and Gunn, 1966; Nathan et al., 1969). There is also a good positive correlation between the severity of the disease in β thalassemia and the size of the free α-chain pool and the degree of α to non-α globin chain imbalance (Bargellesi et al., 1968; Weatherall et al., 1969).

These findings serve to emphasize the relationship of the α-chain inclusions to the hemolytic process and the beneficial role of γ-

chain synthesis in lessening the imbalance of globin-chain synthesis, decreasing the formation of α-chain inclusions and thus increasing the red cells' survival. In β thalassemia, the α-chain inclusions are found in large quantities in the bone marrow erythroid precursors (Fessas, 1963; Yataganas and Fessas, 1969) and are probably the cause of the marked ineffective erythropoiesis or intramedullary destruction of erythroid cells which is observed in homozygous β thalassemia (Finch et al., 1970). Prior to splenectomy, these inclusion bodies are practically never seen in peripheral red blood cells, but following splenectomy they appear in large numbers (Fessas, 1963). This observation correlates well with the demonstrated role of the spleen (and reticuloendothelial system) in removing inclusion bodies of the Heinz body type from red cells, thereby damaging and/or destroying these cells (Rifkind and Danon, 1965; Slater et al., 1968; Wennberg and Weiss, 1968). This phenomenon can be dramatically observed, under phase microscopy, in fresh wet preparations obtained from scrapings of β-thalassemic spleens removed at surgery (Fig. 2–8) and is probably the main basis of the hemolytic anemia observed in β thalassemia. In β thalassemia, the α-chain inclusions result from decreased β-chain synthesis. Another inclusion-body

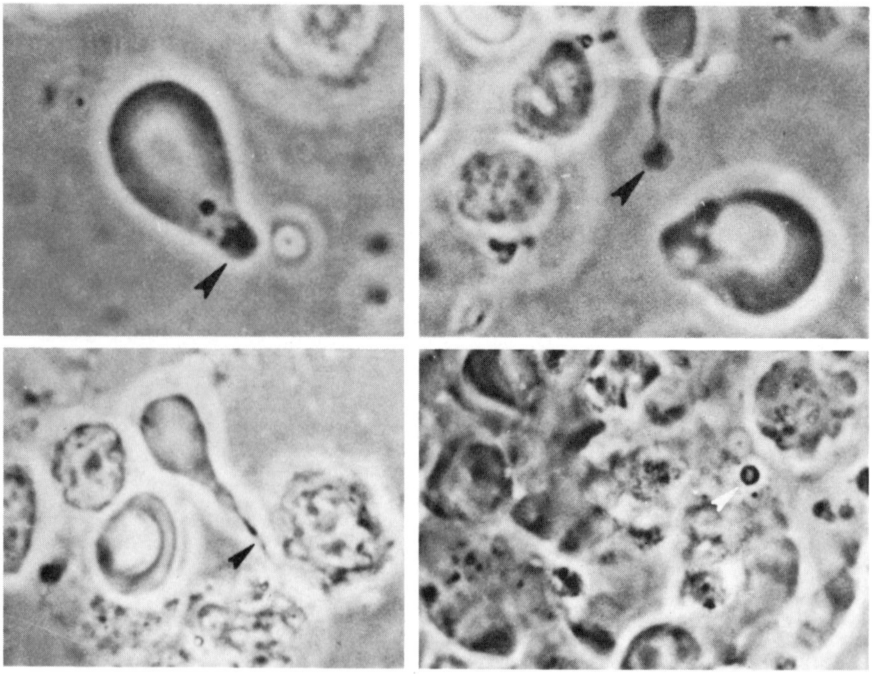

Figure 2–8. Phase microscopy of a wet preparation of scrapings from the spleen of a patient with homozygous beta thalassemia. Note alpha-chain inclusion bodies (arrows) within teardrop-shaped red cells, inclusions being pulled out or "pitted" from the red cell by reticuloendothelial cell action (lower left), and inclusions free in the splenic pulp (white arrow). (From Nathan, D. G.: N. Engl. J. Med. *286*:586, 1972.)

syndrome has recently been reported in which the inclusions apparently result from an absolute increase in α-chain production (Weatherall et al., 1973).

In the α-thalassemia syndrome of Hb H disease, the resulting β_4 tetramers (Hb H) are more stable than α-chain aggregates and precipitate more slowly. One does not observe, therefore, marked ineffective erythropoiesis and intramedullary destruction of erythroid cells as seen in β thalassemia, although some Hb H inclusions are seen in marrow normoblasts (Fessas and Yataganas, 1968). The β_4 inclusions form more gradually and occur mainly in mature red cells rather than in erythroid precursor cells. The spleen removes these inclusions and thus damages the red blood cells, as in β thalassemia (Rigas and Koler, 1961; Nathan and Gunn, 1966; Wennberg and Weiss, 1968; Nathan et al., 1969). Prior to splenectomy, no preformed Hb H inclusions are seen in the peripheral red blood cells, although soluble Hb H is present and can be made to precipitate in the form of small, stippled inclusions by in-vitro incubation of the blood with brilliant cresyl blue (BCB). After splenectomy, large, usually single, round, preformed inclusions are seen in the red cells by staining with BCB (as well as by methyl violet staining and by phase microscopy), in addition to the usual multiple, finely stippled inclusions (Nathan and Gunn, 1966; Weatherall and Clegg, 1972).

A number of secondary abnormalities also occur in thalassemia which can worsen the anemia. Excess iron stores accumulate because of repeated blood transfusions and increased gastrointestinal absorption (Erlandson et al., 1962; Bannerman et al., 1964; Necheles et al., 1969; Heinrich et al., 1973). This iron cannot be utilized owing to the decreased globin synthesis. It therefore accumulates in excess within the erythroid cells and is deposited in the mitochondria of these cells. This phenomenon may lead to decreased function of mitochondrial enzymes, including those which are necessary for heme synthesis. Decreased heme synthesis may contribute to an even further decrease in Hb A synthesis, but the more important cause of impaired heme synthesis is feedback inhibition due to accumulation of heme intermediates because of decreased globin synthesis (Bannerman, 1964).

The anemia of thalassemia may also be aggravated by folic acid deficiency which can easily develop in the thalassemic homozygote because of the high folic acid requirement resulting from the massive marrow erythroid hyperplasia and cellular turnover (Jandl and Greenberg, 1959; Luhby and Cooperman, 1961; Luhby et al., 1961). The splenomegaly invariably associated with homozygous thalassemia also contributes to the anemia by simply acting as a third space, by increasing intravascular volume and causing hemodilution (Prankerd, 1963), or by causing true hypersplenic destruction of red blood cells. After splenectomy the liver may act in a similar fashion but less effectively. Finally, since red cells containing fetal hemoglobin have high oxygen affinity (Chapter 1) there may exist actual tissue hypoxia at hemoglobin levels which would otherwise seem adequate to provide proper tissue oxygenation, if the hemoglobin were all normal adult Hb A (Maurer et al., 1970; DeFuria et al., 1974). In fact, thalassemic red cells appear to adapt poorly to anemia, as reflected by inappropriately low levels of red cell 2,3-DPG and relatively increased oxygen affinity (DeFuria et al., 1974; Pearson, 1975).

Classification of the Thalassemia Syndromes

The thalassemia syndromes are usually classified according to the type of the globin chain which is absent or present in decreased amount. The different types of thalassemia syndromes are listed in

***TABLE 2–2.** Classification of the Thalassemia Syndromes*

A. Alpha Thalassemia Syndromes
  1. Heterozygous alpha thalassemia 1
  2a. Heterozygous alpha thalassemia 2, or "silent carrier"
  2b. Hb Constant Spring trait
  3. Hb H disease: the combination of 1 with 2a or 2b
  4. Hydrops fetalis with Hb Bart's: homozygous alpha thalassemia 1

B. Beta Thalassemia Syndromes
  1. Heterozygous beta thalassemia
    a. With elevated Hb A_2 ± elevated Hb F (total absence of or reduced β-chain synthesis)
    b. With normal Hb A_2 and elevated Hb F: $\delta\beta$-thalassemia or F-thalassemia (total absence of β-chain synthesis)
    c. With normal Hb A_2 and Hb F (? "silent carrier")
    d. Hb Lepore trait
  2. "Homozygous" beta thalassemia or Cooley's anemia
    a. True homozygosity for one or another beta thalassemia gene
    b. Double heterozygosity for any two different beta thalassemia genes
    c. Thalassemia intermedia: certain doubly heterozygous combinations

C. Alpha + Beta Thalassemia
  1. Thalassemia of intermediate severity

D. Rare Forms of Thalassemia
  1. Gamma thalassemia
  2. Delta thalassemia

E. Interacting Thalassemia
  1. Alpha thalassemia + alpha chain variant
    a. Hb Q/alpha thalassemia
  2. Beta thalassemia + beta chain variant
    a. Sickle/beta thalassemia
    b. Hb C/beta thalassemia
    c. Hb E/beta thalassemia

F. Hereditary Persistence of Fetal Hemoglobin (not really a thalassemic disorder)
  1. Heterozygous
  2. Homozygous
  3. In association with beta chain structural variants

Table 2–2. Each type can occur in either the heterozygous or homozygous form. We will first consider the α-thalassemia syndromes. Heterozygous α thalassemia can occur in two forms: a phenotypically detectable form, referred to as α-thalassemia 1 trait, and a very mild defect, the α-thalassemia 2 trait, the existence of which is undectable, except by family studies and by its interaction with the α-thalassemia 1 gene. The latter is frequently referred to as the "silent carrier" state for α thalassemia. The heterozygous state for hemoglobin Constant Spring is phenotypically similar to α-thalassemia 2 trait or the silent carrier state, except that small amounts (1 to 2 per cent) of the abnormal hemoglobin are detectable. The homozygous state for the α-thalassemia 1 gene is the hydrops fetalis or hemoglobin Bart's syndrome. The doubly heterozygous state for the α-thalassemia 1 and α-thalassemia 2 genes is the less severe syndrome of hemoglobin H disease.

In the β-thalassemia syndromes, the heterozygous state for β thalassemia (thalassemia minor or minima) is quite heterogeneous, as indicated by the variations in the amounts of the minor components of hemoglobin present in the affected individual. The various heterozygous states include (1) high hemoglobin A_2-β thalassemia; (2) δβ thalassemia, or F thalassemia, characterized by normal hemoglobin A_2 but elevated hemoglobin F; (3) β-thalassemia trait with normal amounts of Hb F and Hb A_2 (? γδβ thalassemia); and (4) hemoglobin Lepore trait, which is phenotypically similar to heterozygous β thalassemia but is characterized by normal levels of Hb A_2, the presence of small amounts (10 to 15 per cent) of the abnormal hemoglobin, and some elevation of Hb F. "Homozygous" β thalassemia (thalassemia major or Cooley's anemia) may result from the combination of any two of these genes. Occasionally, a child will inherit a β-thalassemia gene of standard severity from one parent and a mild gene (in some cases a "silent carrier" gene) from the other parent. The resulting syndrome is usually less severe clinically than in the usual cases of homozygous β thalassemia and is termed thalassemia intermedia. Finally, β and α thalassemia may interact with each other and with a variety of other hemoglobinopathies. These will all be discussed in the following section.

The Alpha Thalassemia Syndromes

Four clinical syndromes are associated with alpha thalassemia:

(1) Ordinary heterozygous α thalassemia: α-thalassemia 1.

(2a) Mild heterozygous α thalassemia: α-thalassemia 2, or "silent carrier."

(2b) Hb Constant Spring trait.

(3) Hemoglobin H disease: the result of combination of (1) and (2a) or (2b).

(4) Hydrops fetalis associated with hemoglobin Bart's: homozygosity for the α-thalassemia 1 gene.

Two alternate hypotheses have been proposed to explain the two types of α-thalassemia genes (Koler and Rigas, 1961; Wasi et al., 1964; Kattamis and Lehmann, 1970; Lehmann, 1970; Wasi, 1970; Koler et al., 1971; Weatherall and Clegg, 1972). In the first ("one gene") theory, it is believed that only one locus on each chromosome controls α-chain synthesis and that the two types of α-thalassemia genes are allelic but of different severity: one being associated with absent α-chain synthesis, the other with mildly decreased synthesis. In the alternate ("two gene") theory, duplication of the α-chain structural gene is postulated: in α-thalassemia 2, only one of the four genes would be affected, whereas in α-thalassemia 1, two genes, usually on the same chromosome (in cis), would be involved. Hemoglobin H disease, therefore, would be the result of α thalassemia affecting three of the four α-chain genes, and hydrops fetalis with Hb Bart's would be the result of α thalassemia affecting all four α-chain genes. The proposed genotypes of the various α-thalassemia syndromes, according to both theories, are diagrammatically illustrated in Figure 2–9.

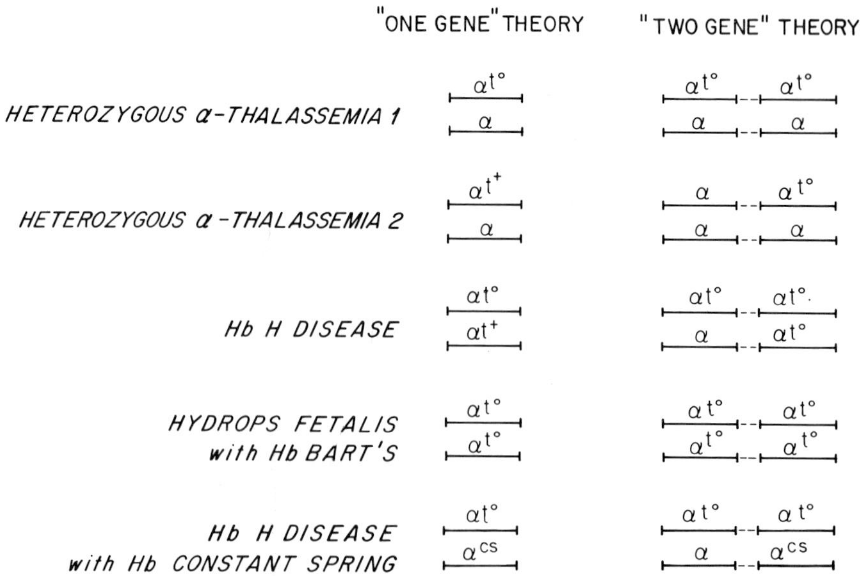

Figure 2–9. Genotypes of various α-thalassemia syndromes according to the "one gene" and "two linked genes" hypotheses. α, normal α-chain gene; α^{t^0}, α-thalassemia gene with total absence of α-chain synthesis; α^{t^+}, α-thalassemia gene with reduced α-chain synthesis; α^{CS}, gene for α-Constant Spring chain. The "one gene" hypothesis does not adequately explain the syndrome of Hb H disease with Hb Constant Spring (see text).

Heterozygous Alpha Thalassemia

Heterozygosity for both types of α-thalassemia genes is benign. Affected patients are usually of Oriental or Mediterranean ancestry. These carriers are detected usually on routine hematological examination, or during family studies of patients with the symptomatic thalassemic disorders. In α-thalassemia 1 trait, there is microcytosis and hypochromia of the red blood cells, with a mild degree of aniso- and poikilocytosis (Fig. 2–10). The hemoglobin level may be slightly depressed (10 to 12 g/100 ml) or near normal as a result of an elevated red cell count (greater than 5 million). Alpha-thalassemia 1 trait can be distinguished from beta-thalassemia trait by the presence of normal levels of hemoglobin A_2 and F. In the adult, the diagnosis is often difficult; iron deficiency and other causes of hypochromia and microcytosis must be ruled out before the diagnosis can be accepted. In some patients, incubation of the peripheral blood with 1 per cent brilliant cresyl blue (BCB) reveals occasional red cells (one in several thousand) bearing typical hemoglobin H inclusions similar to those shown in Figure 2–11A.

The hematological findings in patients heterozygous for α-thalassemia 2 are entirely normal. Diagnosis can only be inferred from family study.

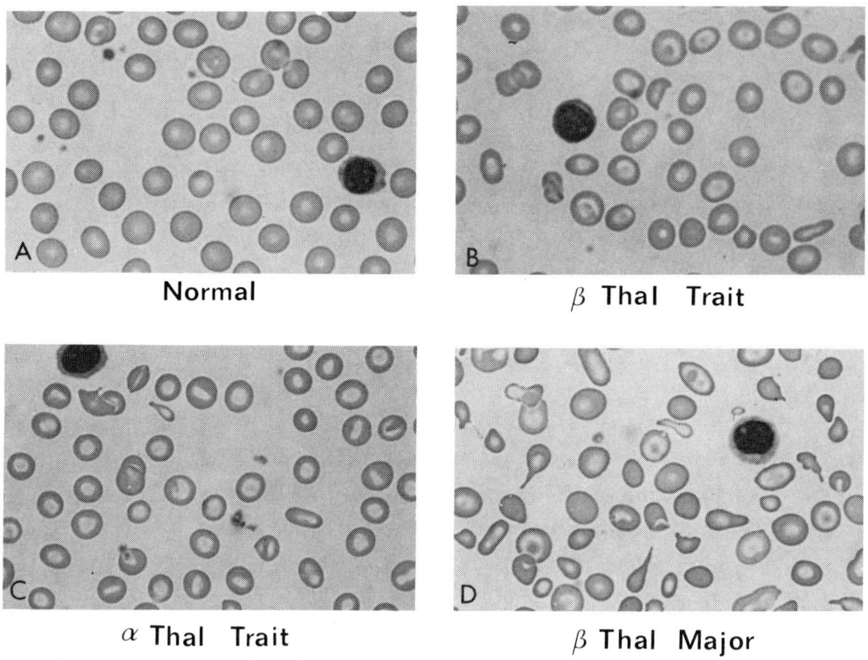

Figure 2–10. Peripheral blood smears of a normal individual (*A*) and patients with heterozygous β thalassemia (*B*), heterozygous α thalassemia (*C*), and homozygous β thalassemia (*D*).

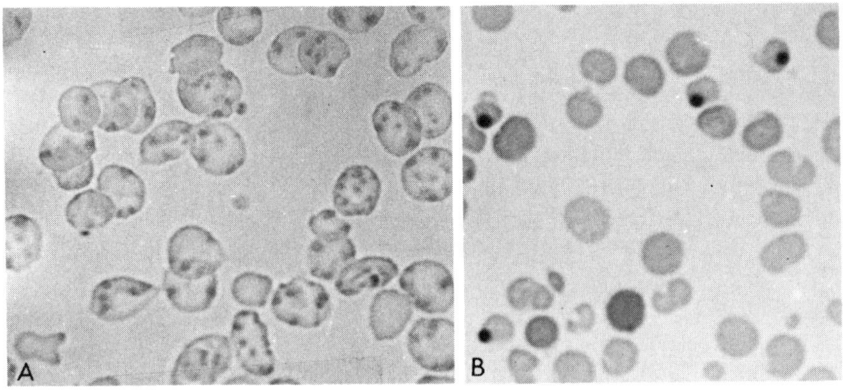

Figure 2–11. Red cell inclusions in Hb H disease. *A*, Inclusions induced by incubating peripheral blood in 1 per cent brilliant cresyl blue (BCB) and 0.4 per cent citrate for 30 minutes at 37° C (patient not splenectomized). *B*, Preformed inclusions, in peripheral blood of a splenectomized patient, stained by new methylene blue reticulocyte stain.

During the neonatal period, the two types of heterozygous α thalassemia can be distinguished by the level of hemoglobin Bart's (γ_4) present in cord blood. This has been most thoroughly studied in Thailand (Pootrakul et al., 1967b, 1970; Na-Nakorn et al., 1969; Na-Nakorn and Wasi, 1970). In patients with α-thalassemia 1 trait there is approximately 5 to 6 per cent hemoglobin Bart's, whereas in those with α-thalassemia 2 trait there is only 1 to 2 per cent hemoglobin Bart's. These components disappear by about the sixth month of life. Alpha-thalassemia 1 can also be detected with certainty in later life by the study of globin-chain synthesis in the peripheral blood reticulocytes of these individuals, as previously discussed in the section on globin synthesis in intact thalassemic erythroid cells. In α-thalassemia 1, there is approximately a 25 per cent reduction in α-chain synthesis relative to β-chain synthesis (Kan et al., 1968). A less significant decrease in α-chain synthesis can be detected by this technique in a group of patients with α-thalassemia 2, but the difference from normal is not great enough for precise identification of individual patients (Kan et al., 1968; Fig. 2–7).

It should be emphasized that the results obtained from analysis of Hb Bart's in cord blood and globin synthetic studies apply only to the α thalassemia found in the Mediterranean and Oriental populations. The findings in patients of African origin are much less well defined. Although α-thalassemia trait occurs in blacks, hemoglobin H disease is very rare, and when it occurs it is usually mild and has atypical features. Hydrops fetalis with Hb Bart's has never been described in blacks (and only once in a Mediterranean family [Diamond et al., 1965]). Hence, the existence of different types of α-thalassemia genes in different populations has been postulated (Lehmann, 1970; Schwartz and Atwater, 1972; Weatherall and Clegg,

1972). It has been proposed that in blacks the α-thalassemia gene is characterized by only slight reduction in α-chain synthesis and never total absence of α-chain synthesis. However, it is possible to propose a unified model for the causation of α thalassemia by gene deletion which in the context of the "two gene" theory can nevertheless account for the findings in blacks: blacks with the phenotype of "heterozygous" α thalassemia may have two deleted α-chain genes but with the deletions on different chromosomes (in trans) rather than on the same chromosome (in cis), as is apparently the case in the Oriental type of α thalassemia. Thus, because each chromosome bearing an α-thalassemia gene deletion would be linked to a second normal α-chain gene, it would be impossible, in a mating of two heterozygotes, for an offspring to inherit three or four deleted genes. Rare cases of Hb H disease in blacks would be due to rare crossing-over events leading to deletion of two α-chain genes on the same chromosome. There is no definitive evidence yet to favor this type of deletion model over the model proposing the presence of a nondeleted but low output α-chain gene in the black type of α thalassemia. Actual quantitation of gene numbers by molecular hybridization assays may soon resolve this question.

HEMOGLOBIN H DISEASE

This condition is characterized by a chronic hemolytic anemia of variable severity (Rigas and Koler, 1961). Most patients have a hemoglobin level of approximately 8 to 10 g/100 ml, with moderate reticulocytosis (5 to 10 per cent). However, the variation is wide and one can see patients either with severe anemia or with very mild anemia. Mongoloid facies similar to that which is associated with homozygous beta thalassemia has occasionally been described. Splenomegaly is usually present and hepatomegaly is not uncommon. Anemia may become more severe during pregnancy, during infection, or after ingestion of oxidant drugs which accelerate the oxidation and precipitation of the Hb H (β_4). The peripheral blood smear typically shows hypochromia, microcytosis, poikilocytosis, polychromasia, and targeting of the red cells. Incubation of blood with 1 per cent brilliant cresyl blue (BCB) causes in-vitro precipitation of Hb H which is seen in the form of multiple speckled bodies (Fig. 2–11*A*). After splenectomy, large Hb H inclusion bodies, formed in vivo during red blood cell aging, can also be seen by supravital staining; they are usually single and round (Rigas and Koler, 1961; Nathan and Gunn, 1966) (Fig. 2–11*B*). The bone marrow typically shows erythroid hyperplasia. Punctate hemoglobin H inclusions can be demonstrated by BCB incubation in nucleated marrow precursor cells, but large, single, round, preformed inclusion bodies, though present in some late normoblasts (Fessas and Yataganas, 1968), are much less abundant than the numerous α-chain inclusion bodies found in homozygous β-thalassemic marrow cells.

The diagnosis can be confirmed by hemoglobin electrophoresis (Fig. 2–12*A*). In the newborn, approximately 20 to 40 per cent hemoglobin Bart's (γ_4) is found. This is gradually replaced in older children and adults by hemoglobin H (β_4), the level of which varies between 5 and 30 per cent. Both Hb H and Hb Bart's migrate more

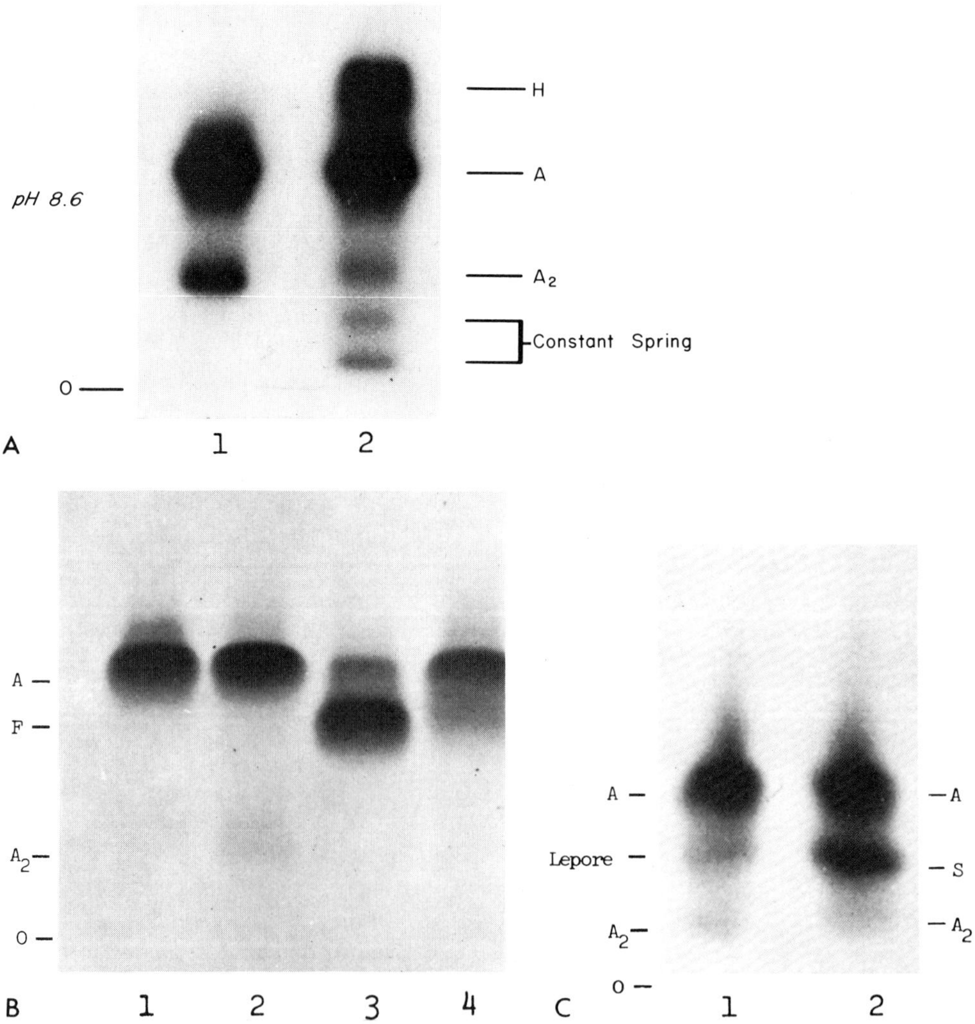

Figure 2–12. Hemoglobin electrophoresis. *A*, Starch-gel electrophoresis at pH 8.6: 1, Normal; 2, Hb H disease with Hb Constant Spring. *B*, Agarose electrophoresis at pH 8.6: 1, Normal; 2, β-thalassemia trait with increased Hb A_2; 3 and 4, homozygous β thalassemia with different relative amounts of Hb A and Hb F. *C*, Starch-gel electrophoresis at pH 8.6: 1, Hb Lepore trait; 2, sickle cell trait. (O indicates the origin and the anode is at the top.)

rapidly than Hb A when electrophoresis is performed at pH 8.6. Hemoglobin A_2 is reduced to about 1 to 1.5 per cent. Biosynthetic studies have shown that in peripheral blood reticulocytes there is approximately a 50- to 75-per cent reduction in α-chain synthesis compared to β-chain synthesis (Clegg and Weatherall, 1967; Kan et al., 1968).

It is noteworthy that assays of globin mRNA isolated from reticulocytes of patients with Hb H disease reveal a much greater deficiency of α mRNA than expected on the basis of the β/α synthetic ratio in the same patient (Benz et al., 1973; Grossbard et al., 1973; Housman et al., 1973; Taylor et al., 1974; Forget et al., 1975a; Kazazian et al., 1975; Ottolenghi et al., 1975). In a thoroughly studied case, biosynthetic studies in intact cells revealed approximately 30 per cent as much α-chain synthesis as β-chain synthesis but there was only 10 to 15 per cent as much α mRNA as β mRNA when mRNA was studied by molecular hybridization, gel electrophoresis, and nucleotide sequence analysis (Housman et al., 1973; Forget et al., 1975a). These results suggest the possible presence of intracellular control mechanisms which can modulate the imbalance of globin-chain synthesis and partially compensate for the mRNA deficiency. Environmental factors can also affect the amount of Hb H which accumulates in red cells. In one of two brothers with Hb H disease, concomitant iron deficiency was asssociated with absence of Hb H (O'Brien, 1973). After therapy with iron, Hb H levels reached 16 per cent, a level similar to that present in the other brother.

Study of the families of patients with Hb H disease usually reveals that one parent has α-thalassemia 1 while the other is hematologically normal and presumably a "silent" carrier of the α-thalassemia 2 gene. Direct transmission of hemoglobin H disease to the offspring of an affected individual has rarely been observed, but in such cases the presence of an α-thalassemia 2 gene in the putatively normal spouse cannot be ruled out. Usually, the offspring of patients with Hb H disease inherit either α-thalassemia 1 trait or α-thalassemia 2 trait (confirmed by analysis of Hb Bart's in cord blood) (Na-Nakorn et al., 1969).

Hemoglobin H has also been described as an acquired defect, usually during the course of erythroleukemia or other myeloproliferative disorders (White et al., 1960; Beaven et al., 1963; Rosenzweig et al., 1968; Hamilton et al., 1971; Andre et al., 1972). In certain of these cases, the abnormality appears to be clonal, or limited to only a certain population of the red cells (Pagnier et al., 1972). The clinical manifestations associated with the primary myeloproliferative disorder easily distinguish this acquired defect from the hereditary variety of Hb H disease. The precise molecular basis of this interesting acquired abnormality remains unknown, but biosynthetic studies have confirmed the presumed decrease in α-chain synthesis relative to β-chain synthesis (Hamilton et al., 1971).

Pathophysiology of Hb H Disease

Deficiency of α-chain synthesis results in overall decreased synthesis of hemoglobin A, hence hypochromia and microcytosis. The excess β chains which accumulate form the β_4 tetramers of hemoglobin H; Hb H has a very high oxygen affinity and lacks the Bohr effect as well as heme-heme interaction. Hence, it is a useless pigment for oxygen transport under physiologic conditions. In addition, hemoglobin H is an unstable tetramer; it is easily oxidized and tends to precipitate as the red cells age. These precipitates, which gradually form in vivo, are normally removed by the spleen and can be demonstrated most abundantly in peripheral blood cells after splenectomy. They cause disturbances in red cell metabolism and interfere with membrane function and deformability (Nathan and Gunn, 1966; Nathan et al., 1969). All these factors lead to shortened red cell survival and the hemolytic component of the disease. Shortened ^{51}Cr-labeled red cell survival and the apparent splenic trapping of ^{51}Cr-labeled red cells is observed in hemoglobin H disease but should be interpreted with caution: ^{51}Cr binds selectively to the β chain, and there is evidence that exchange of β chains can occur between hemoglobin A and Hb H (Gabuzda et al., 1965). The ^{51}Cr can pass from the labeled Hb A to Hb H which then precipitates and is removed from the red cells by the spleen without the cell being destroyed. Thus the cell loses its label without necessarily being destroyed, and this gives a false impression of the actual red cell life span and splenic sequestration (Gabuzda et al., 1965). More recent studies, however, indicate that ^{51}Cr may be a valid label for the determination of red cell life span in Hb H disease (Tso, 1972).

Hemoglobin Constant Spring Syndromes

In as many as 50 per cent of Oriental patients with hemoglobin H disease, hemoglobin electrophoresis shows, in addition to the usual findings, one or two more slowly migrating hemoglobin components, which amount to 3 to 5 per cent of the total hemoglobin (Clegg et al., 1971b; Milner et al., 1971) (Fig. 2–12*A*). This hemoglobin is called hemoglobin Constant Spring (Hb CS) and it has been found in patients of Greek (Sofroniadou et al., 1968), Thai (Pootrakul et al., 1970), and Chinese ancestry (Clegg et al., 1971b; Milner et al., 1971). Hemoglobin CS is made up of two normal β chains and two elongated α chains which have either 28 or 31 additional amino acid residues at their C-terminal ends. The shorter Hb CS chain presumably results from proteolytic digestion of the longer CS chain. Typically, one of the parents of a patient with Hb H–CS disease has α-thalassemia 1 trait, while the other appears to be hematologically normal, except that hemoglobin electrophoresis shows the presence of approximately 1 per cent hemoglobin Constant Spring. Therefore, heterozygotes for Hb Constant Spring are phenotypically similar to individuals with α-thalassemia 2 trait.

The fact that carriers of hemoglobin Constant Spring are phenotypically similar to persons with α-thalassemia 2 and not α-thalassemia 1 has been used to support the theory of α-chain gene duplication. Since the contribution of the α^{CS} gene to the total cell globin is negligible, the absence of hypochromia and other stigmata of thalassemia suggests that there must be more than only one other normal α-chain gene compensating for the deficiency of normal α chains due to the α^{CS} gene. Furthermore, it is difficult to postulate only a single pair of α-chain genes when Hb CS interacts with α-thalassemia 1 to give Hb H disease: there is total absence of α-chain synthesis from the α-thalassemia 1 locus (homozygotes totally lack Hb A and have the Hb Bart's hydrops fetalis syndrome). There must be, therefore, another normal α-chain locus in cis with the α^{CS} locus to account for the presence of some Hb A in these patients (see Figure 2–9). The "one gene" theory can explain the syndrome of Hb H disease associated with Hb CS only if one postulates that (1) the α-thalassemia gene in trans to the CS gene is an α-thalassemia 2 gene (which does not usually fit the clinical or genetic data); or (2) the chain termination mutation hypothesis for the origin of Hb CS is incorrect. An alternate hypothesis is that the abnormal chain arises because of the presence of a suppressor tRNA which reads the chain termination codon as the amino acid glutamine and allows translation to continue (Clegg et al., 1971b). The latter explanation is probably untenable, however, because if it were correct, one should observe other abnormally long proteins in these patients and not simply an abnormality limited to the α globin chain.

The syndrome of Hb H disease has also been described in association with a second α-chain termination mutant, Hb Icaria (Clegg et al., 1974a).

Hydrops Fetalis Associated with Hemoglobin Bart's

The homozygous state for α-thalassemia 1 results in the Hb Bart's hydrops fetalis syndrome. The affected fetus is usually delivered prematurely and either is stillborn or dies within an hour after birth, grossly hydropic with marked hepatosplenomegaly (Lie-Injo and Jo, 1960; Lie-Injo, 1962; Kan et al., 1967; Todd et al., 1967). For reasons yet unknown this syndrome occurs almost exclusively in individuals from Southeast Asia. With the exception of one case observed in a Greek Cypriot (Diamond et al., 1965), no other cases have been reported from the Mediterranean area, and none have been described in people of African ancestry.

The peripheral blood smear is characterized by hypochromia and large numbers of nucleated red blood cells. On hemoglobin electrophoresis, the predominant hemoglobin is hemoglobin Bart's (γ_4) (Lie-Injo and Jo, 1960). In addition, one finds a smaller amount of Hb H and a minor component, hemoglobin Portland-1 ($\zeta_2\gamma_2$) (Todd et al., 1970; Weatherall et al., 1970). Hemoglobin Portland-1 is also found in lower (trace) amounts in normal cord blood (Capp et al., 1970). Studies of globin-chain synthesis in one case of Hb Bart's syndrome revealed total absence of α-chain synthesis (Weatherall et al., 1970).

Hemoglobin Bart's has a very high oxygen affinity similar to that of hemoglobin H. Thus, the bulk of the hemoglobin present in these infants cannot deliver oxygen effectively to the tissues. The cause of death is severe hypoxia. Delivery by cesarian section and exchange transfusion were attempted in one case but were not successful in prolonging life for more than a few hours (Weatherall et al., 1970).

Family studies in such cases usually show the presence of α-thalassemia 1 trait in both parents.

THE BETA THALASSEMIAS

Heterozygous Beta Thalassemia

The hallmark of heterozygous β thalassemia is microcytosis and hypochromia. With the increasing use of electronic cell counting equipment, the diagnosis may first be suspected by the discovery of a low MCV and MCH on routine blood counts (Pearson et al., 1973). Beta-thalassemia heterozygotes are usually not symptomatic and may not be anemic. However, mild anemia with hemoglobin levels of 10 to 11 g/100 ml is usually present in most patients; more pronounced anemia may be found in infancy and during pregnancy. The MCV and MCH are usually decreased well below normal with values of 55 to 70 μ^3 and 16 to 20 pg typically found. Despite the microcytosis, the MCHC is not usually as low as in iron deficiency. The peripheral blood smear typically shows microcytosis, hypochromia, aniso- and poikilocytosis with targeting and basophilic stippling of the red cells (see Figure 2–10). The bone marrow shows mild erythroid hyperplasia with many of the normoblasts showing poor hemoglobinization. Mild to moderate splenomegaly occurs in approximately one third of the cases.

The differential diagnosis between iron deficiency and β- (or α-) thalassemia trait can be difficult in practice. Table 2–3 lists the differentiating features.

In thalassemic heterozygotes, the MCV tends to be lower when related to the red cell count than in iron deficiency. This observation has led to the derivation of various formulas to differentiate thalassemia trait from iron deficiency on the basis of the red cell indices (Torlontano et al., 1972; England and Fraser, 1973; Mentzer, 1973)

TABLE 2–3. Differentiation of β-thalassemia Trait from Iron Deficiency Anemia (Hb 9 to 11 g/100 ml)

	β-THAL TRAIT	IRON DEFICIENCY ANEMIA
I. Definitive Tests		
A. Serum iron	Normal	Decreased
B. TIBC	Normal	Increased
C. % saturation	Normal	Decreased
D. Hb electrophoresis		
$Hb\ A_2$	Increased	Decreased
Hb F	± Increased	Normal
II. Associated Findings		
MCV/RBC*	< 13	> 13
RBC protoporphyrin	Normal	Increased
RBC morphology	3 to 4+ Abnormal	Tr-1+ Abnormal
Serum ferritin	Normal	Low
Dominant inheritance	+	0
Color of plasma	Straw-colored	Colorless

*See Mentzer, 1973.

(see Table 2–3). Although such findings are helpful, they do not provide conclusive evidence of the diagnosis. Precise diagnosis requires hemoglobin electrophoresis and measurement of the serum iron and iron binding capacity. Demonstration of absent stainable iron in bone marrow aspirates may be necessary to identify individuals with combined thalassemia trait and iron deficiency. This combination is quite common in early childhood and during pregnancy. Iron salts should not be withheld when iron deficiency complicates thalassemia trait.

It is noteworthy that the presence of iron deficiency may obscure the diagnosis of concomitant β-thalassemia trait. Iron deficiency causes a decrease in $Hb\ A_2$ synthesis in normals and in β-thalassemia trait as well; with iron deficiency, the usually elevated $Hb\ A_2$ levels in a β-thalassemic heterozygote may fall into the normal range (Wasi et al., 1968; Kattamis et al., 1972). Beta-thalassemia trait should therefore be suspected in cases in which anemia responds only partially and in which hypochromia and microcytosis persist after therapy for iron deficiency. The $Hb\ A_2$ levels will return to their normally elevated values in such patients after replenishment of iron stores.

Moderately severe anemia has occasionally been described in apparent heterozygous β thalassemia (McCarthy et al., 1968; Aksoy, 1970; Stamatoyannopoulos et al., 1974; Friedman et al., 1976a). However, severe anemia is unusual and when it occurs, one should look for associated secondary causes such as concomitant iron or folic acid deficiency. Such cases should also be distinguished by family studies from the milder forms of homozygous β thalassemia or double heterozygosity for β-thalassemia genes of different types and severity. The term thalassemia intermedia has been used to refer to either severe heterozygous β thalassemia or mild homozygous β thalassemia.

There are at least four different types of heterozygous β thalassemia which can be distinguished on the basis of hemoglobin electrophoresis.

1. Ordinary *beta thalassemia,* or high A_2-β thalassemia, by far the commonest variety, is characterized by an increased hemoglobin A_2 level of 4 to 6 per cent (see Figure 2–12*B*) and usually a normal level of hemoglobin F, although in approximately half the cases, a slightly elevated level of hemoglobin F (2 to 5 per cent) may be present (Pootrakul et al., 1973).

2. *In delta-beta thalassemia,* or F thalassemia, the Hb A_2 level is normal or slightly decreased, and the hemoglobin F is increased and varies between 5 and 20 per cent.

3. *Delta-beta thalassemia with normal levels of hemoglobins* A_2 *and F*(?$\gamma\delta\beta$ thalassemia). This type of heterozygous β thalassemia is difficult to distinguish clinically from heterozygous α thalassemia. It is usually suspected by the finding of a clinically significant beta-thalassemia syndrome in an offspring. Globin synthesis studies in peripheral blood reticulocytes may be the only laboratory means to make this diagnosis.

4. *Hb Lepore trait* is characterized by normal Hb A_2, slight elevation of Hb F, and the finding of 5 to 15 per cent Hb Lepore (see Figure 2–12*C*).

The clinical picture in all four types of heterozygous β thalassemia is rather similar except perhaps in types 2 and 3 where anemia and morphological abnormalities of the red blood cells may be minimal. The findings in type 3 may be virtually normal and the term "silent carrier" state has been applied to such cases.

The presence or absence of elevated Hb F in heterozygous A_2-β thalassemia is usually of no prognostic significance with regard to the severity of disease in a homozygous offspring. One exception to this rule is a rare variety of A_2-β thalassemia in which the heterozygote, in addition to an elevated Hb A_2 level, has an unexpectedly high Hb F level—5 to 15 per cent (Weatherall, 1964a; Schokker et al., 1966). The homozygous state for this rare disorder is much milder than homozygosity for the usual A_2-β thalassemia (Schokker et al., 1966).

The results of globin chain biosynthetic studies in heterozygous β thalassemia have been discussed in the section on the molecular pathology of thalassemia. The β/α synthetic ratio is 0.5 in the peripheral blood reticulocytes. In contrast, the ratio in the bone marrow is close to 1.0. As discussed previously, this finding of apparently balanced globin-chain synthesis in the bone marrow is not yet fully explained but it appears to be due to accelerated turnover (? proteolysis) of newly synthesized excess α chains.

The double inheritance of β thalassemia and a β-chain structural variant makes it possible to evaluate the amount of β^A-chain synthesis directed by the β-thalassemia gene. In high A_2-β thalassemia, there is some β^A-chain synthesis directed by the defective gene in approximately two thirds of the cases (β^+ thalassemia), whereas the other one third of the cases show totally absent β^A-chain synthesis (β^0 thalassemia). Total absence of β^Asynthesis is especially characteristic of the A_2-β thalassemia found in Ferrara, Italy (Bargellesi et al., 1967; Conconi et al., 1970) and in Thailand (Weatherall et al., 1969a). In $\delta\beta$ thalassemia, there is almost always total absence of β^A-chain synthesis directed by the $\delta\beta$-thalassemia gene.

Homozygous β Thalassemia (A_2-β Thalassemia)

Clinical Manifestations

The clinical course in most cases is severe. At birth, anemia is not evident, and examination of the peripheral blood smear shows only occasional hypochromic red cells. Diagnosis, however, can be established by study of globin-chain synthesis in the cord blood (Gaburro et al., 1970). Within a few months, hypochromic, microcytic hemolytic anemia develops, and a regular transfusion program must be undertaken to maintain an adequate hemoglobin level. The spleen and liver become progressively enlarged. A typical facies develops in many patients, with prominent frontal bossing, prominent cheek bones, and protruding upper jaw due to expansion of the marrow in the skull and facial bones. Skull x-ray demonstrates the typical "hair on end" appearance (Fig. 2–13*A*). The long bones may also become rarefied from the marrow expansion (Fig. 2–13*B*) and become subject to repeated pathologic fractures. Occasionally, the expanding marrow extrudes from ribs or vertebrae and forms large intrathoracic masses. Gallstones and leg ulcers are frequent complications, as they are in other severe hemolytic anemias.

Intercurrent infection is extremely common and, along with neglected anemia, is the most common cause of death in early childhood. With modern antibiotic therapy and proper transfusion therapy, these causes of death have become less frequent and many patients survive to their twenties. A benign form of pericarditis with pericardial effusion frequently occurs and is usually self-limited. Secondary hypersplenism may develop in some patients and cause thrombocytopenia, leukopenia, and rapid destruction of transfused red cells. This complication may pose a severe management problem, and splenectomy may be required to control it. However, the incidence of overwhelming infection (septicemia) following splenec-

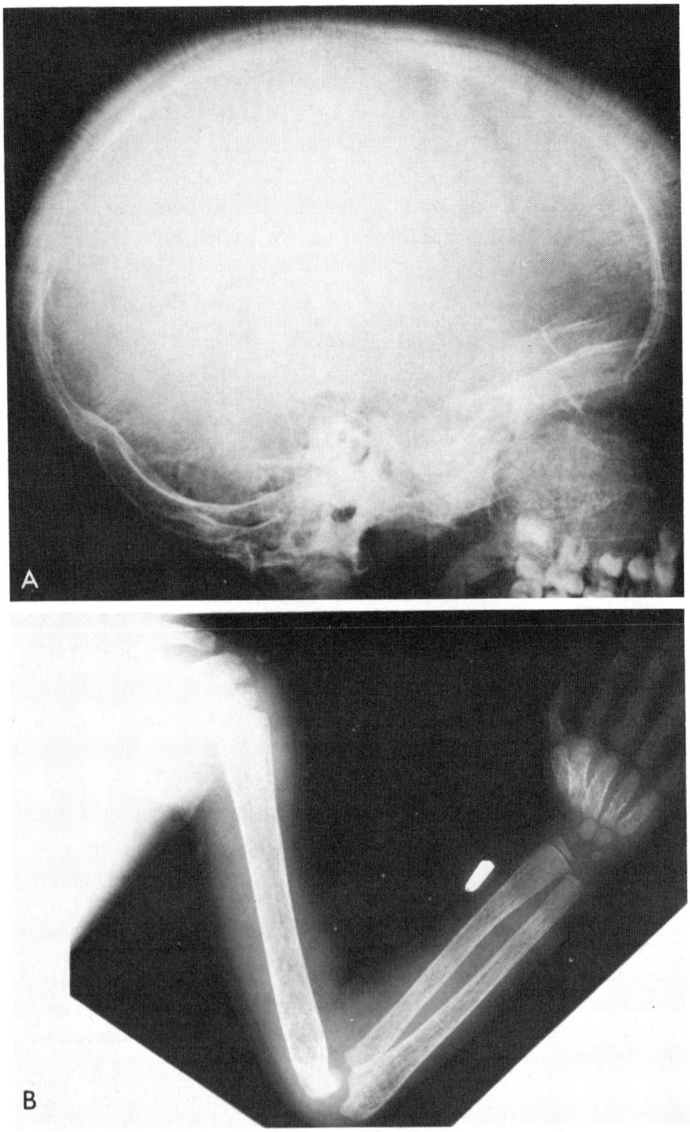

Figure 2–13. Bone changes in severe homozygous β thalassemia. *A*, Skull x-ray. (From Beck, W. S. (ed.): Hematology. 2nd ed. Boston, MIT Press, 1976.) *B*, X-ray of forearm and hand. (From Nathan, D. G.: N. Engl. J. Med. *286*:586, 1972.)

tomy is very high in thalassemic patients (Smith et al., 1962, 1964), and such patients should be observed carefully during febrile episodes.

Physical growth and development of these children are usually below normal. Menarche and secondary sexual characteristics are usually absent, and the final stature of these patients tends to be short. This problem has been well reviewed by Logothetis et al. (1972). Growth retardation begins approximately at 4 years of age and reaches its most significant and noticeable levels at 9 to 10 years of age. There is no associated retardation in intellectual development. No good correlation exists between the degree of anemia (pretransfusion Hb level) and the degree of growth retardation. However, this finding does not rule out the possibility that the degree of anemia in the first few years of life may be related to the degree of growth retardation in later years. Although growth retardation is more pronounced in splenectomized patients, it is believed that this phenomenon simply reflects the correlation between severity of growth retardation and severity of the clinical course of the disease as manifested by hepatomegaly, cutaneous siderosis, and cephalofacial deformities (Logothetis et al., 1972).

Iron absorption is usually increased in thalassemia major (Erlandson et al., 1962; Bannerman et al., 1964; Necheles et al., 1969a; Heinrich et al., 1973). Additional iron overload is supplied by the frequent transfusions. Iron overload is probably responsible for damage to the heart, liver, pancreas, endocrine glands, and other organs. In addition, chronic anemia and hypoxia are believed to play an important role in contributing to the myocardial damage from hemosiderosis (Necheles et al., 1969b). Cardiac failure and arrhythmias are the most common causes of death as these patients survive to their twenties. Diabetes mellitus (Lassman et al., 1974) and hepatic insufficiency may also pose difficult management problems.

Some of the complications and associated manifestations of Cooley's anemia can be prevented or at least lessened by maintaining a near normal hemoglobin level in the children by a high transfusion regimen, as will be discussed in the section on management.

Although the preceding description applies to most patients with homozygous β thalassemia, a small number of patients have a much milder clinical course (so-called thalassemia intermedia) and may require few or no blood transfusions. This is especially true of homozygous β thalassemia in blacks, which appears to be a much milder disease.

Laboratory Findings

Anemia is severe, with marked hypochromia. The findings on peripheral blood smear are striking (see Figure 2–10): the red blood cells show severe hypochromia and microcytosis, marked anisocytosis and poikilocytosis with teardrop-shaped red cells, polychromasia, and basophilic stippling. Poorly hemoglobinized normoblasts are frequently found in the peripheral blood, and their number increases markedly following splenectomy. Even when anemia is severe, the reticulocyte count is usually not very high because of massive destruction of erythroid cells in the marrow, termed ineffective erythropoiesis.

The red cell osmotic fragility is decreased, a phenomenon explained by the marked hypochromia. The bone marrow is hypercellular with marked erythroid hyperplasia characterized by normoblasts which are poorly hemoglobinized (micronormoblastic). Storage cells resembling Gaucher cells are frequently found in the marrow (and spleen) (Beltrami et al., 1973). Examination of the marrow under phase microscopy or after supravital staining reveals the presence of many inclusion bodies (α-chain aggregates) in the normoblasts. This finding can be used as a diagnostic test for homozygous β thalassemia (Fessas, 1963; Yataganas and Fessas, 1969). The α-chain inclusions are also seen in peripheral blood red cells after splenectomy.

Increased nonconjugated bilirubin levels and other biochemical evidence of hemolysis can usually be found. Dipyrroles resulting from increased heme catabolism give the urine a dark brown color (Kreimer-Birnbaum et al., 1966b). The findings on hemoglobin electrophoresis vary from patient to patient and with the type of thalassemia (see Figure 2–12*B*). In the homozygous form of the usual variety of β thalassemia (high A_2-β^+ thalassemia) there is usually a variable amount of Hb A present. Hemoglobin F is usually elevated and may represent from 10 to 90 per cent of the patient's total hemoglobin and is heterogeneously distributed in the red cells. The total amount of circulatory Hb A_2 may be low, normal, or increased, but the ratio of Hb A_2 to Hb A is usually higher than the normal ratio of 1 to 40, suggesting more efficient synthesis of Hb A_2 relative to Hb A in homozygous β thalassemia even if the absolute Hb A_2 level is below normal. Free α chains can also be seen in trace amounts as a slow moving component on the hemoglobin electrophoresis (Fessas and Loukopoulos, 1964). Hemoglobin A is totally absent in patients with homozygous β^0 thalassemia. Patients doubly heterozygous for high A_2-β thalassemia and $\delta\beta$ thalassemia in general have a higher level of Hb F and lower level of Hb A_2 than homozygotes for high A_2-β thalassemia. The former also tend to have a milder clinical course.

Delta-Beta Thalassemia or F Thalassemia

Heterozygous F thalassemia or $\delta\beta$ thalassemia is a condition characterized by mild hypochromia and microcytosis. The changes may be barely noticeable. Hemoglobin electrophoresis reveals low or normal Hb A_2 and elevation of Hb F (5 to 20 per cent). The condition is found mainly in Greeks (Stamatoyannopoulos et al., 1969), although it has also been found in blacks and in other racial groups. In association with the usual variety of high A_2-β thalassemia, a thalassemia intermedia syndrome usually results and is characterized by high levels of Hb F and only mild or moderate anemia and hemolysis (Kattamis et al., 1973). The homozygous form of $\delta\beta$ thalassemia is also a relatively mild disorder and may be barely symptomatic. The affected individuals usually have mild to moderate anemia (Hb 9 to 10 g/100 ml), mild or moderate splenomegaly, and no transfusion requirement. They have 100 per cent Hb F, with no Hb A or Hb A_2. The relatively benign nature of $\delta\beta$ thalassemia seems to be related to the fact that, although it is associated with totally absent β- and δ-chain synthesis, it is also associated with more efficient preservation of γ-chain synthesis than the usual form of β thalassemia: the overall degree of globin-chain imbalance (α vs. non-α) is not as pronounced (Mann et al., 1972) and therefore there is less α-chain inclusion-body formation and less hemolysis. Although $\delta\beta$ thalassemia is almost always associated with absent δ- and β-chain synthesis in cis, there is one black family in which double heterozygosity for $\delta\beta$ thalassemia and Hb S was associated with some β^A synthesis (Russo and Mollica, 1962). In a Chinese family with $\delta\beta$ thalassemia, the only type of γ chain found was $^G\gamma$ suggesting that, in that family, the thalassemia also affected the $^A\gamma$ gene (Mann et al., 1972).

Delta-Beta Thalassemia with Normal Levels of Hb A_2 and Hb F

In the study of parents of children with apparent homozygous β thalassemia, one occasionally encounters a parent in whom both Hb A_2 and Hb F levels are normal. Some of these cases may be heterozygous for the ordinary type of $\delta\beta$ or F thalassemia in which, for unknown reasons, the Hb F level is only at the upper limits of normal instead of constituting over 5 per cent of the total hemoglobin. Such cases have been well documented (Fessas, 1965), and the low level of Hb F is not usually constant within the family; other members in the family with thalassemia trait usually have the expected elevated Hb F levels (Stamatoyannopoulos et al., 1969a; Fessas, 1965).

There is a report of a family in which two children had β thalassemia of intermediate severity. One parent had typical A_2-β thalassemia trait, whereas the other parent was hematologically normal, having normal red cell morphology and normal levels of Hb A_2 and Hb F but an abnormal β/α synthetic ratio of 0.6 characteristic of mild heterozygous β thalassemia (Schwartz, 1969). This latter form of heterozygous β thalassemia was found in a number of relatives of the affected parent and has been termed the "silent carrier" state for β thalassemia.

Heterozygous β thalassemia with normal Hb A_2 and Hb F, however, may also be phenotypically similar to heterozygous high A_2-β thalassemia, and the offspring of such an individual and another individual with typical high Hb A_2–β thalassemia trait may have homozygous β thalassemia (thalassemia major) of usual severity instead of a milder thalassemia intermedia syndrome (Bernini et al., 1962; Aksoy and Erdem, 1969).

Finally, in another family a thalassemia-like disorder was observed in a neonate. A number of family members were found to have typical thalassemic red cell morphology, normal levels of Hb A_2 and Hb F, and a β/α synthetic ratio of 0.5 characteristic of heterozygous β thalassemia (Kan et al., 1972b). The findings suggest that the thalassemia defect in this family may involve the γ-, δ-, and β-chain genes on the same chromosome. Such an occurrence would explain the normal levels of Hb F as well as Hb A_2.

Hemoglobin Lepore Syndrome

Hemoglobin Lepore is composed of two α chains and two abnormal non-α chains which have the structure of the δ chain at their N terminus and that of the β chain at their C terminus (Baglioni, 1962). The Lepore chain is believed to have resulted from nonhomologous crossing over, at meiosis, of the δ and β loci, as previously discussed (see Figure 2–2*A*). At least three different Lepore hemoglobins have been described which vary by the point at which the crossing over occurred between the δ- and β-chain structural genes (see Figure 2–2*B* and Table 3–2).

Hemoglobin Lepore is produced at a markedly reduced rate and, in the heterozygote, it accounts for only about 5 to 15 per cent of the total hemoglobin. Hemoglobin Lepore is easily detected by standard hemoglobin electrophoresis and has approximately the same mobility as Hb S (see Figure 2–12*C*). Clinically, the peripheral blood findings are similar to those of heterozygous high A_2-β thalassemia. Hemoglobin electrophoresis, in addition to the finding of the abnormal hemoglobin, reveals low or normal Hb A_2 and slight elevation of Hb F. Homozygosity for Hb Lepore and the combination of heterozygous high A_2-β thalassemia with hemoglobin Lepore are clinically indistinguishable from true homozygous β thalassemia (Weatherall and Clegg, 1972). In homozygous Hb Lepore, there is no normal Hb A or Hb A_2, only Hb F (approximately 75 per cent) and Hb Lepore (10 to 20 per cent). These findings indicate that the chromosome bearing the Lepore gene has no normal δ or β gene associated with it and thus confirms the crossing-over hypothesis and the location of the δ gene to the N-terminal side of the β gene in the normal.

Mild Homozygous Thalassemia (Thalassemia Intermedia)

There is some evidence that certain forms of β thalassemia are milder and produce a less severe clinical syndrome in the homozygous state (Weatherall and Clegg, 1972). This is especially true of homozygous β thalassemia in the black, which is usually a mild disease (Weatherall, 1964). The mild form of β thalassemia called the "silent carrier" state (Schwartz, 1969) results in a mild disease in association with the usual variety of A_2-β thalassemia. Homozygous $\delta\beta$ thalassemia (F thalassemia) also tends to be relatively mild because of the higher level of hemoglobin F synthesis in each cell resulting in less imbalance between α and non-α chains. Combination of $\delta\beta$ and high A_2-β thalassemia produces a disease of intermediate severity (Stamatoyannopoulos et al., 1969a; Kattamis et al., 1973). In addition, when a patient with homozygous β thalassemia also inherits an α-thalassemia gene, the disease will be milder because the associated α-thalassemia gene results in decreased synthesis of α chains and therefore less accumulation of free α chains. There will result less inclusion-body formation and less hemolysis (Kan and Nathan, 1970). The reverse is also true: a patient who has the α-thalassemia syndrome of hemoglobin H disease and who also inherits a β-thalassemia gene has much less hemolysis than patients with simple Hb H disease (Kan and Nathan, 1970; Knox-Macauley et al., 1972).

Interaction of Thalassemia with Abnormal Hemoglobins

When a patient acquires a thalassemia gene for a given globin chain on one chromosome and a gene for a structural variant of the same type of globin chain on the other chromosome, the percentage of the structurally abnormal hemoglobin observed is increased over the level found in a simple heterozygote for the structural variant, and the clinical severity of the condition approaches that of homozygosity for the abnormal hemoglobin (so-called interacting thalassemia). On the other hand, when a patient acquires the combination of thalassemia for one chain (i.e., β) and a structural variant for another globin chain (i.e., α), no increase in the abnormal hemoglobin is observed and the clinical severity of the condition is similar to that of the heterozygous state for the structural variant (noninteracting thalassemia). In fact, when α thalassemia is combined with a β-chain structural abnormality, the amount of the abnormal hemoglobin observed is sometimes less than in the simple heterozygous state. The precise molecular basis of this phenomenon is not understood. The common feature in all these syndromes is hypochromia and microcytosis of the red cells, as in thalassemia trait, in addition to the finding of the abnormal hemoglobin. Only the clinically important combinations will be briefly described here.

Beta Thalassemia in Association with Beta-Chain Structural Variants

Sickle Cell-β Thalassemia

This disease is described in detail in Chapter 4. S/β thalassemia primarily affects people of African, Italian, and Greek ancestry. The clinical picture resembles that of sickle cell anemia, but the disease in general tends to run a milder course. Splenomegaly is a common feature and is helpful in differentiating S/β thalassemia from sickle cell anemia in the older children and adults. Occasionally, the disease can be extremely mild, and the diagnosis may be discovered as an incidental finding.

Laboratory findings include targeting, hypochromia, and microcytosis of the red cells and a variable degree of anemia; occasional irreversibly sickled forms may be observed in the blood smear in the more severely affected cases. The hemoglobin electrophoresis reveals 60 to 90 per cent Hb S, 0 to 30 per cent Hb A, 1 to 20 per cent Hb F, and increased levels of Hb A_2. The clinical severity of the disease cannot be correlated well with the level of hemoglobin A.

HEMOGLOBIN C-β THALASSEMIA

This condition occurs mainly in blacks. A mild to moderate hemolytic anemia with splenomegaly is present.

HEMOGLOBIN E-β THALASSEMIA

This is a common disease in Thailand. For reasons that are poorly understood, it is almost as severe as homozygous β thalassemia. Hemoglobin electrophoresis shows hemoglobin E, a high percentage of Hb F (approximately 50 per cent) and usually no hemoglobin A. The abnormal physico-chemical properties of Hb E (see Chapter 3) may be in part responsible for the severity of this syndrome.

Alpha Thalassemia in Association with Alpha-Chain Structural Variants

HEMOGLOBIN Q-α THALASSEMIA

This condition is also found mainly in Thailand. The clinical picture is similar to that of Hb H disease. This syndrome is of interest mainly because of the associated hemoglobin electrophoresis findings. The affected individuals have total absence of Hb A. This finding is extremely difficult to explain if one assumes the presence of duplicated α-chain genes: one would expect some α-chain synthesis from the second α-chain gene in cis to the Hb Q, even if the two α-chain genes of the other (α-thalassemia 1) chromosome are totally inactive. One must postulate, therefore, that the second α gene in cis with Hb Q is always affected by α thalassemia in the Hb Q heterozygote.

HEMOGLOBIN G-PHILADELPHIA AND HB I-α THALASSEMIA

The α-chain variant Hb G-Philadelphia has been found in a number of blacks, in the heterozygous state alone and in association with other Hb variants or α thalassemia. Heterozygotes for Hb G-Philadelphia show variability in the amount of the variant present in hemolysates: there is a trimodal distribution in the percentage of the variant in heterozygotes. Individuals have approximately 22, 30, or 41 per cent Hb G-Philadelphia (Baine et al., 1976). The differences have been attributed to two possible mechansims: (1) the association of an $\alpha^{\text{G-Philadelphia}}$ gene with variable numbers (1, 2, or 3) of α^{A} loci due to heterogeneity in the duplication of α-chain loci in blacks, or (2) the association of an α-thalassemia gene in cis with $\alpha^{\text{G-Philadelphia}}$ in some individuals (Rucknagel and Winter, 1974; Rucknagel and Rising, 1975; Baine et al., 1976). In one study, biosynthetic studies revealed no imbalance between α- and β-chain synthesis in Hb G-Philadelphia heterozygotes (Baine et al., 1976), but in another study, heterozygotes for $\alpha^{\text{G-Philadelphia}}$ (alone or in association with Hb S or C) did manifest a deficit in α-chain synthesis compatible with an α-thalassemia–like syndrome (McCurdy et al., 1975). These findings, however, do not help distinguish between the two hypotheses (variable number of α-chain genes versus α thalassemia in cis with $\alpha^{\text{G-Philadelphia}}$). One black individual has been described, however, who is doubly heterozygous for $\alpha^{\text{G-Philadelphia}}$ and α thalassemia (Rieder et al., 1976). This individual has a syndrome analogous to Hb H disease. On hemoglobin electrophoresis there was 3.5 to 8 per cent Hb H and total absence of Hb A and Hb A_2; the α^{G}/β synthetic ratio was 0.63. The mother, two half-siblings, and one offspring had hematological evidence of heterozygous α thalassemia (without Hb G) with α/β synthetic ratios of 0.76 to 0.84. The father was not studied. This case illustrates definitely that, at least in some cases, $\alpha^{\text{G-Philadelphia}}$ is not associated with a functional α^{A} gene in cis, and that some forms of heterozygous α thalassemia in blacks are associated with totally absent α-chain synthesis from the chromosome bearing the α-thalassemia gene. In another black family, an individual inherited Hb G-Philadelphia from one parent and from the other parent Hb Seal Rock, a variant with an elongated α chain analogous to that of Hb Constant Spring (Bradley et al., 1975). The parent heterozygous for $\alpha^{\text{G-Philadelphia}}$ had 28 per cent Hb G-Philadelphia, whereas the doubly heterozygous individual had 39 per cent Hb G-Philadelphia, 2 per cent Hb Seal Rock, and the rest Hb A and Hb A_2, but had no Hb H. The α-thalassemia syndrome in this family is milder than in the previous one and the findings indicate that in this family either the $\alpha^{\text{G-Philadelphia}}$ gene or the $\alpha^{\text{Seal Rock}}$ gene (or both) is associated with a functional α^{A} gene in cis. Finally, one black individual has been described who inherited both α thalassemia and the α-chain variant Hb I (Atwater et al., 1960). This individual did not have Hb H and had 30 per cent Hb A.

These various family studies illustrate that α thalassemia in blacks is quite heterogeneous in the degree of suppression of α-chain synthesis and that there is probably heterogeneity in the number of α-chain loci in blacks.

Gamma Thalassemia

An infant with hemolytic anemia at birth was found to have hypochromic microcytic red cells (Kan et al., 1972b). Heterozygous β thalassemia, with normal levels of hemoglobin A_2 and F, was found in the father and many of his relatives. Globin-chain synthesis studies revealed a decrease in γ- and β-chain synthesis in the reticulocytes of this infant. The disease became self-limited as the baby grew older. The hemolytic anemia disappeared, and the child developed the phenotype of simple heterozygous β thalassemia. It is believed that this child represents an example of heterozygous $\gamma\beta$ (+ δ) thalassemia. The disease should be suspected in cases of hypochromic hemolytic disease in the newborn. Homozygous γ thalassemia would probably not be compatible with life (Stamatoyannopoulos, 1971).

Delta Thalassemia

Isolated delta thalassemia has been described as an incidental finding in both the heterozygous (Frazer et al., 1964) and homozygous (Ohta et al., 1970) forms. In the former, there is decreased Hb A_2; in the latter, total absence of Hb A_2 is noted. In neither situation are hypochromia, anemia, or red cell morphological changes observed. The doubly heterozygous state for δ thalassemia plus $\delta\beta$ thalassemia (Fessas and Stamatoyannopoulos, 1962) and δ thalassemia plus HPFH (Thompson et al., 1965a) have also been described and are clinically similar to simple heterozygosity for $\delta\beta$ thalassemia or HPFH except that there is total absence of Hb A_2.

Hereditary Persistence of Fetal Hemoglobin (HPFH) And HB Kenya

HPFH is found primarily in blacks and in Greeks (Conley et al., 1963; Fessas and Stamatoyannopoulos, 1964). In blacks, there is absence of β- and δ-chain synthesis in cis to the HPFH gene. Heterozygous HPFH differs from heterozygous thalassemia in that non-α (γ + β) chain production is usually equal to α-chain synthesis (Sofroniadou et al., 1975; Natta et al., 1973b). There is no globin-chain imbalance and no microcytosis or hypochromia of the red blood cells. Furthermore, the most important difference is that the fetal hemoglobin is evenly distributed in all the red blood cells in contrast to the heterogeneous distribution of Hb F observed in thalassemic red cells. In most blacks with HPFH the fetal hemoglobin which is present has the typical adult $^{G}\gamma$:$^{A}\gamma$ ratio of 2:3 (Huisman et al., 1971b). However, in some blacks with HPFH, all the Hb F present is of the $^{G}\gamma$ type and these individuals usually have a lower level of Hb F (15 per cent vs. 30 per cent) than other blacks with HPFH. In most Greeks with HPFH, all the Hb F is of the $^{A}\gamma$ type. Rare blacks with HPFH may also have predominantly Hb F of the $^{A}\gamma$ type (Huisman et al., 1971b). These findings indicate that the molecular defect leading to HPFH is quite heterogeneous.

In the heterozygous state, HPFH is asymptomatic. The hemoglobin F level is about 15 to 35 per cent of the total hemoglobin in the black and 10 to 20 per cent in the Greek type. Hemoglobin A_2 is decreased. The homozygous form of HPFH has been found only in the black (reviewed by Weatherall and Clegg, 1972). These individuals have 100 per cent fetal hemoglobin and have mild hypochromia, microcytosis, and red cell morphological changes but no anemia. In fact, mild erythrocytosis is present because of the high oxygen affinity of the blood resulting in relative tissue hypoxia. In two homozygous individuals globin synthesis has been studied and has revealed a mild to moderate deficit in γ-chain synthesis: γ/α 0.52 and 0.70 (Charache et al., 1975b; Forget et al., 1976b). These individuals therefore, have a degree of imbalanced globin-chain synthesis similar to that seen in β-thalassemia trait. Imbalance has also been observed in rare heterozygotes (Huisman et al., 1975; Friedman et al., 1976b).

In association with beta-chain structural variants, such as Hb S, HPFH gives hemoglobin electrophoresis findings similar to those found in Hb S/β^0 thalassemia or homozygous sickle cell anemia, but with an unusually high level of Hb F: absent Hb A, 65 to 85 per cent Hb S, and 15 to 35 per cent Hb F. Clinically, however, this disorder is benign with no anemia, hemolysis, hypochromia, or painful crises. The benign nature of this disorder is probably related to the fact that the Hb F is evenly distributed among the red cells, and it is known that Hb F inhibits the sickling of Hb S (see Chapter 4).

More recently, there have been reports of Hb S/HPFH in blacks in which there is synthesis of Hb A, presumably from an active β^A gene in cis to the HPFH gene (Huisman et al., 1975; Stamatoyannopoulos et al., 1975; Friedman and Schwartz, 1976). In two of these families the HPFH was of the $^{G}\gamma$ types. Similarly, in the Greek type ($^{A}\gamma$) of HPFH (Fessas and Stamatoyannopoulos, 1964), the British type (Weatherall et al., 1975a), and the Swiss type (Marti, 1963) there is convincing evidence for activity of the β-chain locus in cis to the HPFH gene (reviewed by Weatherall and Clegg, 1975).

As previously discussed, the ordinary type of HPFH in the black appears to be associated with gene deletion of β (and δ) structural genes. Obviously, the finding of some forms of HPFH with β-chain synthesis in cis indicates that the HPFH phenotype is not necessarily associated with δ- and *β-structural* gene deletions and that some other common feature must be present such as deletion of control gene elements situated between γ and δ or β structural loci. There is, however, no direct experimental evidence to support the latter hypothesis.

Hemoglobin Kenya is a newly discovered abnormal hemoglobin (Huisman et al., 1972b; Kendall et al., 1973) which is associated with an HPFH phenotype and has provided a more detailed understanding of the relationship between the $^{G}\gamma$-, $^{A}\gamma$-, δ-, and β-chain genes. The non-α chain of Hb Kenya consists of a fusion product containing the N terminus of the γ chain and the C terminus of the β chain, presumably the result of nonhomologous crossing over between a γ-chain gene and the β-chain gene (Fig. 2–3). The crossover from γ to β sequence occurred before position 136 (between residues 81 and 86) of the γ chain, so that it is not possible to tell whether it is an $^{A}\gamma$ or a $^{G}\gamma$ gene which is involved in the fusion product. However, individuals with Hb Kenya have increased levels of Hb F in their red cells and it is all of the $^{G}\gamma$ type. If one assumes that this Hb F comes from the γ-chain gene(s) in cis to the Kenya gene, and if the $^{G}\gamma\ ^{g}\gamma\ ^{A}\gamma\ ^{a}\gamma$ model of the γ-chain genes is correct (see above), then the crossover must involve either the $^{g}\gamma$ or $^{A}\gamma$ genes. In addition, one must conclude from this finding that the $^{A}\gamma$ gene is situated to the N-terminal side of the δ- and β-chain genes and is closer to these genes than is the $^{G}\gamma$ chain gene. The arrangement of the non-α chain genes would therefore be (going from N- to C-terminal): $^{G}\gamma\ ^{g}\gamma\ ^{A}\gamma\ ^{a}\gamma\ \delta\ \beta$. The finding of Hb Kenya, however, does not rule out the possibility that the $^{G}\gamma$ (and $^{g}\gamma$) genes are situated to the C-terminal side of the β-chain gene.

Of additional importance is the fact that Hb Kenya, unlike Hb Lepore, is not associated with a thalassemic phenotype, but rather an HPFH phenotype. Hemoglobin Kenya has been found in the simple heterozygous state as well as in association with Hb S (Kendall et al., 1973; Smith et al., 1973; Nute et al., 1976). In the simple heterozygote it makes up approximately 5 to 10 per cent of the total hemoglobin, but in association with Hb S it accounts for 17 to 19 per cent of the total. Rare simple heterozygotes have as much as 20 to 30 per cent Hb Kenya (Nute et al., 1976). All the patients are asymptomatic. There is no hypochromia or microcytosis and there are no morphological changes in the red cells. In all cases, the elevated fetal hemoglobin is uniformly distributed within the red cells and is of the $^{G}\gamma$ type (Kendall et al., 1973; Smith et al., 1973; Nute et al., 1976). Unlike the situation in the Hb Lepore and anti-Lepore syndromes, the synthesis of the Kenya fusion product is active in reticulocytes (Clegg et al., 1974b).

Management of the Thalassemia Syndromes

Prevention

An important step in the prevention of the occurrence of severely affected children with homozygous α or β thalassemia is the detection of the heterozygous state in adults. Physicians should be aware of the possibility of thalassemia trait occurring in individuals with hypochromic anemias which are refractory to iron therapy and should perform the necessary diagnostic studies to confirm the diagnosis. In areas where there is a high incidence of thalassemia trait, general population screening surveys could be established. Once identified, the affected individuals could be educated and counseled with respect to the disease process and its genetics. Two affected heterozygotes contemplating marriage and planning to have a family should be aware that chances of having a severely affected homozygous child are one in four.

Prenatal diagnosis of thalassemia is now feasible but is still considered an experimental procedure which is done only in a limited number of centers. The procedure involves obtaining a fetal blood sample and incubating it with radioactive leucine to determine the relative amounts of synthesis of γ, β, and α chains. The fetal blood sample can be obtained in one of two ways: (1) needle aspiration of a placental blood vessel without direct visualization, after localization of the placenta by ultrasound (Kan et al., 1974d); or (2) needle aspiration of a placental blood vessel (when the placenta is in a posterior or fundal position) under direct visualization using an amnioscope or fetoscope (Hobbins and Mahoney, 1974, 1975). Although fetal blood sampling has been successfully done a number of times by these techniques without fetal complications, the procedure cannot be considered totally safe: in a few cases fetal loss has occurred owing to infection, hemorrhage, premature labor, or undetermined causes (Alter et al., 1976b; Kan and Globus, 1976).

Another difficulty is obtaining a pure or relatively pure fetal sample. There may be variable contamination of the fetal blood with maternal placental blood. One can overcome the latter difficulty by various techniques which either concentrate and purify the fetal red cells by differential agglutination (Kan et al., 1974b), or correct for the maternal contamination by calculations based on differences in specific activity between fetal and maternal samples or by determining globin synthesis in various known mixtures of fetal plus maternal blood (Cividalli et al., 1974a; Chang et al., 1975). Another approach to the problem of maternal blood contamination is to transfuse the mother prior to the procedure in order to suppress erythropoiesis and thereby reduce the proportion of synthetically active reticulocytes in the maternal peripheral blood (Nathan and Alter, 1975). Finally, for the diagnosis of α-thalassemia syndromes due to gene deletions, prenatal diagnosis can be achieved by measurement of α-chain genes by molecular hybridization, using DNA obtained from cultured amniotic fluid fibroblasts (Kan and Globus, 1976; Kan et al., 1976a).

From the biochemical point of view, prenatal diagnosis of α and β thalassemia and structural hemoglobinopathies should pose no major obstacles. In the case of α thalassemia and α-chain structural variants, the detection of a quantitative or qualitative abnormality in α-chain synthesis should be feasible, since the α chain is normally fully expressed in the first trimester (see Figure 2–4). With respect to β thalassemia and β-chain structural variants, the β gene is normally expressed at only a very low level in the first and second trimesters, but there is still sufficient β-chain synthesis in utero to allow detection of an abnormal β chain or the determination, from the study of a large number of cases, of the range of normal fetal β-chain synthesis, below which β thalassemia should fall (Kazazian et al., 1973; Cividalli et al., 1974a; Chang et al., 1974, 1975). In fact, heterozygosity for Hb S (Kan et al., 1972a), α thalassemia (Kan et al., 1974a, and β thalassemia (Chang et al., 1975) has been diagnosed in studies of abortuses of pregnancies at risk. Prospective prenatal diagnosis attempts have been performed in a number of cases (Kan et al., 1975b, 1975c; Nathan and Alter, 1975; Alter et al., 1976a, 1976b; Kan et al., 1976a, 1976b). Prospective diagnoses have been made of homozygous β thalassemia (Kan et al., 1975c), homozygous sickle cell anemia (Alter et al., 1976a; Kan et al., 1976b), heterozygous α and β thalassemia (Alter et al., 1976b; Kan et al., 1976a), and, incidentally, heterozygosity for Hb G-Philadelphia (Alter et al., 1976a). Some diagnostic errors, however, have occurred (Alter et al., 1976b).

It is not certain, however, that prenatal diagnosis will significantly reduce the incidence of homozygous individuals. Such cases will still arise in instances in which the parents are unaware, before the birth of their first affected child, that they have thalassemia trait. Furthermore, some parents may object to abortion yet wish to attempt having other (hopefully unaffected) children. In individual cases, however, the availability of precise prenatal diagnosis will be of great value.

Supportive Therapy

There is no specific therapy for the severely affected homozygous thalassemic patient. The treatment is mainly supportive and consists of a regular transfusion program to control the anemia. There are two general types of transfusion programs which can be undertaken. Until recently the standard program consisted of transfusing the patient in order to maintain a "safe" hemoglobin level. This usually meant transfusing the patient when his hemoglobin dropped to a level of 7 or 8 g/100 ml, hopefully before the patient became symptomatic.

The second type of transfusion program is the so-called high or hyper-transfusion (HT) regimen. This approach consists of transfusing the patients as frequently as necessary to maintain a "normal" hemoglobin level, which is not allowed to drop below a minimum of 10 g/100 ml. Such a program usually entails a transfusion of 2 to 3 units of packed red cells at intervals of every two to four weeks. The HT regimen has the obvious disadvantage that the patient receives a much larger total body burden of iron which cannot be naturally excreted by the body. Calculations of this excess infusion of iron, in comparison with a more standard transfusion regimen, give minimum values in the range of 1 to 2 grams of elemental iron per year for the net increment of iron accumulated (Necheles, 1969a; Piomelli et al., 1969). If one does not subtract iron removed by chelation therapy and the decreased iron absorbed from food, the increment may be as high as 3 to 4 grams of elemental iron per year in the HT regimen (Beard et al., 1969). Since the major cause of death in these children is related to the effects of iron overload in the second or third decade, many physicians have been reluctant to adopt this HT program. However, there is good evidence that children who are maintained on an HT regimen do as well as, if not better than, children maintained on a more standard regimen. The children in the HT group, in general, have fewer intercurrent illnesses and infections, are more active, and lead more normal and happy lives (Wolman, 1964; Wolman and Ortolani, 1969). There are fewer instances of cardiomegaly and hepatosplenomegaly and fewer bone changes and orthodontic problems (Beard et al., 1969; Piomelli et al., 1969). There is some dispute as to whether the HT regimen actually improves the growth and development of these children. Some studies claim that hypertransfusion does improve growth (Wolman, 1964; Beard et al., 1969; Piomelli et al., 1969; Kattamis et al., 1970), whereas other studies did not show improved growth (Johnston et al., 1966; Wolff and Luke, 1969; Wolman and Ortolani, 1969; Logothetis et al., 1972). One study even found some decrease in growth in the HT group (Brook et al., 1969). The discrepancy is probably related to the age at which HT is started: HT started after the first few years of life probably does not improve growth and development, but HT started in infancy may prevent growth retardation (Beard et al., 1969; Piomelli et al., 1969). The most recent follow-up studies on such patients have still not resolved the issue (Piomelli et al., 1974; Necheles et al., 1976).

It will be some time before one will be able to assess with certainty whether the HT program affects the longevity of the patients who receive it. Thus far, it appears that longevity may not be prolonged (Wolman and Ortolani, 1969) but is probably not shortened, and that the HT regimen seems to contribute to happier lives for the thalassemic children. Certainly one should not limit transfusions in thalassemic children for fear of iron overload. Because the HT regimen does not, in general, appear to shorten longevity, it seems reasonable generally to transfuse a child as frequently as necessary to maintain a minimum hemoglobin of 9 or 10 g/100 ml, if the facilities to do so are available. It seems important to institute such a program from an early age if one wishes to lessen the development of severe facial deformities, bone changes, cardiomegaly, and splenomegaly in these patients.

Any transfusion regimen, and especially the HT regimen, is associated with a certain incidence of transfusion-related complications. Hepatitis and other viral diseases, such as cytomegalovirus infections, are always a risk and are treated symptomatically. Isoimmunization to minor blood groups (Kell, Duffy, C. c, E), although relatively rare (Economidou et al., 1971), may cause difficulties in cross-matching and in survival time of the transfused red cells. This may be avoided by careful, full minor blood-group typing of the patient before the institution of transfusions and by careful selection of blood donors. Urticarial reactions usually respond to epinephrine or antihistamines and may be avoided in some cases by treatment with antihistamines prior to the transfusion. A more difficult problem is the febrile reaction due to prior sensitization of the patient to white blood cell or plasma protein antigens (Economidou et al., 1971). These may be avoided (or prevented) by use of white cell–free blood: frozen red cells or blood passed through Leuko-Pak(R) filters (Fenwal Laboratories). Antipyretics and occasionally steroids are necessary to treat severe febrile reactions.

Splenectomy

Splenectomy has an important place in the management of patients with homozygous β thalassemia. If a child is maintained on a good hypertransfusion regimen from an early age, marked splenomegaly may not develop (Beard et al., 1969; Piomelli et al., 1969) because of decreased production and thus decreased RE destruction of abnormal red cells. Even established splenomegaly may be reversible following institution of HT (O'Brien et al., 1971). However, many patients, in spite of adequate transfusions, do develop significant splenomegaly which may cause problems. Progressive splenomegaly usually aggravates the anemia and increases the transfusion requirement by causing a dilutional type of anemia due to the sequestration of transfused red cells in the large third space provided by the spleen's size.

Thalassemic children with splenomegaly have a greatly increased intravascular blood volume which can be reversed by splenectomy (Blendis et al., 1974). In addition, the patients may develop true hypersplenism, with evidence of destruction in the spleen of red cells and of other formed blood elements such as white cells and platelets. Rapid onset of splenomegaly and splenic destruction of transfused red cells may be triggered by isoimmunization to minor blood-group antigens. Such an occurrence is usually associated with difficulty in cross-matching the blood and development of a positive Coombs' test. In some instances, however, the only sign may be a sudden increase in the child's transfusion requirement and a sudden increase in spleen size. Splenomegaly, on the other hand, may be symptomatic simply by the sheer size of the spleen, causing pressure discomfort in the abdomen or pain from splenic infarcts. In cases in which splenomegaly is symptomatic or causes difficulty in maintaining adequate hemoglobin levels despite appropriate maintenance transfusions, splenectomy should be recommended. Splenectomy will usually result in a lessening of the transfusion requirement and, in combination with a good transfusion program, will usually make it possible to maintain the patient's hemoglobin at a near normal level much more easily than before splenectomy and thus achieve the maximum benefits of HT.

Splenectomy is rarely necessary before the child reaches the age of five or six years, but in certain instances splenectomy at an earlier age may be necessary. The decision to perform splenectomy may be aided by doing a chromium-51 tagged red cell survival study, with scanning of the spleen to demonstrate sequestration of labeled red cells. Splenectomy is rarely indicated before the age of three or four years, because of the demonstration of increased instances of rapidly fatal septicemia in children who have had splenectomy before that age (Eraklis et al., 1967). Thalassemic children, even those over the age of three or four, are particularly susceptible to this type of fatal gram-positive septicemia (Smith et al., 1962, 1964). The reasons for this high incidence are not known. The spleen and the reticuloendothelial (RE) system in general probably function as bacterial filters of the circulation. In the asplenic thalassemic individual, the loss of splenic filter function is probably aggravated, in addition, by some degree of RE system blockade due to the iron overload. A more recent study, however, did not show a high incidence of septicemia in a large series of thalassemic patients who had splenectomy after the age of two years (Englehard et al., 1975). The spleen probably has a function in antibody synthesis, the absence of which may also put the thalassemic patient at a disadvantage in handling infections. Indeed, immunoglobulin levels are low in some splenectomized thalassemic patients (Wasi et al., 1971) but not in all (Englehard et al., 1975). Because of the increased risk of infection, it is probably advisable, after splenectomy, to maintain thalassemic children on prophylactic doses of penicillin for at least two years (the time of peak incidence of postsplenectomy septicemia), if not indefinitely. Another postsplenectomy complication is the occasional development of marked thrombocytosis with thromboembolic phenomena which may require anticoagulation. Most patients, however, improve following splenectomy (Englehard et al., 1975) and some may even have improved growth and development (Blendis et al., 1974).

Use of Iron-Chelating Agents

Because of the marked iron overload which occurs in β thalassemia, it should be clinically advantageous to remove the excess iron stores, especially in patients maintained on high transfusion regimens, by the long-term administration of iron-chelating agents. There are two such agents which are currently available and have been extensively used in Britain and Europe. The first is desferrioxamine B, which is usually administered by intramuscular injection; the second is diethylenetriamine pentacetate (DTPA), which must be given by intravenous infusion, usually at the time of transfusion (Smith, 1962, 1964; Keberle, 1964). It should be theoretically possible to maintain a near balance of iron stores if one uses the following doses of the two agents concomitantly: 6 mg of I.V. DTPA with each transfusion and 0.5 to 1.0 g of desferrioxamine I.M. daily (Weatherall and Clegg, 1972).

The initial studies of urinary iron excretion in response to these drugs demonstrated that not all patients respond equally well. In some patients, concomitant use of vitamin C improved urinary iron excretion in response to desferrioxamine (Wapnick et al., 1969). However, the amount of iron excretion induced by desferrioxamine usually decreased in time and the drug became relatively ineffective (Smith, 1962, 1964; Beard et al., 1969). The reason for this loss of effectiveness is probably that desferrioxamine may only chelate iron which is in certain labile pools: the bulk of the storage iron may not be chelatable when desferrioxamine is administered in the usual manner (Lipschitz et al., 1971). Therefore, in practice, it is not usually possible to achieve a state of sustained negative iron balance in most thalassemic patients by administering desferrioxamine by daily intramuscular injections alone (Beard et al., 1969; Weatherall and Clegg, 1972). Exceptions may, however, exist: in a child with congenital hypoplastic anemia treated for 5 years with intramuscular desferrioxamine, 30 per cent of the amount of transfused iron was recovered in the urine (Lukens and Neuman, 1971). Desferrioxamine has rarely been associated with certain undesirable side effects: patients developed presumed allergic reactions (Beard et al., 1969) and the daily intramuscular injections caused local discomfort. Finally, cataracts have been described in experimental animals and in three individuals after long-term use of desferrioxamine. DTPA is generally considered quite toxic and its usefulness is very limited.

Subsequently, more optimistic reports have appeared on the use of desferrioxamine in thalassemia (Constantoulakis et al., 1974; Modell and Beck, 1974; O'Brien, 1974). These more recent studies have shown that with higher doses of desferrioxamine, including intravenous desferrioxamine at the time of transfusion, and with concomitant daily oral vitamin C, sustained high levels of urinary iron excretion and near normal iron balance can be achieved. More recently, preliminary studies have shown that slow continuous subcutaneous infusions of desferrioxamine (using portable devices) achieve significantly greater urinary iron excretion than single daily intramuscular injections (Propper et al., 1976). In general, however, significant iron excretion occurs only with increasing age and only after considerable iron overload has already occurred as determined by measurements of liver iron. It has not been demonstrated that desferrioxamine can actually prevent the occurrence of this initial iron accumulation: iron stores usually must reach levels nearly 10 times greater than normal before significant chelation is achieved. Although it appears that tissue siderosis cannot be totally prevented by chelation, it is possible that long-term chelation therapy may be of some benefit by eliminating additional increments of more reactive and potentially toxic iron, especially in patients on high transfusion regimens. Recently, Barry et al. (1974) demonstrated that liver iron stores stabilized and hepatic fibrosis failed to progress on long-term use of desferrioxamine. Growth and sexual development were also improved in these patients.

The role and mode of action of vitamin C in chelation therapy are not clear. Thalassemic patients are usually deficient in vitamin C (and E), both nonspecific and anti-oxidant substances, presumably because of the oxidant stress of iron overload. It seems, therefore, theoretically advantageous to replenish these vitamins in the thalassemic patient, both to counteract the tissue toxic oxidant stress of iron and to facilitate mobilization of iron. At one time there was some concern that vitamin C might act by increasing gastrointestinal tract absorption of iron, thus increasing the labile pool of chelatable iron and urinary excretion of iron. However, careful balance studies have ruled out this possibility (Nienhuis et al., 1975).

New iron-chelating drugs, especially orally effective agents, are being sought. One such agent, 2,3-dihydroxybenzoic acid, initially seemed to have some promise (Graziano et al., 1974); however, clinical trials in humans have failed to demonstrate substantial urinary iron excretion (Jones et al., 1975), although the drug seems to be effective as a free radical scavenger and thus may help counteract tissue iron toxicity (Graziano et al., 1976).

Other General Measures

The medical management of a child with homozygous β thalassemia otherwise involves good general pediatric and medical care, which includes a close relationship among physician, patient, and parents and education of parents and child with regard to seeking early medical attention for any illness, especially febrile episodes. Because of the propensity of these children to develop severe and frequently fatal infections, it is probably wise to treat any febrile illness, after taking appropriate cultures, with antibiotics until a specific diagnosis becomes apparent. In addition to the fatal septicemias, other infections which these patients develop include a *benign pericarditis*, believed to be of viral etiology (Engle, 1964); however, it may also be the result of streptococcal infection (Wasi, 1971) or due to an iron-induced pericardial irritation analogous to the arthritis of hemochromatosis. It usually subsides spontaneously, although pericardiocentesis may rarely be necessary to relieve tamponade. Other infections include *transfusion-related infections* such as hepatitis and cytomegalovirus infection, which must be treated symptomatically. The latter may be avoided by use of blood which is over 48 hours old.

Because of the marked marrow hyperplasia due to the hemolytic component of the disease, thalassemic children should be maintained on daily folic acid replacement (1 mg daily) to prevent the development of relative *folic acid deficiency* and a megaloblastic crisis, which may aggravate the anemia. Such a crisis may occasionally present as thrombocytopenia and a bleeding diathesis.

Certain children develop severe *cephalofacial deformities and malocclusion* because of marrow expansion in the maxilla. This complication can usually be avoided by proper transfusion from an early age and early splenectomy (Logothetis et al., 1971). Once the deformity is established, surgical management is possible (Jurkiewicz et al., 1969).

The consequences of *iron overload* must be treated as they develop: diabetes, with appropriate diet and insulin therapy; hepatic dysfunction, by dietary and other supportive means. Frequently, thalassemic children may have a prolonged prothrombin time which, despite its probable hepatocellular basis, may respond to vitamin K therapy. Some malabsorption of vitamin K may occur because of chronic pancreatic insufficiency due to pancreatic siderosis and fibrosis.

As previously discussed in the section on chelation therapy, vitamin C and vitamin E supplementation may be beneficial to counteract the oxidant effects of iron overload (Rachmilewitz et al., 1976).

The most serious and life-threatening complication is that of *cardiac hemosiderosis*, resulting in arrhythmia and chronic congestive heart failure (Engle, 1964). When these complications develop, the patients must be treated vigorously with low salt diet, digitalis, diuretics, and antiarrhythmic medications. Fatal Stokes-Adams attacks may occur from arrhythmias which are presumably due to iron deposition in the conducting system of the heart. In a child who develops recurrent arrhythmias, a cardiac pacemaker may be required to prevent a fatal arrhythmia.

Finally, androgen therapy (oxymetholone) has been reported to improve the anemia in a case of thalassemia intermedia (Craddock et al., 1972), although secondary causes may have contributed to the anemia in that particular case. Hormonal replacement therapy has been used in certain patients in an attempt to treat various *endocrine deficiencies*, presumably due to hemosiderosis, and improve development of secondary sexual characteristics. The therapy is not usually effective because sexual underdevelopment may be due in large part to target organ unresponsiveness (related to siderotic or hypoxic damage) rather than to hormonal deficiency.

Future Treatment

The future may offer more definitive forms of therapy for thalassemia. Two possible means of therapy may one day become available for the child with thalassemia major: (1) bone marrow transplantation, and/or (2) correction of the biochemical defect by genetic engineering and manipulation.

The art of bone marrow transplantation is being developed in a number of centers. It has been successfully carried out in the treatment of aplastic anemia and in certain cases of acute leukemia in relapse, using as a source of bone marrow that of an unaffected sibling who is histocompatible with the patient (Thomas et al., 1975). The major problem, however, is immunological: rejection of the graft by the recipient and graft-versus-host reaction have been difficult problems which have led to many failures and fatalities. In thalassemia, one would have to destroy the patient's own marrow before such a transplantation in order to prevent proliferation of the abnormal erythroid cells. This would be impossible to do without destroying the patient's own granulocyte precursors and megakaryocytes as well. Rejection of the marrow graft by the thalassemic patient is a very likely complication, even with proper immunosuppression and good histocompatibility, because of prior sensitization of the patient to various tissue antigens from the many previous blood transfusions. Rejection of the graft would leave the patient totally aplastic. If marrow engraftment is to be successful in thalassemic patients, transplantation should probably be done in infancy before transfusions are initiated. Finally, even if the transplanted marrow becomes engrafted, a graft-versus-host reaction could lead to a rapidly fatal outcome. Until the current problems of bone marrow transplantation are resolved, and one can offer the patient a good possibility of a successful outcome, bone marrow transplantation cannot be advised at this time in cases of thalassemia in which, with good medical management, the patient can be given some 20 or more years of useful life.

If one could suppress the excessive production of the normally produced globin chain in thalassemia, one would eliminate the precipitation of globin-chain aggregates which leads to much of the pathophysiology and disability in thalassemia. Research is proceeding in a search for drugs or other agents which might specifically inhibit the synthesis of one or another globin chain. In β thalassemia, if one could induce γ-chain synthesis, or prevent the neonatal γ to β chain switchover, one would increase the relative amount of γ chain in the thalassemic red cell. This would decrease the disability of the patients by decreasing or eliminating the formation of α-chain aggregates, which are so important in the development of the hemolytic component of the disease: the γ chains could combine with the excess α chains and balance would be achieved. Research is also under way in this area.

In the not too distant future, actual gene therapy for thalassemia may be feasible. Methods for isolating, purifying, and replicating eukaryotic genes are being rapidly developed as well as techniques for insertion of foreign DNA into eukaryotic cells. The technical scientific difficulties of such an approach are formidable but not insurmountable. A considerable amount of controversy exists, however, concerning the ethical and moral aspects of such an approach. A number of scientists and geneticists strongly oppose the idea of tampering with human genomes because of the potentially harmful consequences which could ensue. It is conceivable that the technical capability of gene therapy will be achieved before the ethical issues are resolved.

These types of therapeutic approaches are not imminent but remain likely future possibilities. Once the genetic defect is known more precisely at the messenger RNA and DNA levels, one may have more insight into ways to approach the treatment of thalassemia at the molecular level. In the meantime, the cornerstone of the treatment of thalassemia must remain good general medical care and proper supportive management of the patient in a center which is equipped to make this possible.

Chapter 3

HUMAN HEMOGLOBIN VARIANTS

To the nonspecialist, perhaps the most bewildering aspect of "hemoglobinology" is the number and variety of human hemoglobin variants. This topic continues to expand logarithmically. At present there are over 250 variants of known structure (Table 3–1). It is not surprising that the first human hemoglobin variants to be recognized were those that attracted clinical attention. Hörlein and Weber (1948) reported the first hemoglobinopathy. They studied a family with congenital cyanosis and demonstrated that affected family members had hemoglobin with abnormal spectral properties. Later, it was shown that they had one of the M hemoglobins. In the early 1950's, sickle cell anemia was found to be due to an electrophoretically abnormal hemoglobin having a single amino acid substitution in the β chain (β6 Glu→Val). Thereafter, electrophoresis became widely employed in the search for other human hemoglobin variants. Those having relatively high gene frequencies were discovered quite readily. Hemoglobins C, D, and E were identified within two years following the structural identification of hemoglobin S. Large-scale screening programs were initiated to find other abnormal hemoglobins. Initially, new variants were named by successive letters of the alphabet. By the time hemoglobin Q was encountered, it became apparent that the letters of the alphabet would soon be exhausted. To add to the confusion, some hemoglobins with identical electrophoretic properties were shown to have different structures. Gradually, investigators agreed to give new hemoglobins a specific name, most often reflecting the origin of the patient. Many colorful and provocative names have appeared in the literature, some exotic (Hb Aida), others chauvinistic (Hb Brigham), parochial (Hb

*TABLE 3–1. Human Hemoglobin Variants: 1976**

	Total	Unstable	Abnormal O_2 Affinity	Hbs M	No Clinical Manifestations
α Chain	80	9	4	2	65
β Chain	166	65	30	3	70
γ Chain	14	1			
δ Chain	9				
Total	269				

*Compiled from Table 3–2.

Riverdale-Bronx), or patriotic (Hb Abraham Lincoln). For a while the naming of hemoglobin variants was treated somewhat lightly because many believed the hemoglobin would be more often remembered by its structure rather than by its eponym. However, just as people naturally tend to call their friends by name rather than by social security number, the names of the variants have stuck. As Table 3–2 shows, the same variant (with a specific structural abnormality) is often "rediscovered" in different laboratories all over the world: $\alpha_2^{47\ Asp \rightarrow Gly}\beta_2$ has nine interesting names, but it is generally called Hb L-Ferrara, after the place where it was first described.

CLINICAL CLASSIFICATION

The large list of human hemoglobin variants shown in Table 3–2 is more readily comprehended if the variants are classified according to their clinical manifestations (Table 3–3). The majority of known variants are unassociated with any apparent clinical sequelae. Many of these were discovered accidentally or during the survey of large populations. Although they may be of genetic or anthropological interest, they have no apparent functional abnormalities.

The clinically significant human hemoglobin variants are classified in Table 3–3. Disorders due to the presence of sickle hemoglobin constitute the most important group both in the United States and worldwide. (The sickle syndromes are discussed in detail in Chapter 4.) Hb C is the second most commonly encountered variant. Like Hb S, Hb C has decreased solubility within the red cell. The pathogenesis of homozygous Hb C disease is discussed at the end of this chapter. Approximately 65 unstable hemoglobin variants have been described to date. They constitute an important form of congenital nonspherocytic hemolytic anemia. (This entity is discussed in Chapter 5.) Variants with abnormal oxygen binding are described in Chapter 6. This group has provided a considerable amount of relevant physiological and biochemical information. Individuals with congenital methemoglobinemia may have one of the so-called M he-

Text continued on page 112.

TABLE 3–2. Human Hemoglobin Variants*

ALPHA CHAIN

Residue and Helical Number	*Amino Acid Substitution*	*Name*	*Major Abnormal Property*	*Reference*
5(A3)	Ala→Asp	Hb J-Toronto		1
6(A4)	Asp→Ala	Hb Sawara		2
11(A9)	Lys→Glu	Hb Anantharaj		3
12(A10)	Ala→Asp	Hb J-Paris-I, J-Aljezur		4,70
15(A13)	Gly→Asp	Hb I-Interlaken, J-Oxford, N-Cosenza		5,6
	Gly→Arg	Hb Ottawa, Siam		7,8
16(A14)	Lys→Glu	Hb I, I-Philadelphia, I-Texas, I-Burlington, I-Skamania		9
21(B2)	Ala→Asp	Hb J-Nyanza		10
22(B3)	Gly→Asp	Hb J-Medellin		11
23(B4)	Glu→Gln	Hb Memphis		12
	Glu→Lys	Hb Chad		13
	Glu→Val	Hb G-Audhali		14
27(B8)	Glu→Gly	Hb Fort Worth		15
27(B8)	Glu→Val	Hb Spanish Town		268
30(B11)	Glu→Lys	Hb O-Padova		16
	Glu→Gln	Hb G-Honolulu, G-Singapore, G-Chinese, G-Hong Kong		17
43(CE1)	Phe→Val	Hb Torino	Unstable; ↓ O_2 affinity	18
	Phe→Leu	Hb Hirosaki		19
47(CE5)	Asp→Gly	Hb L-Ferrara, Umi, Kokura, Michigan-I, Michigan-II, Yukuhashi-II, L-Gaslini, Tagawa-II, Beilinson, Mugino		20
	Asp→His	Hb Hasharon, Sinai, Sealy	Unstable	21,22
	Asp→Asn	Hb Arya	Slightly unstable	23
48(CE6)	Leu→Arg	Hb Montgomery		24
50(CE8)	His→Asp	Hb J-Sardegna		25
51(CE9)	Gly→Asp	Hb J-Abidjan		26
	Gly→Arg	Hb Russ		27
53(E2)	Ala→Asp	Hb J-Rovigo	Unstable	28
54(E3)	Gln→Arg	Hb Shimonoseki		29
	Gln→Glu	Hb J-Mexico, J-Paris-II, Uppsala		30
57(E6)	Gly→Arg	Hb L-Persian Gulf		31
	Gly→Asp	Hb J-Norfolk, Kagoshima, Nishik-I, II, III		32
58(E7)	His→Tyr	Hb M-Boston, M-Osaka, M-Gothenburg, M-Kiskunhalos	Ferri-Hb; ↓ O_2 affinity	33
60(E9)	Lys→Asn	Hb Zambia		34
61(E10)	Lys→Asn	Hb J-Buda	↓ O_2 affinity	35
64(E13)	Asp→Asn	Hb G-Waimanalo, Hb-Aida		36,37
	Asp→His	Hb Q-India		38
68(E17)	Asn→Asp	Hb Ube-2		39
	Asn→Lys	Hb G-Philadelphia, G-Knoxville-II, Stanleyville-I, G-Bristol, G-Uzuakoli, D-Baltimore, D-Washington, D-St. Louis		40
71(E20)	Ala→Glu	Hb J-Habana		41
72(EF1)	His→Arg	Hb Daneshgah-Teheran		42
74(EF3)	Asp→His	Hb Mahidol, G-Taichung, Q-Thailand		43,44
	Asp→Asn	Hb G-Pest		35
	Asp→Gly	Hb Chapel Hill	↑ O_2 affinity	280
75(EF4)	Asp→His	Hb Q-Iran		44
	Asp→Tyr	Hb Winnipeg		45
78(EF7)	Asn→Lys	Hb Stanleyville-II		46
80(F1)	Leu→Arg	Hb Ann Arbor	Unstable	47,48
84(F5)	Ser→Arg	Hb Etobicoke	Unstable	49
85(F6)	Asp→Asn	Hb G-Norfolk	↑ O_2 affinity	50,51
	Asp→Tyr	Hb Atago		52
	Asp→Val	Hb Inkster		53

*Kindly supplied by the Director of the International Hemoglobin Information Center, Augusta, Georgia.

Table continued on following page.

TABLE 3–2. ***Human Hemoglobin Variants*** **—Continued**

ALPHA CHAIN

Residue and Helical Number	*Amino Acid Substitution*	*Name*	*Major Abnormal Property*	*Reference*
87(F8)	His→Tyr	Hb M-Iwate, M-Kankakee, M-Oldenburg	Ferri-Hb; ↓ O_2 affinity	54
90(FG2)	Lys→Asn	Hb J-Broussais, Tagawa-I		55
	Lys→Thr	Hb J-Rajappen		56
92(FG4)	Arg→Gln	Hb J-Cape Town	↑ O_2 affinity	57
	Arg→Leu	Hb Chesapeake	↑ O_2 affinity	58,59
94(G1)	Asp→Tyr	Hb Setif	Unstable	60
	Asp→Asn	Hb Titusville	↓ O_2 affinity	61
95(G2)	Pro→Leu	Hb G-Georgia	↑ Dissociation	62,63
	Pro→Ser	Hb Rampa	↑ Dissociation	63,64
	Pro→Ala	Hb Denmark Hill	↑ O_2 affinity	65
	Pro→Arg	Hb St. Lukes	↑ Dissociation	66
100(G7)	Leu			
102(G9)	Ser→Arg	Hb Manitoba		67
112(G19)	His→Gln	Hb Dakar*	Unstable	68
	His→Asp	Hb Hopkins-2	Unstable; ↑ O_2 affinity	69
	His→Arg	Hb Strumica, Serbia		70,71
114(GH2)	Pro→Arg	Hb Chiapas		30
115(GH3)	Ala→Asp	Hb J-Tongariki		72
116(GH4)	Glu→Lys	Hb O-Indonesia, Buginese-X, Oliviere		73
118(H1)	Thr→Gly	Hb Hopkins-2-II		74
120(H3)	Ala→Glu	Hb J-Meerut (J-Birmingham)		75,76
127(H10)	Lys→Thr	Hb St. Claude		77
136(H19)	Leu→Pro	Hb Bibba	Unstable; ↑ dissociation	78
141(HC3)	Arg→Pro	Hb Singapore		79
	Arg→His	Hb Suresnes	↑ O_2 affinity, ↓ Bohr	281

*Hb Dakar has recently been shown to be identical to Hb Grady rather than having the substitution shown above (see ref. 269).

BETA CHAIN

Residue and Helical Number	*Amino Acid Substitution*	*Name*	*Major Abnormal Property*	*Reference*
2(NA1)	His→Arg	Hb Deer Lodge		80
6(A3)	Glu→Val	Hb S	Sickling	81
	Glu→Lys	Hb C		82
	Glu→Ala	Hb G-Makassar		83
7(A4)	Glu→Gly	Hb G-San Jose		84
	Glu→Lys	Hb C-Siriraj		85
9(A6)	Ser→Cys	Hb Porto Alegre	Polymerization	86
10(A7)	Ala→Asp	Hb Ankara		87
14(A11)	Leu→Arg	Hb Sögn	Unstable	88
	Leu→Pro	Hb Saki	Unstable	89
15(A12)	Trp→Arg	Hb Belfast	Unstable	90
16(A13)	Gly→Asp	Hb J-Baltimore, J-Trinidad, J-Ireland, J-Georgia		91
	Gly→Arg	Hb D-Bushman		92
17(A14)	Lys→Glu	Hb Nagasaki		93
19(B1)	Asn→Lys	Hb D-Ouled Rabah		94
20(B2)	Val→Met	Hb Olympia	↑ O_2 affinity	95
	Val→Asp	Hb Strasbourg	Unstable	285
22(B4)	Glu→Lys	Hb E-Saskatoon		96
	Glu→Gly	Hb G-Taipei		97
	Glu→Ala	Hb G-Saskatoon, Hsin Chu, G-Coushatta, G-Taegu		98,99
	Glu→Gln	Hb D-Iran		100

TABLE 3–2. *Human Hemoglobin Variants*—Continued

BETA CHAIN

Residue and Helical Number	*Amino Acid Substitution*	*Name*	*Major Abnormal Property*	*Reference*
24(B6)	Gly→Arg	Hb Riverdale-Bronx	Unstable	101
	Gly→Val	Hb Savannah	Unstable	102
	Gly→Asp	Hb Moscva	Unstable; ↓ O_2 affinity	103
25(B7)	Gly→Arg	Hb G-Taiwan-Ami		104
26(B8)	Glu→Lys	Hb E		105
	Glu→Val	Hb Henri Mondor	Unstable	286
27(B9)	Ala→Asp	Hb Volga, Drenthe	Unstable	106,107
28(B10)	Leu→Gln	Hb St. Louis	Unstable; ferri-Hb	108
	Leu→Pro	Hb Genova	Unstable; ↑ O_2 affinity	109
30(B12)	Arg→Ser	Hb Tacoma	Unstable; ↓ Bohr; normal O_2 affinity	110
32(B14)	Leu→Pro	Hb Perth, Abraham Lincoln	Unstable	111,112
	Leu→Arg	Hb Castilla	Unstable	113
35(C1)	Tyr→Phe	Hb Philly	Unstable	114
37(C3)	Trp→Ser	Hb Hirose	↑ O_2 affinity	115
39(C5)	Gln→Lys	Hb Alabama		24
40(C6)	Arg→Lys	Hb Athens-Georgia	↑ O_2 affinity	116
41(C7)	Phe→Tyr	Hb Mequon	Unstable	117
42(CD1)	Phe→Ser	Hb Hammersmith, Chiba	Unstable; ↓ O_2 affinity	118
	Phe→Leu	Hb Louisville, Bucuresti	Unstable; ↓ O_2 affinity	119,120
43(CD2)	Glu→Ala	Hb G-Galveston, G-Port Arthur, G-Texas		121
46(CD5)	Gly→Glu	Hb K-Ibadan		122
47(CD6)	Asp→Asn	Hb G-Copenhagen		123
48(CD7)	Leu→Arg	Hb Okaloosa	Unstable; ↓ O_2 affinity	124
50(D1)	Thr→Lys	Hb Edmonton		125
51(D2)	Pro→Arg	Hb Willamette	Unstable; ↑ O_2 affinity	270
52(D3)	Asp→Asn	Hb Osu-Christiansborg		126
	Asp→Ala	Hb Ocho-Rios		127
56(D7)	Gly→Asp	Hb J-Bangkok, J-Meinung, J-Korat, J-Manado		58
	Gly→Arg	Hb Hamadan		128
57(E1)	Asn→Lys	Hb G-Ferrara		129
58(E2)	Pro→Arg	Hb Yukuhashi, Dhofar		130,131
59(E3)	Lys→Glu	Hb I-High Wycombe		132
	Lys→Thr	Hb J-Kaohsiung, J-Honolulu		133
61(E5)	Lys→Glu	Hb N-Seattle		134
	Lys→Asn	Hb Hikari		135
62(E6)	Ala→Pro	Hb Duarte	Unstable; ↑ O_2 affinity	136
63(E7)	His→Arg	Hb Zürich	Unstable; ↑ O_2 affinity	137
	His→Tyr	Hb M-Saskatoon, M-Emory, M-Kurumi, M-Hida, M-Radom, M-Arhus, M-Chicago, Leipzig, Hörlein-Weber, Novi Sad, M-Erlangen	Ferri-Hb; ↑ O_2 affinity	33
	His→Pro	Hb Bicetre	Unstable; ferri-Hb	282
64(E8)	Gly→Asp	Hb J-Calabria, J-Bari, J-Cosenza	Unstable	138
65(E9)	Lys→Asn	Hb Sicilia		139
	Lys→Gln	Hb J-Cairo		271
66(E10)	Lys→Glu	Hb I-Toulouse	Unstable; ferri-Hb	140
67(E11)	Val→Asp	Hb Bristol	Unstable	141
	Val→Glu	Hb M-Milwaukee-I	Ferri-Hb; ↓ O_2 affinity	33
	Val→Ala	Hb Sydney	Unstable	142
69(E13)	Gly→Asp	Hb J-Cambridge, J-Rambam		123
70(E14)	Ala→Asp	Hb Seattle	↓ O_2 affinity	143
71(E15)	Phe→Ser	Hb Christchurch	Unstable	144
73(E17)	Asp→Asn	Hb Korle-Bu, G-Accra		145,146
	Asp→Val	Hb Mobile		147
74(E18)	Gly→Val	Hb Bushwick		148
	Gly→Asp	Hb Shepherds Bush	Unstable; ↑ O_2 affinity	149
75(E19)	Leu→Pro	Hb Atlanta	Unstable	150
76(E20)	Ala→Asp	Hb J-Chicago		151
77(EF1)	His→Asp	Hb J-Iran		152

Table continued on following page.

TABLE 3–2. Human Hemoglobin Variants—Continued

BETA CHAIN

Residue and Helical Number	*Amino Acid Substitution*	*Name*	*Major Abnormal Property*	*Reference*
79(EF3)	Asp→Gly	Hb G-Hsi-Tsou	↑ O_2 affinity	153,154
80(EF4)	Asn→Lys	Hb G-Szuhu, Gifu	↑ O_2 affinity	154
81(EF5)	Leu→Arg	Hb Baylor	Unstable; ↑ O_2 affinity	272
82(EF6)	Lys→Asn (Asp)	Hb Providence	↓ O_2 affinity	155,156
	Lys→Thr	Hb Rahere	↑ O_2 affinity	157
	Lys→Met	Hb Helsinki	↑ O_2 affinity	287
83(EF7)	Gly→Cys	Hb Ta-Li		158
	Gly→Asp	Hb Pyrgos		159
85(F1)	Phe→Ser	Hb Bryn Mawr, Buenos Aires	Unstable; ↑ O_2 affinity	160,161
87(F3)	Thr→Lys	Hb D-Ibadan		162
88(F4)	Leu→Arg	Hb Borås	Unstable	163
	Leu→Pro	Hb Santa Ana	Unstable	164
89(F5)	Ser→Asn	Hb Creteil	↑ O_2 affinity	165
90(F6)	Glu→Lys	Hb Agenogi	↓ O_2 affinity	166
91(F7)	Leu→Pro	Hb Sabine	Unstable	167
	Leu→Arg	Hb Caribbean	Unstable; ↓ O_2 affinity	283
92(F8)	His→Tyr	Hb M-Hyde Park, M-Akita	Normal O_2; ferri-Hb	168
	His→Gln	Hb Istanbul, Hb-St. Etienne	Unstable; ↑ O_2 affinity; ↑ dissociation	169,170
	His→Asp	Hb J-Altgeld Gardens	Normal O_2 affinity	171
	His→Pro	Hb Newcastle		172
95(FG2)	Lys→Glu	Hb N-Baltimore, Hopkins-I, Jenkins, N-Memphis, Kenwood		173
97(FG4)	His→Gln	Hb Malmö	↑ O_2 affinity	174
	His→Leu	Hb Wood	↑ O_2 affinity	175
98(FG5)	Val→Met	Hb Köln, San Francisco (Pacific), Ube-I	Unstable; ↑ O_2 affinity	176
	Val→Gly	Hb Nottingham	Unstable; ↑ O_2 affinity	177
	Val→Ala	Hb Djelfa	Unstable	178
99(G1)	Asp→Asn	Hb Kempsey	↑ O_2 affinity	179
	Asp→His	Hb Yakima	↑ O_2 affinity	180
	Asp→Tyr	Hb Ypsilanti (Ypsi)	↑ O_2 affinity	181
100(G2)	Pro→Leu	Hb Brigham	↑ O_2 affinity	182
101(G3)	Glu→Gln	Hb Rush	Unstable	183
	Glu→Lys	Hb British Columbia	↑ O_2 affinity	273
	Glu→Gly	Hb Alberta	↑ O_2 affinity	274
102(G4)	Asn→Lys	Hb Richmond	Asymmetrical hybrids	184
	Asn→Thr	Hb Kansas	↓ O_2 affinity; ↑ dissociation	185
	Asn→Ser	Hb Beth Israel	↓ O_2 affinity	186
103(G5)	Phe→Leu	Hb Heathrow	↑ O_2 affinity	187
104(G6)	Arg→Ser	Hb Camperdown	Slightly unstable	188
106(G8)	Leu→Pro	Hb Casper	↑ O_2 affinity	189
	Leu→Pro	Hb Southampton		190
	Leu→Gln	Hb Tübingen		191
107(G9)	Gly→Arg	Hb Burke	Unstable; ↓ O_2 affinity	284
108(G10)	Asn→Asp	Hb Yoshizuka	↓ O_2 affinity	192
109(G11)	Val→Met	Hb San Diego	↑ O_2 affinity	193
111(G13)	Val→Phe	Hb Peterborough	Unstable; ↓ O_2 affinity	194
113(G15)	Val→Glu	Hb New York		195
115(G17)	Ala→Pro	Hb Madrid	Unstable	196
117(G19)	His→Arg	Hb P-Galveston		197
119(GH2)	Gly→Asp	Hb Fannin-Lubbock	Unstable	288, 289
120(GH3)	Lys→Glu	Hb Hijiyama		198
	Lys→Asn	Hb Riyadh		275
121(GH4)	Glu→Gln	Hb D, D-Chicago, D-Punjab, D-North Carolina, D-Los Angeles, D-Portugal, Oak Ridge	↑ O_2 affinity	199
	Glu→Lys	Hb O-Arab, Egypt		73
	Glu→Val	Hb Beograd		200
124(H2)	Pro→Arg	Hb Khartoum	Unstable	79
126(H4)	Val→Glu	Hb Hofu		201
127(H5)	Gln→Glu	Hb Hacettepe		202

TABLE 3–2. ***Human Hemoglobin Variants*****—Continued**

BETA CHAIN

Residue and Helical Number	*Amino Acid Substitution*	*Name*	*Major Abnormal Property*	*Reference*
129(H7)	Ala→Asp	Hb J-Taichung		203
	Ala→Glu or Asp	Hb K-Cameroon		122
130(H8)	Tyr→Asp	Hb Wien	Unstable	204
131(H9)	Gln→Glu	Hb Camden, Tokuchi		205,206
132(H10)	Lys→Gln	Hb K-Woolwich		122
135(H13)	Ala→Pro	Hb Altdorf	Unstable	276
136(H14)	Gly→Asp	Hb Hope	Unstable	207
141(H19)	Leu→Arg	Hb Olmsted		174
143(H21)	His→Arg	Hb Abruzzo	↑ O_2 affinity	208
	His→Gln	Hb Little Rock	↑ O_2 affinity	209
	His→Pro	Hb Syracuse	↑ O_2 affinity	210
144(HC1)	Lys→Asn	Hb Andrew-Minneapolis	↑ O_2 affinity	211
145(HC2)	Tyr→His	Hb Bethesda	↑ O_2 affinity	212
	Tyr→Cys	Hb Rainier	↑ O_2 affinity; alkali resistant	212
	Tyr→Asp	Hb Fort Gordon, Osler, Nancy	↑ O_2 affinity	213,214
	Tyr→Term	Hb McKees Rocks	↑ ↑ O_2 affinity	215
146(HC3)	His→Asp	Hb Hiroshima	↑ O_2 affinity	216
	His→Pro	Hb York	↑ O_2 affinity	217
	His→Arg	Hb Cochin, Port Royal		218

DELTA CHAIN

Residue and Helical Number	*Amino Acid Substitution*	*Name*	*Reference*
2(NA2)	His→Arg	Hb A_2-Sphakiá	219
12(A9)	Asn→Lys	Hb A_2-NYU	220
16(A13)	Gly→Arg	Hb $A_2'(B_2)$	221
20(B2)	Val→Glu	Hb A_2-Roosevelt	277
22(B4)	Ala→Glu	Hb A_2-Flatbush	222
43(CD2)	Glu→Lys	Hb A_2-Melbourne	223
69(E13)	Gly→Arg	Hb A_2-Indonesia	224
116(G18)	Arg→His	Hb A_2-Coburg	225
136(H14)	Gly→Asp	Hb A_2-Babinga	226

GAMMA CHAIN

Residue and Helical Number	*Amino Acid Substitution*	*Name*	*Reference*
1(NA1)	Gly→Cys (136 Gly)	Hb F-Malaysia	227
5(A2)	Glu→Lys (136 Ala)	Hb F-Texas-I	228,229
6(A3)	Glu→Lys	Hb F-Texas-II	230
7(A4)	Asp→Asn	Hb F-Auckland	231
12(A9)	Thr→Lys	Hb F-Alexandra	232
22(B4)	Asp→Gly (136 Ala)	Hb F-Kuala Lumpur	233
61(E5)	Lys→Glu (136 Ala)	Hb F-Jamaica	234
75(E19)	Ile→Thr	Hb F-Sardinia	235
80(EF4)	Asp→Tyr (136 Ala)	Hb F-Victoria Jubilee	236
97(FG4)	His→Arg	Hb F-Dickinson	237
117(G19)	His→Arg (136 Gly)	Hb F-Malta-I	238
121(GH4)	Glu→Lys (136 Ala)	Hb F-Hull	239
125(H3)	Gly→Ala	Hb F-Port Royal	240
130(H8)	Trp→Gly (136 Gly)	Hb F-Poole	241

Table continued on following page.

TABLE 3–2. ***Human Hemoglobin Variants*** **—Continued**

FUSION HEMOGLOBINS

	A6 9	A9 12	B4 22	D1 50	F2 86	F3 87	G18 116	G19 117	H2 124	H4 126	Reference
δ Chain →→→→→→→→→→	Thr	Asn	Ala	Ser	Ser	Gln	Arg	Asn	Gln	Met	
β Chain →→→→→→→→→→	Ser	Thr	Glu	Thr	Ala	Thr	His	His	Pro	Val	
Lepore-Hollandia			δ	β							242
Lepore-Baltimore				δ	β						243
Lepore-Washington-Boston							δ	β			244
Miyada		β	δ								130
P-Congo			β				δ				245
P-Nilotic			β	δ							246

	NA1 1	EF4 80	EF5 81	F2 86	F3 87	HC3 146	Reference
γ Chain →→→→→→→→→→	Gly	Asp	Leu	Ala	Gln	His	
β Chain →→→→→→→→→→	Val	Asn	Leu	Ala	Thr	His	
Kenya			γ	β			247

DELETED RESIDUES

Residue Number	*Amino Acid Substitution*	*Name*	*Major Abnormal Property*	*Reference*
β6 or 7	Glu→0	Hb Leiden	Unstable; slightly ↑ O_2 affinity	255
β17-18	(Lys-Val)→0	Hb Lyon	↑ O_2 affinity	256
β23	Val→0	Hb Freiburg	↑ O_2 affinity	257
β42-44 or 43-45	(Phe-Glu-Ser)→0 or (Glu-Ser-Phe)→0	Hb Niteroi	↓ O_2 affinity; unstable	258
β56-59	(Gly-Asn-Pro-Lys)→0	Hb Tochigi	Unstable; not known	259
β74-75	(Gly-Leu)→0	Hb St. Antoine	Unstable; normal O_2 affinity	260
β87	Thr→0	Hb Tours	↑ O_2 affinity; unstable	260
β91-95	(Leu-His-Cys-Asp-Lys)→0	Hb Gun Hill	Unstable; ↑ O_2 affinity	261
β131	Gln→0	Hb Leslie, Deaconess	Unstable; normal O_2 affinity	262,263
β141	Leu→0	Hb Coventry	Unstable	278
β145-146	(Tyr-His)→0	Hb McKees Rock	↑ O_2 affinity	279

MORE THAN ONE POINT MUTATION IN THE SAME POLYPEPTIDE CHAIN

Residue and Helical Number	*Amino Acid Substitution*	*Name*	*Major Abnormal Property*	*Reference*
β6(A3)	Glu→Val, 73 Asp→Asn	Hb C-Harlem, G-Georgetown	Normal O_2 affinity	264
	Glu→Lys, 95 Lys→Glu	Hb Arlington Park	Not done	265
α78(EF7)	Asn→Asp 79 Ala→Gly	Hb J-Singapore	Not done	266
β6(A3)	Glu→Val 58 Pro→Arg	Hb C-Ziguinchor		267

TABLE 3–2. *Human Hemoglobin Variants*—Continued

	Residue	Name	Major Abnormal Property	Reference
EXTENDED CHAINS				
α141	(31 additional residues) Tyr(140)-Arg-Gln-Ala-Gly-Ala-Ser- Val(150)-Ala-Val-Pro-Pro-Ala-Arg-Trp-Ala-Ser-Gln-Arg-Ala- Leu(160)-Leu-Pro(His,Ser,Leu)-Arg-Pro-Phe-Leu-Val(170)-Phe-Glu	Hb Constant Spring		248
α141	31 additional residues—identical to Hb Constant Spring except for residue 142, which is lysine instead of glutamine	Hb Icaria		249
α141	Probably 31 additional residues—identical to Hb Constant Spring except for residue 142, which is serine instead of glutamine	Hb Koya Dora		250
α139–141	Thr-Ser-Asn(140)-Thr-Val-Lys-Leu-Glu-Pro-Arg (Frame shift)	Hb Wayne		251
β145	Lys(144)-Ser-Ile-Thr-Lys-Leu-Ala-Phe-Leu-Leu-Ser-Asn-Phe- Tyr(157)-COOH (Frame shift)	Hb Cranston	Unstable; ↑ O_2 affinity	252
β147	Lys(144)-Tyr-His-Thr-Lys-Leu-Ala-Phe-Leu-Leu-Ser-Asn-Phe- Tyr(157)-COOH (Frame shift)	Hb Tak	↑ O_2 affinity	253
α115–118	Ala(115)-Glu(116)-Phe(117)-Thr(118)-*Glu-Phe-Thr*-Pro(119) (Insertion)	Hb Grady	Normal	254

REFERENCES FOR TABLE 3–2

1. Crookston, J. H., Beale, D., Irvine, D., and Lehmann, H.: Nature (London) *208*:1059, 1965.
2. Sumida, I., Ohta, Y., Imamura, T., and Yanase, T.: Biochim. Biophys. Acta *322*:23, 1973.
3. Pootrakul, S., Kematorn, B., Na-Nakorn, S., and Suanpan, S.: Biochim. Biophys. Acta *405*:161, 1975.
4. Rosa, J., Maleknia, N., Vergoz, D., and Dunet, R.: Nouv. Rev. Fr. Hematol. *6*:423, 1965.
5. Marti, H. R., Pik, C., and Mosimann, P.: Acta Haematol. *32*:9, 1964.
6. Liddell, J., Brown, D., Beale, D., Lehmann, H., and Huntsman, R. G.: Nature (London) *204*:269, 1964.
7. Vella, F., Casey, R., Lehmann, H., Labossiere, A., and Jones, T. G.: Biochim. Biophys. Acta *336*:25, 1974.
8. Pootrakul, S., Srichiyanont, S., Wasi, P., and Suanpan, S.: Humangenetik *23*:199, 1974.
9. Beale, D., and Lehmann, H.: Nature (London) *207*:259, 1965.
10. Kendall, A. G., Barr, R. D., Lang, A., and Lehmann, H.: Biochim. Biophys. Acta *310*:357, 1973.
11. Gottlieb, A. J., Restrepo, A., and Itano, H. A.: Fed. Proc. *23*:172, 1964.
12. Kraus, A. P., Miyaji, T., Iuchi, I., and Kraus, L. M.: J. Lab. Clin. Med. *66*:886, 1965.
13. Boyer, S. H., Crosby, E. F., Fuller, G. F., Ulenurm, L., and Buck, A. A.: Am. J. Hum. Genet. *20*:570, 1968.
14. Marengo-Rowe, A. J., Beale, D., and Lehmann, H.: Nature (London) *219*:1164, 1968.
15. Schneider, R. G., Brimhall, B., Jones, R. T., Bryant, R., Mitchell, C. B., and Goldberg, A. I.: Biochim. Biophys. Acta *243*:164, 1971.
16. Vettore, L., DeSandre, G., Dilorio, E. E., Winterhalter, K. H., Lang, A., and Lehmann, H.: Blood *44*:869, 1974.
17. Swenson, R. T., Hill, R. L., Lehmann, H., and Jim, R. T. S.: J. Biol. Chem. *237*:1517, 1962.
18. Beretta, A., Prato, V., Gallo, E., and Lehmann, H.: Nature (London) *217*:1016, 1968.
19. Ohba, Y., Miyaji, T., Matsuoka, M., Yokoyama, M., Numakura, H., Nagata, K., Takebe, Y., Izumi, Y., and Shibata, S.: Biochim. Biophys. Acta *405*:155, 1975.
20. Bianco, J., Modiano, G., Bottini, E., and Lucci, R.: Nature (London) *198*:395, 1963.
21. Halbrecht, I., Isaacs, W. A., Lehmann, H., and Ben-Porat, F.: Isr. J. Med. Sci. *3*:827, 1967.
22. Ostertag, W., and Smith, E. W.: Humangenetik *6*:377, 1968.
23. Rahbar, S., Mahdavi, N., Nowzari, G., and Mostafavi, I.: Biochim. Biophys. Acta *386*:525, 1975.
24. Brimhall, B., Jones, R. T., Schneider, R. G., Hosty, T. S., Tomlin, G., and Atkins, R.: Biochim. Biophys. Acta *379*:28, 1975.
25. Tangheroni, W., Zorcolo, G., Gallo, E., and Lehmann, H.: Nature (London) *218*:470, 1968.
26. Cabannes, R., Renaud, R., Mauran, A., Pennors, H., Charlesworth, D., Price, B. G., and Lehmann, H.: Nouv. Rev. Fr. Hematol. *12*:289, 1972.
27. Reynolds, C. A., and Huisman, T. H. J.: Biochim. Biophys. Acta *130*:541, 1966.
28. Alberti, R., Mariuzzi, G. M., Artibani, L., Bruni, E., and Tentori, L.: Biochim. Biophys. Acta *342*:1, 1974.
29. Miyaji, T., Iuchi, I., Takeda, I., and Shibata, S.: Acta Haematol. Jap. *26*:531, 1963.
30. Jones, R. T., Brimhall, B., and Lisker, R.: Biochim. Biophys. Acta *154*:488, 1968.
31. Rahbar, S., Kinderlerer, J. L., and Lehmann, H.: Acta Haematol. *42*:169, 1969.
32. Baglioni, C.: J. Biol. Chem. *237*:69, 1962.
33. Gerald, P. S., and Efron, M. L.: Proc. Nat. Acad. Sci. (Wash.) *47*:1758, 1961.
34. Barclay, G. P. T., Charlesworth, D., and Lehmann, H.: Brit. Med. J. *4*:595, 1969.
35. Brimhall, B., Duerst, M., Hollán, S. R., Stenzel, P., Szelényi, J., and Jones, R. T.: Biochim. Biophys. Acta *336*:344, 1974.
36. Blackwell, R. Q., Jim, R. T. S., Tan, T. G. H., Weng, M.-I., Liu, C.-S., and Wang, C. L.: Biochim. Biophys. Acta *322*:27, 1973.

37. Ramot, B., Kinderlerer, J. B., and Lehmann, H.: Cited in WHO Technical Report Series No. 509, Annex 1, Geneva, 1972.
38. Sukumaran, P. K., Merchant, S. M., Desai, M. P., Wiltshire, B. G., and Lehmann, H.: J. Med. Genet. 9:436, 1972.
39. Miyaji, T., Iuchi, I., Yamamoto, K., Ohba, Y., and Shibata, S.: Clin. Chim. Acta *16*:347, 1967.
40. Baglioni, C., and Ingram, V. M.: Biochim. Biophys. Acta *48*:253, 1961.
41. Colombo, B., Vidal, H., Kamuzora, H., and Lehmann, H.: Biochim. Biophys. Acta *351*:1, 1974.
42. Rahbar, S., Nowzari, G., and Daneshmand, P.: Nature [New Biol.] *245*:268, 1973.
43. Pootrakul, S., and Dixon, G. H.: Canad. J. Biochem. *48*:1066, 1970.
44. Lorkin, P. A., Charlesworth, D., Lehmann, H., Rahbar, S., Tuchinda, S., and Lie-Injo, L. E.: Brit. J. Haematol. *19*:117, 1970.
45. Vella, F., Wiltshire, B. G., Lehmann, H., and Galbraith, P.: Clin. Biochem. *6*:66, 1973.
46. Van Ros, G., Beale, D., and Lehmann, H.: Brit. Med. J. *4*:92, 1968.
47. Rucknagel, D. L., Brandt, N. J., and Spencer, H. H.: Proc. First Inter-American Symp. Hemoglobins, Caracas, 1969.
48. Adams, J. G., III, Winter, W. P., Rucknagel, D. L., and Spencer, H. H.: Science *176*:1427, 1972.
49. Crookston, J. H., Farquharson, H. A., Beale, D., and Lehmann, H.: Canad. J. Biochem. *47*:143, 1969.
50. Lorkin, P. A., Huntsman, R. G., Ager, J. A. M., Lehmann, H., Vella, F., and Darbre, P. D.: Biochim. Biophys. Acta *379*:22, 1975.
51. Cohen-Solal, M., Manesse, B., Thillet, J., and Rosa, J.: FEBS Lett. *50*:163, 1975.
52. Fujiwara, N., Maekawa, T., and Matsuda, G.: Int. J. Pept. Protein Res. *3*:35, 1971.
53. Reed, R. E., Winter, W. P., and Rucknagel, D. L.: Brit. J. Haematol. *26*:475, 1974.
54. Miyaji, T., Iuchi, I., Shibata, S., Takeda, I., and Tamura, A.: Acta Haematol. Jap. *26*:538, 1963.
55. DeTraverse, P. M., Lehmann, H., DeCoquelet, M. L., and Isaacs, W. A.: Compt. R. Scéanc. Soc. Biol. *160*:2270, 1966.
56. Hyde, R. D., Kinderlerer, J. L., Lehmann, H., and Hall, M. D.: Biochim. Biophys. Acta *243*:515, 1971.
57. Botha, M. C., Beale, D., Isaacs, W. A., and Lehmann, H.: Nature (London) *212*:792, 1966.
58. Clegg, J. B., Naughton, M. A., and Weatherall, D. J.: J. Mol. Biol. *19*:91, 1966.
59. Charache, S., Weatherall, D. J., and Clegg, J. B.: J. Clin. Invest. *45*:813, 1966.
60. Wajcman, H., Belkhodja, O., and Labie, D.: FEBS Lett. *27*:298, 1972.
61. Schneider, R. G., Atkins, R. J., Hosty, T. S., Tomlin, G., Casey, R., Lehmann, H., Lorkin, P. A., and Nagai, K.: Biochim. Biophys. Acta *400*:365, 1975.
62. Huisman, T. H. J., Adams, H. R., Wilson, J. B., Efremov, G. D., Reynolds, C. A., and Wrightstone, R. N.: Biochim. Biophys. Acta *200*:578, 1970.
63. Smith, L. L., Plese, C. L., Barton, B. P., Charache, S., Wilson, J. B., and Huisman, T. H. J.: J. Biol. Chem. *247*:1433, 1972.
64. DeJong, W. W. W., Bernini, L. F., and Khan, P. M.: Biochim. Biophys. Acta *236*:197, 1971.
65. Wiltshire, B. G., Clark, K. G. A., Lorkin, P. A., and Lehmann, H.: Biochim. Biophys. Acta *278*:459, 1972.
66. Bannister, W. H., Grech, J. L., Plese, C. F., Smith, L. L., Barton, B. P., Wilson, J. B., Reynolds, C. A., and Huisman, T. H. J.: Eur. J. Biochem. *29*:301, 1972.
67. Crookston, J. H. Farquharson, H., Kinderlerer, J., and Lehmann, H.: Canad. J. Biochem. *48*:911, 1970.
68. Rosa, J., Oudart, J. L., Pagnier, J., Belkhodja, O., Boigne, J. M., and Labie, D.: 12th Congress Internat. Soc. Haemat., New York, 1968, Abstracts, p. 72.
69. Charache, S., and Ostertag, W.: Blood *36*:852, 1970.
70. Niazi, G. A., Efremov, G. D., Nikolov, N., Hunter, E., Jr., and Huisman, T. H. J.: Biochim. Biophys. Acta *412*:181, 1975.
71. Beksedic, D., Rajevska, T., Lorkin, P. A., and Lehmann, H.: FEBS Letters *58*:226, 1975.
72. Gajdusek, D. C., Guiart, J., Kirk, R. L., Carrell, R. W., Irvine, D., Kyn-

och, P. A. M., and Lehmann, H.: J. Med. Genet. *4*:1, 1967.
73. Baglioni, C., and Lehmann, H.: Nature (London) *196*:229, 1962.
74. Ostertag, W., von Ehrenstein, G., and Charache, S.: Nature [New Biol.] *237*:90, 1972.
75. Blackwell, R. Q., Wong, H. B., Wang, C.-L., Weng, M.-L., and Liu, C.-S.: Biochim. Biophys. Acta *351*:7, 1974.
76. Kamuzora, H., Lehmann, H., Griffiths, K. D., Mann, J. R., and Raine, D. N.: Ann. Clin. Biochem. *11*:53, 1974.
77. Vella, F., Galbraith, P., Wilson, J. B., Wong, S. C., Folger, G. C., and Huisman, T. H. J.: Biochim. Biophys. Acta *365*:318, 1974.
78. Kleihauer, E. F., Reynolds, C. A., Dozy, A. M., Wilson, J. B., Moores, R. R., Berenson, M. P., Wright, C.-S., and Huisman, T. H. J.: Biochim. Biophys. Acta *154*:220, 1968.
79. Clegg, J. B., Weatherall, D. J., Wong, H. B., and Mustafa, D.: Nature (London) *222*:379, 1969.
80. Labossiere, A., Vella, F., Hiebert, J., and Galbraith, P.: Clin. Biochem. *5*:46, 1972.
81. Ingram, V. M.: Biochim. Biophys. Acta *36*:402, 1959.
82. Hunt, J. A., and Ingram, V. M.: Biochim. Biophys. Acta *42*:409, 1960.
83. Blackwell, R. Q., Oemijati, S., Pribadi, W., Weng, M.-I., and Liu, C.-S.: Biochim. Biophys. Acta *214*:396, 1970.
84. Hill, R. I., Swenson, R. T., and Schwartz, H. C.: J. Biol. Chem. *235*:3182, 1960.
85. Tuchinda, S., Beale, D., and Lehmann, H.: Brit. Med. J. *1*:1583, 1965.
86. Bonaventura, J., and Riggs, A.: Science *158*:800, 1967.
87. Arcasoy, A., Casey, R., Lehmann, H., Cavdar, A. O., and Berki, A.: FEBS Lett. *42*:121, 1974.
88. Monn, E., Gaffney, P. J., and Lehmann, H.: Scand. J. Haematol. *5*:353, 1968.
89. Beuzard, Y., Basset, P., Braconnier, F., Gammal, H. E., Martin, L., Oudard, J. L., and Thillet, J.: Biochim. Biophys. Acta *393*:182, 1975.
90. Kennedy, C. C., Blundell, G., Lorkin, P. A., Lang, A., and Lehmann, H.: Brit. Med. J. *4*:324, 1974.
91. Baglioni, C., and Weatherall, D. J.: Biochim. Biophys. Acta *78*:637, 1963.
92. Wade, P. T., Jenkins, T., and Huehns, E. R.: Nature (London) *216*:688, 1967.
93. Maekawa, M., Maekawa, T., Fujiwara, N., Tabara, K., and Matsuda, G.: Int. J. Pept. Protein Res. *II:* 147, 1970.
94. Elion, J., Belkhodja, O., Wajcman, H., and Labie, D.: Biochim. Biophys. Acta *310*:360, 1973.
95. Stamatoyannopoulos, G., Nute, P. E., Adamson, J. W., Bellingham, A. J., Funk, D., and Hornung, S.: J. Clin. Invest. *52*:342, 1973.
96. Vella, F., Lorkin, P. A., Carrell, R. W., and Lehmann, H.: Canad. J. Biochem. *45*:1385, 1967.
97. Blackwell, R. Q., Yang, H. J., and Wang, C. C.: Biochim. Biophys. Acta *175*:237, 1969.
98. Vella, F., Isaacs, W. A., and Lehmann, H.: Canad. J. Biochem. *45*:351, 1967.
99. Bowman, B. H., Barnett, D. R., and Hite, R.: Biochim. Biophys. Acta *26*:466, 1967.
100. Rahbar, S.: Brit. J. Haematol. *24*:31, 1973.
101. Ranney, H. M., Jacobs, A. S., Udem, L., and Zalusky, R.: Biochim. Biophys. Acta *33*:1004, 1968.
102. Huisman, T. H. J., Brown, A. K., Efremov, G. D., Wilson, J. B., Reynolds, C. A., Uy, R., and Smith, L. L.: J. Clin. Invest. *50*:650, 1971.
103. Idelson, L. I., Didkovskii, N. A., Casey, R., Lorkin, P. A., and Lehmann, H.: Nature (London) *249*:768, 1974.
104. Blackwell, R. Q., and Liu, C.-S.: Biochem. Biophys. Res. Commun. *30*:690, 1968.
105. Hunt, J. A., and Ingram, V. N.: Biochim. Biophys. Acta *49*:520, 1961.
106. Idelson, L. I., Didkovskiĭ, N. A., Filippova, A. V., Casey, R., Kynoch, P. A. M., and Lehmann, H.: FEBS Lett. *58*:122, 1975.
107. Kuis-Reerink, J. D., Jonxis, J. H. P., Niazi, G. A., Wilson, J. B., Bolch, K. C., Gravely, M., and Huisman, T. H. J.: Biochim. Biophys. Acta. *439*:63, 1976.
108. Cohen-Solal, M., Seligmann, M., Thillet, J., and Rosa, J.: Abstract 408, 14th Int. Congress of Hematology, Sao Paulo, Brazil, 1972. FEBS Lett. *33*:37, 1973.

109. Sansone, G., Carrell, R. W., and Lehmann, H.: Nature (London) *214*:877, 1967.
110. Brimhall, B., Jones, R. T., Baur, E. W., and Motulsky, A. G.: Biochemistry *8*:2125, 1969.
111. Jackson, J. M., Yates, A., and Huehns, E. R.: Brit. J. Haematol. *25*:607, 1973.
112. Honig, G. R., Green, D., Shamsuddin, M., Vida, L. N., Mason, R. G., Gnarra, D. J., and Maurer, H. S.: J. Clin. Invest. *52*:1746, 1973.
113. Garel, M. C., Blouquit, Y., and Rosa, J.: FEBS Lett. *58*:145, 1975.
114. Rieder, R. F., Oski, F. A., and Clegg, J. B.: J. Clin. Invest. *48*:1627, 1969.
115. Yamaoka, K.: Blood *38*:730, 1971.
116. Brown, W. J., Niazi, G. A., Jayakalshmi, M., Abraham, E. C., and Huisman, T. H. J.: Biochim. Biophys. Acta. *437*:70, 1976.
117. Burkert, L. B., Sharma, V. S., Piscotta, A. V., Ranney, H., and Bruckheimer, P.: Blood *48*:645, 1976.
118. Dacie, J. V., Shinton, N. K., Gaffney, P. J., Jr., Carrell, R. W., and Lehmann, H.: Nature (London) *216*:663, 1967.
119. Keeling, M. M., Ogden, L. L., Wrightstone, R. N., Wilson, J. B., Reynolds, C. A., Kitchens, J. L., and Huisman, T. H. J.: J. Clin. Invest. *50*:2395, 1971.
120. Bratu, V., Lorkin, P. A., Lehmann, H., and Predescu, C.: Biochim. Biophys. Acta *251*:1, 1971.
121. Bowman, B. H., Oliver, C. P., Barnett, D. R., Cunningham, J. R., and Schneider, R. G.: Blood *23*:193, 1964.
122. Allan, N., Beale, D., Irvine, D., and Lehmann, H.: Nature (London) *208*:658, 1965.
123. Sick, K., Beale, D., Irvine, D., Lehmann, H., Goodall, P. T., and MacDougall, S.: Biochim. Biophys. Acta *140*:231, 1967.
124. Charache, S., Brimhall, B., Milner, P., and Cobb, L.: J. Clin. Invest. *52*:2858, 1973.
125. Labossiere, A., Hill, J. R., and Vella, F.: Clin. Biochem. *4*:114, 1971.
126. Konotey-Ahula, F. I. D., Kinderlerer, J. L., Lehmann, H., and Ringelhann, B.: J. Med. Genet. *8*:302, 1971.
127. Beresford, C. H., Clegg, J. B., and Weatherall, D. J.: J. Med. Genet. *9*:151, 1972.
128. Rabhar, S., Nowzari, G., Haydari, H., and Daneshmand, P.: Biochim. Biophys. Acta *379*:645, 1975.
129. Tentori, L., Bruni, E., and Marinucci, M.: Int. Istanbul Symposium on Abnormal Hemoglobins and Thalassemia. M. Aksoy, Ed. Ankara.
130. Yanase, T., Hanada, M., Seita, M., Obya, I., Ohta, Y., Imamura, T., Fijimura, T., Kawasaki, K., and Yamaoka, K.: Jap. J. Hum. Genet. *13*:40, 1968.
131. Marengo-Rowe, A. J., Lorkin, P. A., Gallo, E., and Lehmann, H.: Biochim. Biophys. Acta *168*:58, 1968.
132. Boulton, F. E., Huntsman, R. G., Lehmann, H., Lorkin, P., and Romero Herrera, A.: Brit. J. Haematol. *20*:671, 1971.
133. Blackwell, R. Q., Liu, C.-S., and Shih, T.-B.: Biochim. Biophys. Acta *229*:343, 1971.
134. Jones, R. T., Brimhall, B., Huehns, E. R., and Motulsky, A. G.: Biochim. Biophys. Acta *154*:278, 1968.
135. Shibata, S., Miyaji, T., Iuchi, I., Ueda, S., and Takeda, I.: Clin. Chim. Acta *10*:101, 1964.
136. Beutler, E., Lang, A., and Lehmann, H.: Blood *43*:527, 1974.
137. Muller, C. J., and Kingma, S.: Biochim. Biophys. Acta *50*:595, 1961.
138. Tentori, L.: Int. Symp. Abnormal Hemoglobins and Thalassemia. Istanbul, Turkey, Abstracts 68, 1974.
139. Ricco, G., Pich, P. G., Massa, U., Rossi, G., Ajmar, F., Arese, P., and Gallo, E.: FEBS Lett. *39*:200, 1974.
140. Rosa, L., Labie, D., Wajcman, H., Boigne, J. M., Cabannes, R., Bierme, R., and Ruffie, J.: Nature (London) *223*:190, 1969.
141. Steadman, J. H., Yates, A., and Huehns, E. R.: Brit. J. Haematol. *18*:435, 1970.
142. Carrell, R. W., Lehmann, H., Lorkin, P. A., Raik, E., and Hunter, E.: Nature (London) *215*:626, 1967.
143. Kurachi, S., Hermodson, M., Hornung, S., and Stamatoyannopoulos, G.: Nature [New Biol.] *243*:275, 1973.
144. Carrell, R. W., and Owen, M. C.: Biochim. Biophys. Acta *236*:507, 1971.
145. Konotey-Ahulu, F. I. D., Gallo, E., Lehmann, H., and Ringelhann, B.: J. Med. Genet. *5*:107, 1968.

146. Boi-Doku, F. S., Kinderlerer, J., and Lehmann, H.: Atlas of Protein Sequence and Structure, May, 1972, Vol. 5.
147. Schneider, R. G., Hosty, T. S., Tomlin, G., Atkins, R., Brimhall, B., and Jones, R. T.: Biochem. Genet. *13*:411, 1975.
148. Rieder, R. F., Wolf, D. J., Clegg, J. B., and Lee, S. L.: Nature (London) *254*:725, 1975.
149. White, J. M., Brain, M. C., Lorkin, P. A., Lehmann, H., and Smith, M.: Nature (London) *225*:939, 1970.
150. Hubbard, M., Winton, E., Lindeman, J. G., Dessauer, P. L., Wilson, J. B., Wrightstone, R. N., and Huisman, T. H. J.: Biochim. Biophys. Acta *386*:538, 1975.
151. Romain, P. L., Schwartz, A. D., Shamsuddin, M., Adams, J. G., III, Mason, R. G., Vida, L. N., and Honig, G. R.: Blood *45*:387, 1975.
152. Rahbar, S., Beale, D., Isaacs, W. A., and Lehmann, H.: Brit. Med. J. *1*:674, 1967.
153. Blackwell, R. Q., Shih, T.-B., Wang, C.-L., and Liu, C.-S.: Biochim. Biophys. Acta *257*:49, 1972.
154. Blackwell, R. Q., Yang, H. T., and Wang, C.-C.: Biochim. Biophys. Acta *188*:59, 1969.
155. McCurdy, P. R., Fox, J., and Moo-Penn, W.: Am. J. Hum. Genet. *27*:62a, 1975.
156. Charache, S., McCurdy, P., and Fox, J.: 18th Ann. Meeting Am. Soc. Hemat., Dallas, Texas, December, 1975.
157. Lorkin, P. A., Stephens, A. D., Beard, M. E. J., Wrigley, P. F. M., Adams, L., and Lehmann, H.: Brit. Med. J. *4*:200, 1975.
158. Blackwell, R. Q., Liu, C.-S., and Wang, C.-L.: Biochim. Biophys. Acta *243*:467, 1971.
159. Tatsis, B., Sofroniadou, K., and Stergiopoulos, K.: Ann. Meeting Am. Soc. Hemat., Miami, Florida, 1972, Abstract 168.
160. Bradley, T. B., Wohl, R. C., Murphy, S. B., Oski, F. A., and Bunn, H. F.: Ann. Meeting Am. Soc. Hemat., Miami, 1972, Abstract 67.
161. DeWeinstein, B. I., White, J. M., Wiltshire, B. G., and Lehmann, H.: Acta Haematol. *50*:357, 1973.
162. Watson-Williams, E. J., Beale, D., Irvine, D., and Lehmann, H.: Nature (London) *205*:1273, 1965.
163. Hollender, A., Lorkin, P. A., Lehmann, H., and Svensson, B.: Nature (London) *222*:953, 1969.
164. Opfell, R. W., Lorkin, P. A., and Lehmann, H.: J. Med. Genet. *5*:292, 1968.
165. Cohen-Solal, M., Blouquit, Y., Carel, M. C., Reyes, F., Thillet, J., Carburi, J., Beuzard, Y., and Rosa, J.: Int. Symp. Abnormal Hemoglobins and Thalassemia, Istanbul, Turkey, Abstracts 5, 1974.
166. Miyaji, T., Suzuki, H., Ohba, Y., and Shibata, S.: Clin. Chim. Acta *14*:624, 1966.
167. Schneider, R. G., Satoshi, U., Alperin, J. B., Brimhall, B., and Jones, R. T.: N. Engl. J. Med. *280*:739, 1969.
168. Heller, P., Coleman, R. D., and Yakulis, V.: J. Clin. Invest. *45*:1021, 1966.
169. Aksoy, M., Erdem, S., Efremov, G. D., Wilson, J. B., Huisman, T. H. J., Schroeder, W. A., Shelton, J. R., Shelton, J. B., Ulitin, O. N., and Müftüoglu, A.: J. Clin. Invest. *51*:2380, 1972.
170. Beuzard, Y., Courvalin, J. C., Cohen-Solal, M., Carel, M. C., Rosa, J., Brizard, C. P., and Gibaud, A.: FEBS Lett. *27*:76, 1972.
171. Adams, J. G., III, Przywara, K. P., Shamsuddin, M., and Heller, P.: 18th Ann. Meeting Am. Soc. Hemat., Dallas, Texas, December, 1975.
172. Finney, R., Casey, R., Lehmann, H., and Walker, W.: FEBS Lett. *60*:435, 1975.
173. Clegg, J. B., Naughton, M. A., and Weatherall, D. J.: Nature (London) *207*:945, 1965.
174. Lorkin, P. A., Lehmann, H., Fairbanks, V. F., Berglund, G., and Leonhardt, T.: Biochem. J. *119*:68, 1970.
175. Taketa, F., Huang, Y. P., Libnoch, J. A., and Dessel, B. H.: Biochim. Biophys. Acta *400*:348, 1975.
176. Carrell, R. W., Lehmann, H., and Hutchison, H. E.: Nature (London) *210*:915, 1966.
177. Gordon-Smith, E. C., Dacie, J. V., Blecher, T. E., French, E. A., Wiltshire, B. G., and Lehmann, H.: Proc. Roy. Soc. Med. *66*:507, 1973.
178. Gacon, G., Wajcman, H., and Labie, D.: FEBS Lett. *58*:238, 1975.
179. Reed, C. S., Hampson, R., Gordon, S., Jones, R. T., Novy, M. J., Brimhall, B., Edwards, M. J., and Koler, R. D.: Blood *31*:623, 1968.

180. Jones, R. T., Osgood, E. E., Brimhall, B., and Koler, R. D.: J. Clin. Invest. *46*:1840, 1967.
181. Glynn, K. P., Penner, J. A., Smith, J. R., and Rucknagel, R. L.: Ann. Intern. Med. *69*:769, 1968.
182. Lokich, J. J., Mahoney, C., Bunn, H. F., Bruckheimer, S. M., and Ranney, H.: J. Clin. Invest. *52*:2060, 1973.
183. Adams, J. B., Winter, W. P., Tausk, K., and Heller, P.: Blood *43*:261, 1974.
184. Efremov, G. D., Huisman, T. H. J., Smith, L. L., Wilson, J. B., Kitchens, J. L., Wrightstone, R. N., and Adams, H. R.: J. Biol. Chem. *244*:6105, 1969.
185. Bonaventura, J., and Riggs, A.: J. Biol. Chem. *243*:980, 1968.
186. Nagel, R. L., Lynfield, J., Johnson, J., Landau, L., Bookchin, R. M., and Harris, M. B.: N. Engl. J. Med. *295*: 125, 1976.
187. White, J. M., Szur, L., Gillies, I. D. S., Lorkin, P. A., and Lehmann, H.: Brit. Med. J. *3*:665, 1973.
188. Wilkinson, T., Ching Geh Chua, Carrell, R. W., Robin, H., Exner, T., Kit Ming Lee, and Kronenberg. Biochim. Biophys. Acta *393*:195, 1975.
189. Koler, R. D., Jones, R. T., Bigley, R. H., Litt, M., Lovrien, E., Brooks, R., Lahey, M. E., and Fowler, R.: Am. J. Med. *55*:549, 1973.
190. Hyde, R. D., Hall, M. D., Wiltshire, B. G., and Lehmann, H.: Lancet *2*:1170–1172, 1972.
191. Kleihauer, E., Waller, H. D., Benöhr, H. C., Kohne, E., and Gelinsky, P.: Klin. Wochenschr. *48*:651, 1971.
192. Imamura, T., Fujita, S., Ohta, Y., Hanada, M., and Yanase, T.: J. Clin. Invest. *48*:2341, 1969.
193. Nute, P. E., Stamatoyannopoulos, G., Hermodson, M. A., Roth, D., and Hornung, S.: J. Clin. Invest. *53*:320, 1974.
194. King, M. A. R., Wiltshire, B. G., Lehmann, H., and Morimoto, H.: Brit. J. Haematol. *22*:125, 1972.
195. Ranney, H. M., Jacobs, A. S., and Nagel, R. L.: Nature (London) *213*:876, 1967.
196. Outeirino, J., Casey, R., White, J. M., and Lehmann, H.: Acta Haematol. *52*:53, 1974.
197. Schneider, R. G., Alperin, J. B., Brimhall, B., and Jones, R. T.: J. Lab. Clin. Med. *73*:616, 1969.
198. Miyaji, T., Oba, Y., Yamamoto, K., Shibata, S., Iuchi, I., and Hamilton, H. B.: Science *159*:204, 1968.
199. Baglioni, C.: Biochim. Biophys. Acta *59*:437, 1962.
200. Efremov, G. D., Duma, H., Ruvidic, R., Rolovic, Z., Wilson, J. B., and Huisman, T. H. J.: Biochim. Biophys. Acta *328*:81, 1973.
201. Miyaji, T., Ohba, Y., Yamamoto, K., Shibata, S., Iuchi, I., and Takenaka, H.: Nature (London) *217*:89, 1968.
202. Altay, C., Altinoz, N., Wilson, J. B., Bolch, K. C., and Huisman, T. H. J.: Biochim. Biophys. Acta. *434*: 1, 1976.
203. Blackwell, R. Q., Yang, H.-J., and Wang, C.-C.: Biochim. Biophys. Acta *194*:1, 1969.
204. Lorkin, P. A., Pietschmann, H., Braunsteiner, H., and Lehmann, H.: Acta Haematol. *51*:351, 1974.
205. Wade Cohen, P. T., Yates, A., Bellingham, A. J., and Huehns, E. R.: Nature [New Biol.] *243*:467, 1973.
206. Shibata, S.: Personal communication.
207. Minnich, V., Hill, R. J., Khuri, P. D., and Anderson, M. E.: Blood *25*:830, 1965.
208. Tentori, L., Carta Sorcini, M., and Buccella, C.: Clin. Chim. Acta *38*:258, 1972.
209. Bromberg, P. A., Alben, J. O., Bare, G. H., Balcerzak, S. P., Jones, R. T., Brimhall, B., and Padilla, F.: Nature [New Biol.] *243*:177, 1973.
210. Jensen, M., Oski, F. A., Nathan, D. G., and Bunn, H. F.: J. Clin. Invest. *55*:469, 1975.
211. Zak, S. J., Brimhall, B., Jones, R. T., and Kaplan, M. E.: Blood *44*:543, 1974.
212. Hayashi, A., Stamatoyannopoulos, G., Yoshida, A., and Adamson, J.: Nature [*New Biol.*] *230*:264, 1971.
213. Kleckner, H. B., Wilson, J. B., Lindeman, J. G., Stevens, P. D., Niazi, G., Hunter, E., Chen, C. J., and Huisman, T. H. L.: Biochim. Biophys. Acta *400*:343, 1975.
214. Charache, S., Brimhall, B., and Jones, R. T.: Johns Hopkins Med. J. *136*:132, 1975.
215. Winslow, R. M., Swenberg, M., Gross, E., Chervenick, P., Buchman, R. R., and Anderson, W. F.: Am. J. Hum. Genet. *27*:95a, 1975.
216. Perutz, M. F., del Pulsinelli, P., Ten Eyck, L., Kilmartin, J. V., Shibata, S., Iuchi, I., Miyaji, T., and Ham-

ilton, H. B.: Nature [New Biol.] *232*:147, 1971.
217. Bare, G. H., Bromberg, P. A., Alben, J. O., Brimhall, B., Jones, R. T., Mintz, S., and Rother, I.: Nature *259*:155, 1976.
218. Wajcman, H., Kilmartin, J. V., Najman, A., and Labie, D.: Biochim. Biophys. Acta *400*:354, 1975.
219. Jones, R. T., Brimhall, B., Huehns, E. R., and Barnicot, N. A.: Science *151*:1406, 1966.
220. Ranney, H. M., Jacobs, A. S., Ramot, B., and Bradley, T. B., Jr.: J. Clin. Invest. *48*:2057, 1969.
221. Ball, E. W., Meynell, M. J., Beale, D., Kynoch, P., Lehmann, H., and Stretton, A. O. W.: Nature (London) *209*:1217, 1968.
222. Jones, R. T., and Brimhall, B.: J. Biol. Chem. *242*:5141, 1967.
223. Sharma, R. S., Harding, D. L., Wong, S. C., Wilson, J. B., Gravely, M. E., and Huisman, T. H. J.: Biochim. Biophys. Acta *359*:233, 1974.
224. Lie-Injo, L. E., Pribada, W., Boerma, F. W., Efremov, G. D., Wilson, J. B., Reynolds, C. A., and Huisman, T. H. J.: Biochim. Biophys. Acta *229*:335, 1971.
225. Sharma, R. S., Williams, L., Wilson, J. B., and Huisman, T. H. J.: Biochim. Biophys. Acta *393*:379, 1975.
226. DeJong, W. W. W., and Bernini, L. F.: Nature (London) *219*:1360, 1968.
227. Lie-Injo, L. E., Kamuzora, H., and Lehmann, H.: J. Med. Genet. *11*:25, 1974.
228. Jenkins, G. C., Beale, D., Black, A. J., Huntsman, G. R., and Lehmann, H.: Brit. J. Haematol. *13*:252, 1967.
229. Ahern, E. E., Wiltshire, B. G., and Lehmann, H.: Biochim. Biophys. Acta *271*:61, 1972.
230. Larkin, I. L. M., Baker, T., Lorkin, P. A., Lehmann, H., Black, A. J., and Huntsman, R. G.: Brit. J. Haematol. *14*:233, 1968.
231. Carrell, R. W., Owen, M. C., Anderson, R., and Berry, E.: Biochim. Biophys. Acta *365*:323, 1974.
232. Loukopoulos, D., Kaltsoya, A., and Fessas, P.: Blood *33*:114, 1969.
233. Lie-Injo, L. E., Wiltshire, B. G., and Lehmann, H.: Biochim. Biophys. Acta *322*:224, 1973.
234. Ahern, E. J., Jones, R. T., Brimhall, B., and Gray, R. H.: Brit. J. Haematol. *18*:369, 1970.
235. Grifoni, V., Kamuzora, H., Lehmann, H., and Charlesworth, D.: Acta Haematol. *53*:347, 1975.
236. Ahern, E. J., Holder, W., Ahern, V., Serjeant, G. R., Serjeant, B. E., Forbes, M., Brimhall, B., and Jones, R. T.: Biochim. Biophys. Acta *393*:188, 1975.
237. Schneider, R. G., Haggard, M. E., Gustavson, L. P., Brimhall, B., and Jones, R. T.: Brit. J. Haematol. *28*:515, 1974.
238. Cauchi, M. N., Clegg, J. B., and Weatherall, D. J.: Nature (London) *223*:311, 1969.
239. Sacker, L. S., Beale, D., Black, A. J., Huntsman, R. G., Lehmann, H., and Lorkin, P. A.: Brit. Med. J. *3*:531, 1967.
240. Brimhall, B., Vedvick, T. S., Jones, R. T., Ahern, E. J., Palomino, L., and Ahern, V.: Brit. J. Haematol. *27*:313, 1973.
241. Lee-Potter, J. P., Deacon-Smith, R. A., Simpkiss, M. J., Kamuzora, H., and Lehmann, H.: J. Clin. Path. *28*:317, 1975.
242. Barnabas, J., and Muller, C. J.: Nature (London) *194*:931, 1962.
243. Ostertag, W., and Smith, E. W.: Eur. J. Biochem. *10*:371, 1969.
244. Baglioni, C.: Proc. Nat. Acad. Sci. (Wash.) *48*:1880, 1962.
245. Lehmann, H., and Charlesworth, D.: Biochem. J. *119*:43, 1970.
246. Badr, F. M., Lorkin, P. A., and Lehmann, H.: Nature [New Biol.] *242*:107, 1973.
247. Huisman, T. H. J., Wrightstone, R. N., Wilson, J. B., Schroeder, W. A., and Kendall, A. G.: Arch. Biochem. Biophys. *153*:850, 1972.
248. Clegg, J. B., Weatherall, D. J., and Milner, P. F.: Nature (London) *234*:337, 1971.
249. Clegg, J. B., Weatherall, D. J., Contopolou-Griva, I., Caroutsos, K., Poungouras, P., and Tsevrenis, H.: Nature (London) *251*:245, 1974.
250. DeJong, W. W. W., Meera Khan, P., and Bernini, L. F.: Am. J. Hum. Genet. *27*:81, 1975.
251. Seid-Akhaven, M., Winter, W. P., Abramson, R. K., and Rucknagel, D. L.: Ann. Meeting Am. Soc. Hemat., Miami, Florida, 1972, Abstract 9.

252. Bunn, H. F., Schmidt, G. J., Haney, D. N., and Dluhy, R. G.: Proc. Nat. Acad. Sci. (USA) *72*:3609, 1975.
253. Flatz, G., Kinderlerer, J. L., Kilmartin, J. V., and Lehmann, H.: Lancet 10:732, 1971.
254. Huisman, T. H. J., Wilson, J. B., Gravely, M., and Hubbard, M.: Proc. Nat. Acad. Sci. (USA) *71*: 3270, 1974.
255. DeJong, W. W. W., Went, L. N., and Bernini, L. F.: Nature (London) *220*:788, 1968.
256. Cohen-Solal, M., Blouquitt, Y., Garel, M. G., Thillet, J., Gaillard, L., Creyssel, R., Gibaud, A., and Rosa, J.: Biochim. Biophys. Acta *351*:306, 1974.
257. Jones, R. T., Brimhall, B., Huisman, T. H. J., Kleihauer, E., and Betke, K.: Science *154*:1024, 1966.
258. Praxedes, H., and Lehmann, H.: Proc. 14th Int. Congress of Hematology, Sao Paulo, Brazil, 1972.
259. Shibata, S., Miyaji, T., Ueda, S., Matsuoka, M., Iuchi, I., Yamada, K., and Shinkai, N.: Proc. Jap. Acad. *46*:440, 1970.
260. Wajcman, H., Labie, D., and Schapira, G.: Biochim. Biophys. Acta *295*:495, 1973.
261. Bradley, T. B., Wohl., R. C., and Rieder, R. F.: Science *157*:1581, 1967.
262. Lutcher, C. L., and Huisman, T. H. J.: Blood *47*:99, 1976.
263. Moo-Penn, W. F., Jue, D. L., Bechtel, K. C., Johnson, M. H., Bemis, E., Brosious, E., and Schmidt, R. M.: Biochem. Biophys. Res. Commun. *65*:8, 1975.
264. Bookchin, R. M., Nagel, R. L., and Ranney, H. M.: J. Biol. Chem. *242*:248, No. 2., 1967.
265. Adams, J. G., and Heller, P.: Blood *42*:990, 1973.
266. Blackwell, R. Q., Wong, H. B., Liu, C.-S., and Weng, M.-L.: Biochim. Biophys. Acta *278*:482, 1972.
267. Goossens, M., Garel, M. C., Auvinet, J., Basset, P., Gomes, P. F., and Rosa, J.: FEBS Lett. *58*:149, 1975.
268. Ahern, E., Ahern, V., Holder, W., et al.: Biochim. Biophys. Acta *427*:530, 1976.
269. Garel, M. C., Goosens, M., Oudart, J. L., Blouquit, Y., Thillet, J., and Rosa, J.: Biochim. Biophys. Acta *453*:459, 1976.
270. Jones, R. T., Koler, R. D., Duerst, M. L., and Dhindsa, D. S.: Hemoglobin *1*:45, 1976.
271. Garel, M. C., Hassan, W., Coquelet, M. T., et al.: Biochim. Biophys. Acta *420*:97, 1976.
272. Schneider, R. G., Hettig, R. A., Bilunos, M., and Brimhall, B.: Hemoglobin *1*:85, 1976.
273. Jones, T. R., Brimhall, B., and Gray, G.: Hemoglobin *1*:171, 1976.
274. Mant, M. J., Salkie, M. L., Cope, N., et al.: Hemoglobin *1*:183, 1976.
275. El-Hazmi, M. A. F., and Lehmann, H.: Hemoglobin *1*:59, 1976.
276. Marti, H. R., Winterhalter, K. W., di Iorio, E. E., et al.: FEBS Lett. *63*:193, 1976.
277. Rieder, R. F., Clegg, J. B., Weiss, H. J., et al.: Biochim. Biophys. Acta *439*:501, 1976.
278. Casey, R., Lang, A., Lehmann, H., and Shinton, N. K.: Brit. J. Haemat. *33*:143, 1976.
279. Winslow, R. M., Swenberg, M.-L., Gross, E., et al.: J. Clin. Invest. *57*:772, 1976.
280. Orringer, E. P., Wilson, J. B., and Huisman, T. H. J.: FEBS Lett. *65*: 297, 1976.
281. Poyart, C., Krishnamoorthy, R., Bursaux, E., Gacon, G., and Labie, D.: FEBS Lett. *69*:103, 1976.
282. Wajcman, H., Krishnamoorthy, R., Gacon, G., Elion, J., Allard, C., and Labie, D.: J. Mol. Med. *1*:187, 1976.
283. Ahern, E., Ahern, V., Hilton, T., Serjeant, G. R., Serjeant, B. E., Seakins, M., Lang, A., Middleton, A., and Lehmann, H.: FEBS Lett. *69*:99, 1976.
284. Turner, J. W., Jones, R. T., Brimhall, B., DuVal, M. C., and Koler, R. D.: Biochem. Genet. *14*:577, 1976.
285. Garel, M. C., Blouquit, Y., North, M. L., Arous, N., and Rosa, J.: FEBS Lett. *72*:1, 1976.
286. Blouquit, Y., Arous, N., Machado, P. E. A., Perrone, F., and Garel, M. C.: FEBS Lett. *72*:5, 1976.
287. Ikkala, E., Koskela, J., Pikkarainen, P., et al.: Acta Haemat. *56*:257, 1976.
288. Schneider, R. G., Berkman, N. L., Brimhall, B., and Jones, R. T.: Biochim. Biophys. Acta *453*:478, 1976.
289. Moo-Penn, W. F., Bechtel, K. C., Johnson, M. H., Jue, D. L., Therrell, B. L., Morrison, B. Y., and Schmidt, R. M.: Biochim. Biophys. Acta *453*:472, 1976.

TABLE 3–3. Clinically Important Hemoglobin Variants

I. The Sickle Syndromes
   A. Sickle cell trait
   B. Sickle cell disease
      1. SS
      2. SC
      3. SD_{Punjab}
      4. SO_{Arab}
      5. S/Thal
II. The Unstable Hemoglobins (Congenital Heinz Body Anemia)
      (Approx. 64 variants)
III. Hemoglobins with Abnormal Oxygen Affinity
   A. High affinity (familial erythrocytosis)
      (Approx. 24 variants)
   B. Low affinity (Hb Kansas, Hb Beth Israel → familial cyanosis)
IV. The M Hemoglobins (Familial Cyanosis)
      (5 variants)
V. Structural Variants which result in a Thalassemic Phenotype
   A. Lepore hemoglobins (β-thalassemia phenotype)
   B. Chain termination mutants (i.e., Hb Constant Spring: α-thalassemia phenotype)

moglobins. The five M hemoglobins encountered thus far have very interesting properties, which are described in Chapter 7. There are three different Lepore-type hemoglobins which result in a β-thalassemia phenotype (see Chapter 2) and four different α-chain termination mutants which cause α thalassemia (Chapter 2).

GENETIC BASIS OF THE HEMOGLOBIN VARIANTS

Mendelian Inheritance

As Chapter 2 explains, the α and non-α globin polypeptide chains are products of separate genes. Thus, a mutant hemoglobin involves a structural abnormality of a specific globin subunit. Hemoglobin variants are inherited as co-dominant traits, according to classic Mendelian genetics. Figure 3–1 shows two pedigrees. If both parents have sickle trait (AS) (left-hand panel), half of these children will be AS, while one fourth will be AA and the remaining fourth will be homozygotes (SS). If one parent has sickle trait and the other C trait, one fourth of the offspring will be AA, one fourth will be AS, one fourth will be AC, and the remaining fourth will be double heterozygotes (SC).

As Table 3–1 shows, variants have been encountered for each of the four globin chains (α,β,γ, and δ) that are found in human red cells in postnatal life. The relatively small number of γ-chain variants is due in part to the fact that hemoglobin F is barely detectable after the first six months of life. Likewise, δ-chain variants may often escape detection, since they are present in small amounts (1 to

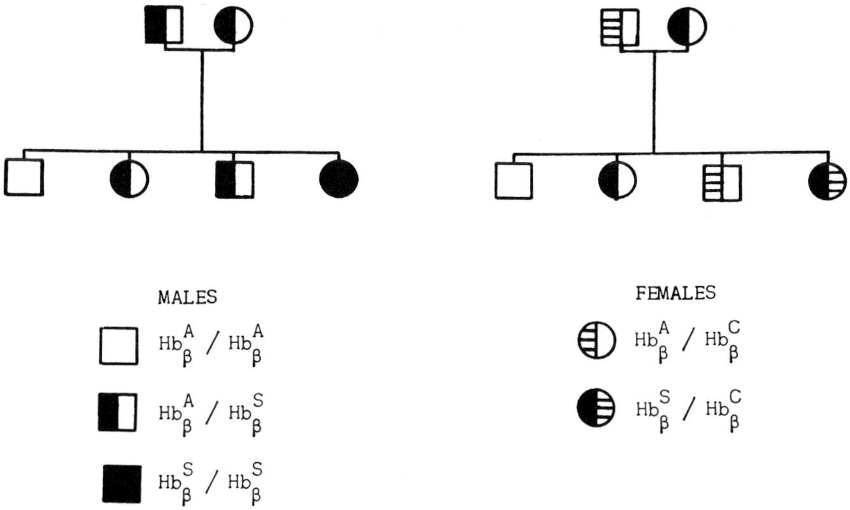

Figure 3–1. Pedigrees showing the inheritance of homozygous sickle cell anemia (SS) (*left*) and Hb SC disease (*right*). (From Rucknagel, D., and Laros, R. K.: Clin. Obst. Gynec. *12*:49, 1969.)

3 per cent). No functional significance has been ascribed to any of the γ-chain variants that have been reported with the exception of Hb F-Poole, an unstable fetal hemoglobin causing hemolytic anemia in the neonatal period (Lee-Potter et al., 1975). Occasionally, individuals may inherit more than one hemoglobin variant. A heterozygote for both an α-chain variant and a β-chain variant will have four major hemoglobin bands on electrophoresis ($\alpha_2^A\beta_2^A$, $\alpha_2^X\beta_2^A$, $\alpha_2^A\beta_2^Y$, and $\alpha_2^X\beta_2^Y$). Figure 3–2 shows an electrophoretic pattern of an individual who has an α-chain variant (HB I) and a β-chain variant (Hb S).

Single Base Substitutions

Of the 269 variants listed in Tables 3–1 and 3–2, the vast majority (238) are single amino acid substitutions in a globin polypeptide chain. The structural alteration can be explained by a single base substitution in the corresponding triplet codon of the globin gene DNA (and its corresponding mRNA).* For example, hemoglobins Rainier ($\alpha_2\beta_2{}^{145\ \mathrm{Tyr}\rightarrow\mathrm{Cys}}$), Bethesda ($\alpha_2\beta_2{}^{145\ \mathrm{Tyr}\rightarrow\mathrm{His}}$), and Fort Gordon

*For descriptive purposes, in the following discussions the mutations are described in terms of the nucleotide sequence changes created in the transcription product of the gene: the globin messenger RNA (mRNA). The actual mutation, of course, occurs in the complementary DNA sequence of the gene at the appropriate corresponding position.

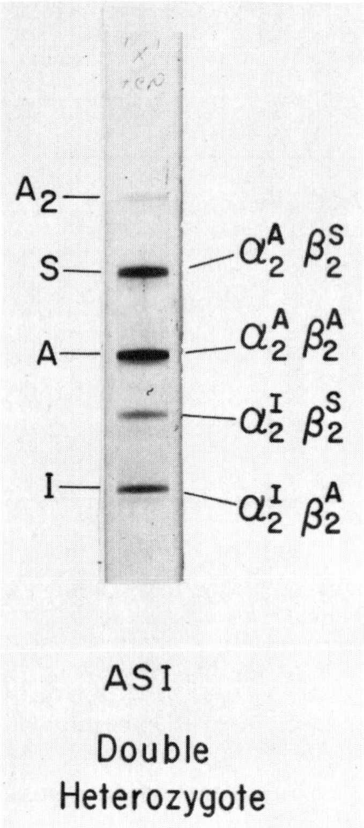

Figure 3–2. Gel electrofocusing pattern of individual doubly heterozygous for an α-chain variant (Hb I) and a β-chain variant (Hb S).

($\alpha_2\beta_2{}^{145\ \mathrm{Tyr}\rightarrow\mathrm{Asp}}$) can all be explained by single base substitutions in the triplet UAU, which is thought to code for tyrosine 145 (Table 3–4).

A few variants have amino acid substitutions at two different sites on the same subunit. These include hemoglobins C-Harlem (β6 Glu→Val, 73 Asp→Asn), Arlington Park (β6 Glu→Lys, 95 Lys→Glu), J-Singapore (α78 Asn→Asp, 79 Ala→Gly), and C-Ziguinchor (β6 Glu→Val, 58 Pro→Arg). These variants also presumably arose by the same mechanism of single base substitutions in the involved triplet codons of the globin gene DNA (and thence the mRNA).

It is presumed that there exist unique "normal" mRNA sequences for the α and β globin chains. This hypothesis is supported by the fact that all the amino acid substitutions thus far described in human hemoglobins can be explained by single nucleotide base substitutions in a single corresponding codon of the normal mRNA, as illustrated in Table 3–4. In fact, the occurrence of multiple variants with different amino acid substitutions at the same site has permitted the hypothetical assignment of specific nucleotide bases in certain positions of many mRNA codons, the full sequence of which

TABLE 3–4. *Single Base Substitutions in Hemoglobin Variants*

β-Chain Variants		Residue Number 144	145	146	Termination Codon
β^A	Base sequence	AAG -	UAU -	CAC -	UAA*
	Amino acid sequence	Lys -	Tyr -	His-	COOH
β Rainier	Base sequence	AAG -	UGU -	CAC -	UAA
	Amino acid sequence	Lys -	Cys -	His-	COOH
β Bethesda	Base sequence	AAG -	CAU -	CAC -	UAA
	Amino acid sequence	Lys -	His -	His-	COOH
β Fort Gordon	Base sequence	AAG -	GAU -	CAC -	UAA
	Amino acid sequence	Lys -	Asp -	His-	COOH

*The nucleotide sequence for this segment of mRNA was proposed by Marotta et al. (1974) on the basis of direct nucleotide sequence studies of normal globin mRNA.

could not otherwise be predicted (Fitch, 1974). Thus far, direct studies of the sequence of normal globin mRNA has not uncovered any contradictions in this general theory (Forget et al., 1974b; Marotta et al., 1974).

There is one possible exception, however, to this general scheme. Three different variants have been described with amino acid substitutions at β-chain residue number 67: Hb Sydney ($\alpha_2\beta_2^{67\ Val\rightarrow Ala}$), Hb M-Milwaukee-1 ($\alpha_2\beta_2^{67\ Val\rightarrow Glu}$), and Hb Bristol ($\alpha_2\beta_2^{67\ Val\rightarrow Asp}$). As illustrated in Table 3–5, Hb M-Milwaukee-1 and Hb Bristol could not arise by a single nucleotide base substitution in a single common normal valine codon: the former must arise from a GUG or GUA valine codon, whereas the latter must arise from a GUC or GUU valine codon. Direct nucleotide sequence analysis of human globin mRNA suggests that the normal codon for $\beta^{67\ Val}$ in the indi-

TABLE 3–5. *Hemoglobin Variants Affecting Residue* β^{67}

Variant	Possible Mutant Codons	Corresponding Normal Valine Codons
Hb Sydney ($\beta^{67\ Val\rightarrow Ala}$)	GCU	GUU
	GCC	GUC
	GCA	GUA
	GCG	GUG
Hb M-Milwaukee ($\beta^{67\ Val\rightarrow Glu}$)	GAA	GUA
	GAG	GUG
Hb Bristol ($\beta^{67\ Val\rightarrow Asp}$)	GAU	GUU
	GAC	GUC

Note that Hb Bristol and Hb M-Milwaukee cannot originate by a single base substitution in a common normal valine codon.

viduals thus far studied is in fact GUG (Marotta et al., 1977). Hemoglobin Bristol could have arisen through a double nucleotide base substitution—GUG→GAU (or GAC)—or perhaps as a mutation in a "normal" gene that had a silent polymorphism (base substitution) in the $\beta^{67\ Val}$ codon—GUC or GUU instead of GUG. The globin mRNA of only a small number of individuals has thus far been studied, and it is certainly feasible that silent polymorphisms may in fact exist in the mRNA sequences of normal α and β mRNA in different individuals or in different ethnic groups. A second example of probable polymorphism has recently been identified at β codon number 20 (see Table 3–2).

ELONGATED SUBUNITS: TERMINATION ERRORS

A second general class of abnormal hemoglobins is that in which the mutant globin chain is abnormally long or short. These seem to have resulted from a variety of different genetic mechanisms. Hb Constant Spring (CS) has abnormally long α chains carrying 28 or 31 extra amino acids at the C-terminal end of the α chain, the sequence of the first 141 amino acid residues being normal (Clegg et al., 1971b; Milner et al., 1971). The shorter form of the α^{CS} chain probably results from post-translational proteolytic cleavage of the last three amino acids of the chain (Clegg et al., 1971b). One can account for the abnormally long α^{CS} chain by a single base substitution in the normal termination codon of the α-chain mRNA (Clegg et al., 1971b). Mutation of the UAA or UAG termination codon of the α-chain mRNA to a CAA or CAG would result in a codon which codes for glutamine, and glutamine is precisely the amino acid in position 142 of the α^{CS} chain (i.e., the first amino acid of the abnormal segment of the α^{CS} chain). In the case of Hb CS, then, a simple base substitution would abolish the termination signal and allow the translation of normally untranslated sequences of the mRNA, which are known to exist (see Chapter 2 and Figure 3–3).

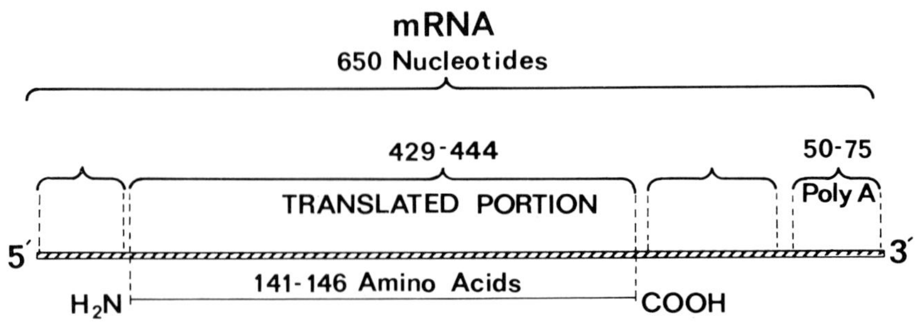

Figure 3–3. Schematic diagram showing the translated and untranslated portions of globin mRNA. Included in the translated portion are the six nucleotides of the initiation and termination codons.

The hypothesis of chain termination mutation as the basis for Hb CS has been strengthened by the finding of three other variants with elongated α chains: Hb Icaria (Clegg et al., 1974a), Hb Seal Rock (Bradley et al., 1975), and Hb Koya Dora (DeJong et al., 1975). These variants both have the same number of extra residues at the C-terminal end of the α chain and they differ only in the nature of the amino acid at position number 142; the other 30 additional C-terminal residues are the same in all four variants. The amino acid present at position 142 is lysine in Hb Icaria, glutamic acid in Hb Seal Rock, and serine in Hb Koya Dora. The presence of these residues can be explained, just as in Hb CS, by base substitutions in the termination codon: UAA (or UAG) to AAA (or AAG) in Hb Icaria, UAA (or UAG) to GAA (or GAG) in Hb Seal Rock, and UAA (or UAG) to UCA (or UCG) in Hb Koya Dora. In fact, direct nucleotide sequence analysis of normal globin mRNA has confirmed the presence of untranslated nucleotide sequences in the mRNA, and some of these nucleotide sequences can be matched to amino acid sequences in the elongated α-chain sequence of Hb CS (Forget et al., 1974b; Marotta et al., 1974). These various findings all support the hypothesis that chain termination mutations can be the cause of certain variant hemoglobins.

Elongated Subunits: Frame-Shift Mutations

Hb Wayne (Seid-Akhavan et al., 1972, 1976) also has an abnormally long α chain with extra amino acids at its C terminus, but it probably arose by a different mechanism. The α chain of Hb Wayne has the normal α-chain amino acid sequence through position 138; then a totally new sequence of eight amino acids is present at the C-terminal end of the α chain. The mechanism of mutation in this case was probably a single nucleotide base deletion which caused a "frame shift," or change in the mRNA reading phase or frame. It can be described as follows: the normal α-chain mRNA sequence coding for the C-terminal α-chain amino acids (numbers 137 to 141) is thought to have been identified (Forget et al., 1974b; Marotta et al., 1974). This mRNA sequence is

137	138	139	140	141	142	143
(ACC)	(UCC)	(AAA)	(UAC)	(CGU)	(UAA)	(GCN).
Thr	Ser	Lys	Tyr	Arg	term.	

In the mRNA of the Hb Wayne α chain, one of the A's of codon 139 (or one of the C's of codon 138) is presumed deleted. The mutant sequence would then be read in the following order:

137	138	139	140	141	142
(ACC)	$(\mathrm{UC}^{\mathrm{C}}_{\mathrm{A}})$	(AAU)	(ACC)	(GUU)	(AAG).
Thr	Ser	Asn	Thr	Val	Lys

Because the translational apparatus can only decode the mRNA by reading successive intact triplet codons, the apparatus cannot detect or correct for deletions. It is readily apparent that a single base deletion will disrupt the normal decoding phase or triplet punctuation built into the mRNA, and as a result the UAA will no longer be read as an intact termination codon. The "U" is now read as part of the codon for position 141 and the "AA", as part of the codon for position 142. Consequently, translation of the mRNA continues until a new stop signal is encountered, and an abnormally long α chain is synthesized.

The nucleotide sequence of the untranslated portion of normal human α-chain mRNA, which is located just distal to (to the 3′ side of) the termination codon, can be predicted by comparing the amino acid sequences of the α Constant Spring and α Wayne chains with reference to the genetic code (Laux et al., 1973). A unique nucleotide sequence of 26 base residues can be derived which contains a new "in phase" termination codon, UAG, at the predicted position to terminate the α Wayne chain. Some of these nucleotide sequences predicted for α-chain mRNA have in fact been found by direct nucleotide sequence analysis of normal human α-chain mRNA (Forget et al., 1974b; Marotta et al., 1974). This finding supports the hypothesis that the α^{CS} and α^{Wayne} chains arose by the mechanisms outlined above.

Two hemoglobins with abnormally long β globin chains have been described: Hb Tak (Flatz et al., 1971) and Hb Cranston (Bunn et al., 1975b). The amino acid sequence of the β^{Tak} chain is normal through position 146, the normal β-chain C-terminal residue, just as the α-chain sequence of hemoglobin Constant Spring is normal through position 141, the normal α-chain C-terminal residue. However, the β^{Tak} chain is not likely to have arisen by the same type of mutation which produced the α^{CS} chain. The first "extra" (147th) amino acid in the β^{Tak} chain is threonine. None of the threonine codons (ACN) can be formed from any of the termination codons (UAA, UAG, or UGA) by a single base substitution: a double base substitution must be postulated. The first two nucleotide bases following the normal β-chain termination codon are thought to be GC– (Forget et al., 1974b; Marotta et al., 1974) (see also Table 3–6). GCN must code for alanine and not lysine, which is the amino acid found in position 148 of the β^{Tak} chain and which must have as its codon

TABLE 3–6. *Frame-Shift Mutations of β-Chain mRNA Giving Rise to Hb Tak and Hb Cranston*

Sequence	Globin Chain
144 145 146 Lys - Tyr - His - Term AAG - UAU - CAC - UAA - GCN	β^{A}
144 145 146 147 148 149 Lys - Ser - Ileu - Thr - Lys - Leu AAG AGU AUC ACU AAG CUN	β^{Cranston}
144 145 146 147 148 149 Lys - Tyr - His - Thr - Lys - Leu AAG UAU CAC ACU AAG CUN	β^{Tak}

The nucleotide sequence of normal β mRNA was determined by Marotta et al. (1974) and Forget et al. (1975); N indicates any of the four nucleotides. The frame shift results from reduplication of the underlined dinucleotides in the normal sequence: AG in codon 144 for β^{Cranston}, and AC in codon 146 for β^{Tak} (Fitch, 1974; Bunn et al., 1975b; Forget et al., 1975b).

AAG or AAA. It is therefore unlikely that Hb Tak arose by simple chain termination mutation (single base substitution in the termination codon the the β mRNA).

Studies of Hb Cranston provide further insight into the probable molecular basis of Hb Tak. The amino acid sequence of the β^{Cranston} chain is normal through residue number 144, where it changes to a different amino acid sequence for 13 additional residues (Bunn et al., 1975b). The sequence of the first five new amino acids can be reconciled to the previously proposed nucleotide sequence for this portion of the normal β-chain mRNA (Forget et al., 1974b; Marotta et al., 1974) by postulating a frame-shift mutation resulting from duplication of the last two nucleotide bases of the codon for amino acid 144, AAG-AGU (Table 3–6 and Bunn et al., 1975b). Such a frame shift would account for the new residues in positions 145 to 147 and result in read-through beyond the normal termination codon (Table 3–6).

Fitch (1974), on the basis of the normal β mRNA sequence, proposed a similar mechanism for the origin of the β^{Tak} chain: duplication of the last two nucleotide bases of the codon for amino acid 146, CAC-ACU, resulting in a frame shift which allows read-through of the normal termination codon and translation of normally untranslated portions of the β mRNA.

The type of frame shifts proposed for the origins of the β^{Tak} and β^{Cranston} chains could have arisen through nonhomologous crossing over of chromosomes at meiosis, with resulting insertion of repeated nucleotide base pairs, although other defects of DNA replication, excision, and repair could result in the same type of mutation.

If Hbs Tak and Cranston arose by the mechanisms just proposed, they should have identical sequences from residue number 148 onward, because this portion of the sequence would result from the read-through (in the same "frame" or order) of the same untranslated portion of the β mRNA. The completed structural analysis of Hb Tak shows that this is indeed true (Lehmann et al., 1975).

Again direct nucleotide sequence analysis of normal globin mRNA has provided support for these hypotheses. Nucleotide sequences have been identified in normal β mRNA which can be correlated to almost the entire elongated amino acid sequence of the β^{Cranston} and β^{Tak} chains, and one long, normally untranslated nucleotide sequence provides a new chain termination codon in the predicted position following the C-terminal Tyr codon (Forget et al., 1975).

Hemoglobin Grady: Crossover in Phase

One last elongated globin chain has been described. In Hb Grady (Huisman et al., 1974) the α chain contains three additional amino acids but the additional residues are not located at the C terminus of the affected globin chain. The α^{Grady} chain contains a "repetition" of the tripeptide sequence normally found at positions 116 to 118; then its sequence continues as the normal α-chain sequence:

114 115 116 117 118 119 120
Pro-Ala-Glu-Phe-Thr-Glu-Phe-Thr-Pro-Ala- etc.

This hemoglobin variant may have arisen by nonhomologous crossing over of complementary globin chain genes, with insertion (reduplication) of three adjacent codons (Huisman et al., 1974). On the other hand, the new codons could have resulted from some other defect in DNA replication or repair.

Shortened Subunits

A few mutant hemoglobins have abnormally short globin chains (Table 3–2). In all cases described, one or a few adjacent amino acids are missing from the abnormal chains. The remainder of the subunit is normal. These variants probably involve deletion of one or more intact codons (of the mRNA) which code for the missing amino acids. If an entire codon is deleted, then no frame shift will result and the remainder of the amino acid sequence will not differ from normal. Such codon deletions could arise by nonhomologous crossing over of complementary globin chain genes or by other mechanisms of faulty

DNA replication, which have been previously alluded to. These variants are generally unstable and are associated with congenital Heinz body hemolytic anemia (see Chapter 5).

One hemoglobin variant, Hb McKees Rocks, has a shortened β subunit that is probably due to a nonsense mutation (Winslow et al., 1976). The β chain of the variant has a structure identical to β^A chains through residue 144, but lacks the two C-terminal residues (-Tyr-His). This mutant hemoglobin may have arisen because of a substitution of A or G for U, at the third base of the codon UA<u>U</u> for tyrosine at position 145, thus producing a termination codon (UAA or UAG). However, the same structure could have resulted from a frame shift or a deletion.

FUSION SUBUNITS

The final class of mutant hemoglobins to be considered are the hemoglobins with fused or hybrid globin chains. Hemoglobin Lepore, for example, contains normal α chains and abnormal non-α chains. These non-α chains have a normal length but an abnormal sequence: the first 50 to 80 amino acids have the normal N-terminal amino acid sequence of δ chains, while the last 60 to 90 residues have the normal C-terminal amino acid sequence of β chains. The Lepore chain is thus a fusion or hybrid NH_2-$\delta\beta$-COOH chain. Three different Lepore chains have been described, in which the switch from δ to β sequences occurs at different points of the sequence (Fig. 2–2*B*). Hemoglobin Kenya is analogous except that the abnormal hybrid chain contains γ and β sequences (NH_2-$\gamma\beta$-COOH) (see Chapter 2).

Hemoglobin Lepore appears to have arisen through nonhomologous crossing over between part of the δ locus on one chromosome and part of the β locus on the complementary chromosome, as illustrated in Figure 2–2*A*. This phenomenon occurs as a consequence of misalignment of a chromosome pair during meiosis, resulting in the pairing of a β gene with a δ gene instead of with its homologous β gene. Such an event should give rise to two abnormal chromosomes: the first, the Lepore chromosome, has no normal intact β or δ loci but has instead only the fused $\delta\beta$ Lepore gene. Because of the absence of a normal β locus in cis and the low output of the Lepore gene product, heterozygous Hb Lepore patients should have the clinical features of β-thalassemia trait while homozygous Hb Lepore syndrome should mimic β thalassemia major. This prediction has proved to be true (see Chapter 2 and Weatherall and Clegg, 1972). The second abnormal chromosome arising from a $\delta\beta$-gene nonhomologous crossing-over event should be an "anti-Lepore" chromosome, which carries normal β and δ loci as well as a gene for an NH_2-$\beta\delta$-COOH anti-

Lepore globin chain (see Figure 2–2*A*). Because of the presence of a normal β locus in cis, patients with this chromosome should be clinically normal except for the presence of the anti-Lepore hemoglobin. Such patients have recently been identified and two different anti-Lepore hemoglobins have been characterized: Hb Miyada and Hb P-Nilotic (see Figure 2–2*B*). The discovery of these anti-Lepore hemoglobins strongly supports the model of nonhomologous crossing over for the origin of Hb Lepore.

Hb Kenya seems to have arisen by nonhomologous crossing over between γ and β loci, giving an NH_2-$\gamma\beta$-COOH fusion product (see Figure 2–3). Because the γ loci are less homologous to the β loci and are situated farther away from the β loci than are the δ loci, the Kenya crossover must have required a greater degree of mispairing during meiosis. Only one type of Hb Kenya has been described so far. The "anti-Kenya" gene has not been identified. The occurrence of both Hb Lepore and Hb Kenya provides strong support for the hypothesis that the γ, δ, and β loci are closely linked on the same chromosome in the order NH_2-$\gamma\delta\beta$-COOH (see Chapter 2).

PATTERN OF SYNTHESIS OF HEMOGLOBIN VARIANTS

From the previous discussions, one can conclude that abnormal hemoglobins probably arise by many different types of mutations in the globin genes which result in the synthesis of a globin mRNA with an abnormal nucleotide sequence. Most of these hemoglobins are made in reduced amounts. It is readily apparent that any of the steps in mRNA metabolism could result in reduced synthesis of the abnormal globin chain. The mutant mRNA could be transcribed, processed, or transported less efficiently. Alternatively, the abnormal mRNA could be unstable and degraded rapidly or translated more slowly than normal because it contains an abnormal codon which requires a transfer RNA which is in short supply in the cell (so-called modulation; see Chapter 2). Finally, the mutant globin chain could be synthesized normally but be structurally unstable or unable to associate normally with other chains to form tetramers; as a result, the abnormal chain could be preferentially lost owing to precipitation or catabolism. All these processes would result in reduced amounts of the abnormal hemoglobin.

White (1971) has reviewed the many studies done to distinguish among the above possibilities. In most cases, the abnormal globin chain is synthesized at a normal rate but is preferentially lost or degraded because of increased catabolism or because of the inadequate capacity of the mutant chain to participate in tetramer assembly. In most cases for which decreased synthesis has been alleged to exist, these post-translational phenomena have not been completely ruled out, nor has the precise mechanism of presumed decreased synthesis been elucidated. Abnormal translation (elongation) times have not been found in such cases. In Hb Gun Hill (Rieder, 1971), the abnormal β chain seems to accumulate 20 to 50 per cent faster than normal, but the assembly time of the chain is normal. This entire area remains poorly understood.

Hemoglobins with abnormal α chains tend to be present in heterozygotes as an even smaller percentage (10 to 25 per cent) of the total hemoglobin than hemoglobins with mutant β chains (35 to 50 per cent) (Fig. 3–4). This is best explained by the independent evidence for duplication of the α-chain loci (see Chapter 2 and Wasi, 1973). A mutant α-chain locus would then constitute only 1 of 4 α-chain loci in the diploid heterozygous state, whereas mutant β-chain loci would constitute 1 of 2 β-chain loci.

The synthesis of Hb Lepore, the anti-Lepore hemoglobins, and Hb Constant Spring (like that of normal Hb A_2) appears to be confined almost entirely to bone marrow and is virtually absent from circulating reticulocytes. The molecular mechanisms responsible for this observation are obscure, but instability of the mRNA has been suggested (see Chapter 2).

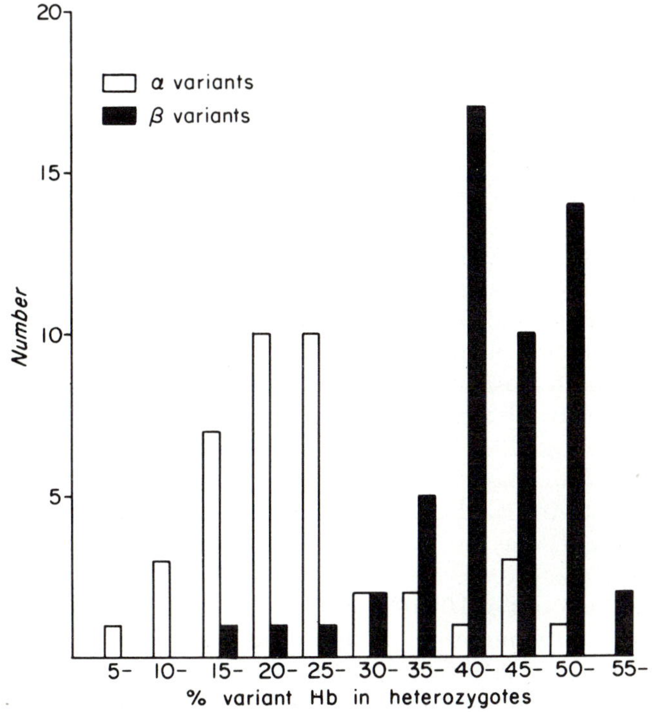

Figure 3–4. Distribution of variant hemoglobins in humans heterozygous for α-chain and β-chain mutant hemoglobin. (From Nute, P., et al.: Ann. N.Y. Acad. Sci. *241*: 39, 1974a.)

Finally, the reasons for the extremely low output of the abnormally long α-chain variants (Wayne, Seal Rock, Icaria, Koya Dora, and Constant Spring) are not understood. These variants constitute only 1 to 3 per cent of the total hemoglobin, and it is not immediately obvious why these frame-shift and chain-termination mutants should be present in such low amounts. Simple translation of normally untranslated sequences of the mRNA cannot be the only factor. The two β-chain frame-shift mutants accumulate in much greater amounts (25 to 40 per cent of the total hemoglobin). The observed low yields of the Lepore and anti-Lepore hemoglobins are also difficult to understand (see Chapter 2).

In summary, the molecular mechanisms by which mutant hemoglobins arise have been reasonably well delineated, but the effects of these mutations on the ultimate amounts of the mutant hemoglobins finally accumulated in the cell remain poorly understood at the molecular level.

COMMON HEMOGLOBIN VARIANTS

Hb S ($\alpha_2\beta_2^{6\ \mathrm{Glu}\rightarrow\mathrm{Val}}$)

Hb S is the most common human hemoglobin variant. The sickle syndromes are an important group of disorders and are discussed in detail in Chapter 4. Representative blood films of the sickle syndromes and some of the other common hemoglobinopathies are shown in Figure 3–5.

Hb C ($\alpha_2\beta_2^{6\ \mathrm{Glu}\rightarrow\mathrm{Lys}}$)

Hb C was the second variant to be identified electrophoretically (Itano and Neel, 1950) and structurally (Hunt and Ingram, 1960). The replacement of lysine for glutamic acid at the sixth position of the β chain (the same site as the substitution in hemoglobin S) gives Hb C a relatively high positive charge. Accordingly, it has slow mobility upon zone electrophoresis at alkaline pH, identical to that of Hb A_2. However, hemoglobins A_2 and C can be separated by column chromatography (Huisman, 1972). Hb C is found primarily in blacks. In areas of West Africa, the gene frequency (and therefore, the incidence of C trait) may be as high as 28 per cent. About 2 per cent of black Americans are AC heterozygotes, while approximately $0.02 \times 0.02 \times 0.25$, or 1 out of 10,000 are CC homozygotes. Hb C is probably the second most commonly encountered variant worldwide.

Individuals who have *Hb C trait* (AC) lack any clinical manifestations. Red cell life span is normal (Prindle and McCurdy, 1969). The red cells contain about 30 to 40 per cent Hb C, 50 to 60 per cent

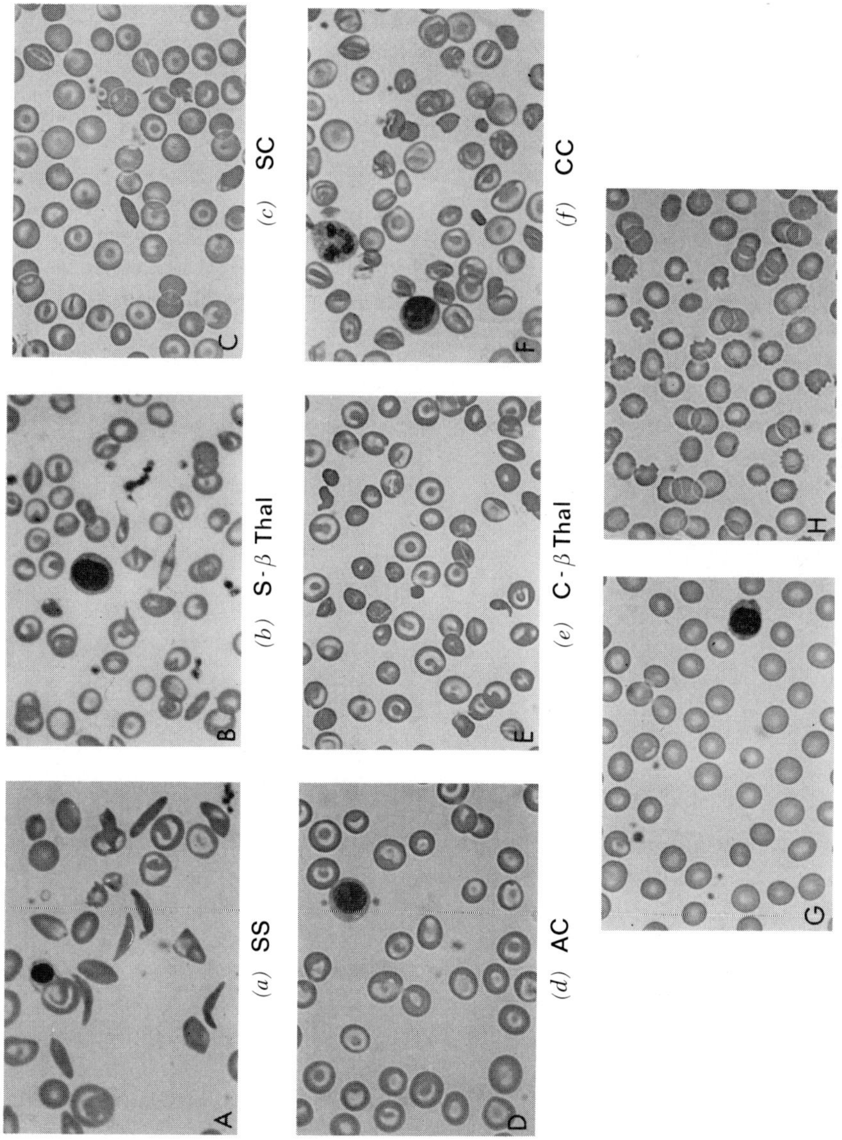

Figure 3–5. Peripheral blood smears of patients with various hemoglobinopathies. (*a*) Homozygous sickle cell anemia; (*b*) sickle/β thalassemia; (*c*) hemoglobin SC disease; (*d*) hemoglobin C trait; (*e*) hemoglobin C/β thalassemia; (*f*) homozygous hemoglobin C disease; (*g*) normal; (*h*) congenital Heinz body hemolytic anemia. (This figure was prepared by Ms. Carola Kapff.)

Hb A, and slightly increased amounts of Hb A_2 (Huisman, 1972). If α thalassemia is also present, the proportion of Hb C will be reduced (Weatherall, 1973). Stained films of AC blood show increased numbers of target cells, but these are much fewer in number than what is seen in homozygotes (Fig. 3–5*d*).

Patients who are doubly heterozygous for Hb C and Hb S have a disease of moderate severity. Hb C participates with Hb S in sickling more readily than does Hb A. Hb SC disease is discussed in detail in Chapter 4.

Patients who are *homozygous for Hb C* have a mild to moderate congenital hemolytic anemia (Ranney, 1953; Spaet et al., 1953; Singer, 1954; Terry, 1954; Hartz and Schwartz, 1955; Jensen et al., 1957; Smith and Krevans, 1959; Redetski et al., 1968). They are usually asymptomatic, although ill-defined arthralgia and abdominal pain and, rarely, hemorrhagic manifestations have been reported. Splenomegaly is generally present. As in other chronic hemolytic disorders, cholelithiasis and "aplastic crises" may occur. Packed cell volume generally ranges between 25 and 37 per cent, accompanied by a moderate reticulocytosis (4 to 8 per cent). Red cell survival is decreased with splenic sequestration (Singer, 1954; Jensen et al., 1957). Erythropoiesis is not sufficient to maintain a normal red cell mass (Jensen et al., 1957; Prindle and McCurdy, 1969). Mean corpuscular hemoglobin is normal but hemoglobin concentration per cell is increased (Murphy, 1968). The majority of erythrocytes on a dried stained blood film are target cells (Fig. 3–5*f*). These are plumper and of smaller diameter than the target cells seen in liver disease or biliary obstruction. Hb CC erythrocytes do not appear targeted when examined in a wet preparation (Murphy, 1968). However, their increased resistance to osmotic hemolysis indicates that these red cells have an increased ratio of surface area to volume (Charache et al., 1967). The mechanism by which red cells containing Hb C (or for that matter Hb S, D, or E) assume a target appearance and have abnormal osmotic fragility is not known. On electrophoresis, Hb C constitutes over 90 per cent of the total. Hb F may be slightly increased. No Hb A is seen.

The shortened life span of CC erythrocytes is probably based on the fact that they are abnormally rigid and therefore may traverse capillaries less readily than normal red cells. Hb CC blood and cell suspensions have increased viscosity and decreased filterability (Charache et al., 1967; Murphy, 1968). This is particularly true of microspherocytes which make up a minor population of CC red cells. The increased viscosity of CC red cells may be due in part to a marked increase in cell water bound to hemoglobin (Murphy, 1968). Deoxy Hb C is less soluble than deoxy Hb A (Charache et al., 1967), although this difference is much less than that for Hb S. The amino acid substitution (β6 Glu$\rightarrow$Lys) may favor intracellular aggregation of

Hb molecules. Hb CC cells will form intracellular crystals when suspended in a hypertonic medium (Kraus and Diggs, 1956; Wheby, 1956). A concentration of about 48 per cent Hb C is required for crystallization (Charache et al., 1967). Formation of these crystals is enhanced if the cells are deoxygenated (Charache et al., 1967). There is ultrastructural evidence that hemoglobin aggregation adjacent to the membrane precedes the formation of intracellular crystals (Lessin et al., 1969). This increased cellular rigidity probably does not require the presence of morphologically demonstrable inclusions.

The oxygen saturation curve of dilute solutions of Hb C is normal. Furthermore, Hb C has normal reactivity to 2,3-DPG and CO_2 (Bunn, 1972). However, the whole blood oxygen affinity of Hb C is reduced (Bellingham and Huehns, 1968). This may be explained in part by increased red cell 2,3-DPG due to decreased mean red cell age. The fact that CC red cells have a decrease of solvent water (Murphy, 1968) may affect intracellular pH and thus oxygen affinity. In addition, the aggregation of Hb C at high concentration, if oxygen-linked, may also influence intracellular oxygen affinity.

Hb D

Itano (1951) encountered a new hemoglobin variant which co-migrated with Hb S on moving-boundary electrophoresis but failed to sickle. It was labeled Hb D and was subsequently found to have the structure $\alpha_2\beta_2^{121\ \mathrm{Glu}\rightarrow\mathrm{Gln}}$ (Hb D-Punjab or D-Los Angeles) (Baglioni, 1962). Since that time, other variants have been found which also co-migrate with Hb S when electrophoresis is run at an alkaline pH. A number of these have been named with the prefix D followed by the locale where they were discovered (e.g., D-Ibadan [$\alpha_2\beta_2^{87\ \mathrm{Thr}\rightarrow\mathrm{Lys}}$], D-Iran [$\alpha_2\beta_2^{22\ \mathrm{Glu}\rightarrow\mathrm{Gln}}$], etc.) or the prefix G (e.g., G-Galveston [$\alpha_2\beta_2^{43\ \mathrm{Glu}\rightarrow\mathrm{Ala}}$], G-San Jose [$\alpha_2\beta_2^{7\ \mathrm{Glu}\rightarrow\mathrm{Gly}}$], etc.). None of these hemoglobins sickle, yet when they co-exist with Hb S in the doubly heterozygous state, they can affect sickling to a varying degree. For example, Hb S/D-Punjab is a much more severe condition than Hb S/D-Ibadan (Watson-Williams et al., 1965). The interaction of S and D hemoglobins is covered in detail in Chapter 4. Note that all the D (and G) hemoglobins involve an increase in one unit of positive charge per affected subunit: either a substitution of a neutral for a negatively charged amino acid or a substitution of a positively charged residue for a neutral one. Although they co-migrate with Hb S under standard electrophoretic conditions at alkaline pH, most of them can be separated from Hb S by electrophoresis on agar gel at pH 6.0 to 6.5. In addition to their failure to sickle, these hemoglobins also differ from Hb S in their solubility properties. Thus, heterozygotes for Hb D (or G) will have negative solubility tests for Hb S.

Hb D-Punjab (D-Los Angeles) is by far the most commonly encountered of the "D" hemoglobins (Vella and Lehmann, 1974). Among Sikhs of the Punjab region of India, Hb D has an incidence of 2 to 3 per cent. A number of homozygotes have been reported from various parts of the world (Bird and Lehmann, 1956; Chernoff, 1958; Stout et al., 1964; Ozsoylu, 1970). These individuals have normal hemoglobin values with no evidence of hemolysis. Red cell indices are generally within normal limits. Some individuals have had target cells and decreased osmotic fragility. Hemoglobin electrophoresis shows 95 per cent Hb D and normal amounts of Hb A_2. Tests for sickling are negative. This condition must be distinguished from the double heterozygous state Hb D/β_0 thalassemia. Appropriate family studies and careful measurement of red cell indices and Hbs A_2 and F are important in establishing the diagnosis. Individuals doubly heterozygous for Hb D and β thalassemia usually have mild anemia and minimal hemolysis (Rieder, 1976) in contrast to those with E/β thalassemia (see below) and S/β thalassemia (see Chapter 4).

Hb E ($\alpha_2\beta_2{}^{26\ \mathrm{Glu}\rightarrow\mathrm{Lys}}$)

Hb E is the third most prevalent hemoglobin variant worldwide. It is found primarily in Orientals, although it has also been reported in blacks (Bunn et al., 1972). The gene frequency in Thailand and Burma is approximately 15 per cent. The maintenance of such a high gene frequency may be a reflection of some type of balanced polymorphism, in which AE heterozygotes have improved fitness. Hb E co-migrates with Hb A_2 and Hb C on electrophoresis.

AE heterozygotes are commonly encountered. They have no hematological abnormalities. Hemoglobin electrophoresis reveals about 30 per cent Hb E; the remainder is Hb A. As in AS and AC heterozygotes, the proportion of Hb E decreases significantly in individuals who also have α thalassemia (Tuchinda et al., 1964; Wasi et al., 1969). In addition, the relative amount of Hb E in AE heterozygotes may decrease if they become iron-deficient (Wasi et al., 1968). Patients who are doubly heterozygous for Hb E and β thalassemia have an anemia which is variable in its severity but is generally more severe than in patients with Hb S/β thalassemia (Sturgeon et al., 1955; Chernoff, 1956).

Individuals homozygous for Hb E may have a mild anemia with somewhat reduced red cell survival. Others have normal hemoglobin levels with no evidence of hemolysis (Lehmann et al., 1956). Most of these individuals have significantly reduced mean corpuscular volume (Lehmann et al., 1956). Red cell indices may be difficult to interpret because both iron deficiency and the thalassemias are very prevalent in Southeast Asia. Target cells are seen on dried peripheral smears and, in keeping with this observation, there is increased resistance to osmotic lysis (Chernoff, 1955; Lehmann et al., 1956). The basis for these morphological abnormalities is unknown. It is curious that homozygotes for hemoglobins S, C, D, and E all have target cells and reduced osmotic fragility, although there are significant differences in red cell indices among these conditions.

Whole blood oxygen dissociation curves of EE homozygotes are shifted slightly to the right (Kolatat, 1964; Bellingham and Huehns, 1968), probably owing to increased red cell 2,3-DPG (Gacon et al., 1974). Purified Hb E has normal oxygen affinity, Bohr effect, and reactivity to 2,3-DPG (Bunn et al., 1972b; Gacon et al., 1974). Hemoglobin E appears to be relatively unstable to an oxidant stress (Frischer and Bowman, 1975) and may behave abnormally in subunit association (Pagnier et al., 1974). However, these phenomena probably have no clinical significance.

Hb G-Accra (Korle-Bu) ($\alpha_2\beta_2^{73\ \mathrm{Asp}\rightarrow\mathrm{Asn}}$)

Hemoglobin Korle-Bu is encountered quite frequently in central Africans. There are no clinical or hematological manifestations associated with either the heterozygous or the homozygous state (Lehmann and Huntsman, 1966). It is interesting that red cells from an individual homozygous for Hb Korle-Bu had a perfectly normal appearance on blood smear. No target cells were seen (Lehmann and Huntsman, 1968). This variant is of additional interest because of its interaction with Hb S. As discussed in detail in Chapter 4, Hb Korle-Bu behaves like Hb F in its failure to participate in the gelation of Hb S (Bookchin et al., 1970). Thus, individuals who are doubly heterozygous for Hb S and Hb Korle-Bu have a mild form of Hb "SD" disease.

Hb H (β_4)

Hb H is a tetramer composed of four normal β chains. This abnormal hemoglobin is seen in some individuals with α thalassemia (see Chapter 2).

Hb I ($\alpha_2^{16\ \mathrm{Lys}\rightarrow\mathrm{Glu}}\beta_2$)

Hb I is probably the most commonly encountered α-chain variant (Schneider et al., 1966). It has been found in individuals of various racial backgrounds. They have no apparent clinical or hematological abnormalities. Heterozygotes have about 25 per cent Hb I and 75 per cent Hb A. This proportion is similar to other α-chain variants (Fig. 3–4) and provides indirect evidence that each parent contributes two α-chain genes (see above). Biosynthetic studies of an AI heterozygote confirm that the reduced amount of Hb I in the red cell is due to a relative decrease in synthesis rather than preferential destruction of Hb I (Esan et al., 1970). The amino acid substitution in Hb I is in one of the invariant residues. Nevertheless, Hb I has perfectly normal functional properties (McDonald et al., 1974).

Chapter 4

SICKLE CELL ANEMIA AND RELATED DISORDERS

Sickling of red blood cells was first described in 1910 by Herrick who observed unusual shapes of red cells in blood smears of a black student. The dependence of sickling and unsickling on deoxygenation and reoxygenation was noted by Hahn and Gillespie in 1927. During the ensuing years this phenomenon was observed not only in patients with chronic hemolytic anemia and recurrent episodes of painful crises, but also in the blood cells of some normal, healthy individuals. According to Konotey-Ahulu (1974), the characteristics and familial incidence of recurrent severe painful crises were recognized for many years in Ghana, where the lowland incidence of sickle cell trait exceeds 20 per cent.

In the late 1940's, interrelationships among the asymptomatic healthy carriers, the severely anemic individuals who had recurrent painful crises, and the less commonly encountered patients who exhibited clinical syndromes intermediate between sickle cell trait and sickle cell anemia were largely clarified by family studies and by analysis of the hemoglobin of affected individuals. Neel (1947, 1949) and Beet (1949) presented formal genetic evidence which indicated that sickle cell trait represented the heterozygous state for a gene which in the homozygous state was manifest as sickle cell anemia.[1]

In-vitro studies by Ham and Castle (1940) established the relationship between sickling and increasing viscosity with decreasing oxygen tension. In the same year, I. J. Sherman demonstrated that

[1]In 1946, Accioly presented a brief but correct genetic analysis in an obscure Brazilian journal (see Azevêdo, 1973).

upon deoxygenation, sickle cells became birefringent. Castle reported these observations to Linus Pauling during a historic train ride in 1948. The following year Pauling, Itano, Singer, and Wells (1949) demonstrated that hemoglobin S differed electrophoretically from normal hemoglobin.

Pauling and his associates showed that most of the hemoglobin of individuals with sickle cell anemia was of the abnormal "S" type, with a greater net positive charge than normal hemoglobin (Hb A). Of the hemoglobin prepared from red cells of asymptomatic individuals with sickle cell trait, about 35 per cent was found to be of the S type while the remainder was normal Hb A. The introduction of zone electrophoresis and its adaptation to use in clinical laboratories led to the delineation of intermediate forms of sickling which resulted from the simultaneous presence of heterozygosity for Hb S and for another abnormal but nonsickling hemoglobin, e.g., Hb C or Hb D; similar syndromes of intermediate severity could also be attributed to the simultaneous presence of single genes for Hb S and for β thalassemia.

In 1950, Harris showed that deoxygenation of a concentrated solution of Hb S resulted in the formation of liquid crystals (or tactoids) accompanied by a marked increase in viscosity. Harris concluded that the sickling of red cells was due to polymerization of the abnormal hemoglobin into elongated fibers. Proof of the structural abnormality of sickle hemoglobin was provided by Ingram (1956, 1959), who demonstrated that Hb S differed from Hb A by the substitution of valine for glutamic acid in the sixth position of the β chain.

THE MOLECULAR BASIS OF SICKLING

The growing knowledge of the stereochemistry of hemoglobin function has allowed a more thorough understanding of how the sickling phenomenon takes place at the molecular level. The primary questions which need to be resolved are (1) What is the structure of the sickle polymer and how are Hb S molecules oriented within the polymer? (2) What is the sequence of events in the formation of the polymer? In order to approach these problems, it is necessary to derive a model which is in agreement with a number of experimental observations.

Structure of the Sickle Fiber

Nature of Intermolecular Bonding

The sickling phenomenon must be explained ultimately by the substitution of the hydrophobic valine residue for glutamic acid at the sixth position of the β chain. This is probably due to a local alteration on the surface of the molecule at this site rather than to any widespread conformational changes. In dilute solution, hemoglobin S has entirely normal functional properties including oxygen affinity, heme-heme interaction, Bohr effect, and reactivity with 2,3-DPG and CO_2 (Allen and Wyman, 1954; Bunn, 1972; Rossi-Bernardi et al., 1975).

The early studies by Murayama (1966) indicated that the aggregation of sickle hemoglobin molecules involved hydrophobic bonding. Evidence supporting this conclusion included the demonstration of a negative temperature coefficient of gelation and the ability of nonpolar molecules such as propane and urea to disrupt sickling. Later studies by Bookchin and Nagel (1973b) showed that electrostatic bonds were also important in the polymerization of sickle hemoglobin molecules in the formation of the sickle fiber. They found that the minimum concentration of deoxygenated S hemoglobin required for gelling decreased progressively at ionic strengths below 0.15. Thus, salt exerted some degree of inhibition upon the aggregation of the hemoglobin molecules. Taken together, these results indicate that the polymerization of sickle hemoglobin is complex and cannot be explained by a simple two-point interaction between neighboring molecules.

Studies on the *interaction of sickle and nonsickle hemoglobins* have provided more specific information about the contact points between neighboring molecules in the sickle polymer. The early studies of Singer and Singer (1953) established that the presence of hemoglobin F increased the minimum concentration of total hemoglobin required for gelation (MGC). In fact, these MGC results suggested that hemoglobin F failed to participate at all in the sickling phenomenon. The Singers (1953) also demonstrated that hemoglobins A and C participated in gelling to an increasing degree, and that these interactions correlated with the clinical severity of the heterozygous states SA and SC.

Bookchin, Nagel, and Ranney extended this experimental approach to other hemoglobin variants having known amino acid substitutions (1967, 1970). They demonstrated that Hb C-Harlem ($\alpha_2\beta_2{}^{6\ \mathrm{Glu \rightarrow Val,\ 73\ Asp \rightarrow Asn}}$) sickled less readily than hemoglobin S. Furthermore, hemoglobin Korle-Bu ($\alpha_2\beta_2{}^{73\ \mathrm{Asp \rightarrow Asn}}$) participated in gelation with hemoglobin S less readily than did hemoglobin A (Bookchin et al., 1970). These observations, summarized in Table 4–1, indicated that the aspartate residue at position 73 of the beta chain is probably an important site in the polymerization of sickle hemoglobin. Subsequently, interaction of other hemoglobin variants with hemoglobin S has also been shown to be different from that of hemoglobin A. For example, hemoglobin O-Arab ($\alpha_2\beta_2{}^{121\ \mathrm{Glu \rightarrow Lys}}$) and hemoglobin D-Punjab ($\alpha_2\beta_2{}^{121\ \mathrm{Glu \rightarrow Gln}}$) both interact strongly with sickle hemoglo-

TABLE 4–1. *Effect of Non-S Hemoglobins and Chemical Modifications on the Gelling of Sickle Hemoglobin*

EXPERIMENT	MGC* (g/100 ml)	REFERENCE
I. *Interaction of S and non-S Hbs (all deoxy)*		
100% S	24	Singer and Singer; 1953; Bookchin et al.; 1970
50% S, 50% O-Arab	21	Milner et al., 1970
50% S, 50% D-Punjab	24	Charache and Conley, 1967
50% S, 50% C	27	Singer and Singer, 1953
50% S, 50% A	30	Singer and Singer, 1953; Bookchin et al., 1970
50% S, 50% Korle-Bu	36	Bookchin et al., 1970
50% S, 50% F	36	" " " "
II. *Asymmetrical Hybrids (all deoxy)*		
40% S, 60% A: half hybrid ($\alpha_2\beta^S\beta^A$)	30	Bookchin et al., 1975
40% S, 60% A: no hybrid	30	" " "
40% S, 60% F: half hybrid ($\alpha_2\beta^S\gamma$)	39	" " "
40% S, 60% F: no hybrid	31	" " "
III. *Valency Hybrids*		
100% deoxy S (no hybrids)	24	Bookchin and Nagel, 1971
50% deoxy S, 50% CNMet-S (no hybrids)	30	" " " "
$\alpha_2^{CNMet}\beta_2^S$	34	Bookchin and Nagel, 1973a
$\alpha_2\beta_2^{S\text{-}CNMet}$	34	" " " "
$\alpha_2^{CNMet}\beta_2^{S\text{-}CNMet}$	No Gel	" " " "
IV. *Chemical Modifications (all deoxy)*		
Native Hb S ($\alpha_2\beta_2^S$)	23	Benesch et al., 1974
Pyridoxal derivatives:		
$\alpha_2^P\beta_2^S$	30	" " "
$\alpha_2\beta_2^{S\text{-}P}$	26	" " "
Native Hb S ($\alpha_2\beta_2^S$)	24	Nigen et al., 1974
Carbamylated derivatives:		
$\alpha_2^{CNO}\beta_2^S$	24	" " "
$\alpha_2\beta_2^{S\text{-}CNO}$	29	" " "
$\alpha_2^{CNO}\beta_2^{S\text{-}CNO}$	29	" " "

*Minimum concentration required for gelation (MGC) measured by method of Singer and Singer (1953) in 0.15 M phosphate, pH 7.35.

bin (McCurdy, 1960; Milner et al., 1970). Thus, β121 Glu may be another important contact point between neighboring molecules in the sickle polymer. The fact that hemoglobin Memphis ($\alpha_2^{23\ Glu\rightarrow Gln}\beta_2^{6\ Glu\rightarrow Val}$) gels less readily than does hemoglobin S (Kraus et al., 1966) indicates that this site on the alpha chain contributes to the polymerization of sickle hemoglobin molecules. Data on several different α-chain variants (Benesch et al., 1976) suggest that other nearby sites on the surface of the α chain are also involved in the aggregation of Hb S.

It is likely that non-S hemoglobins can participate in gelation by the formation of asymmetrical hybrid tetramers such as $\alpha_2\beta^S\beta^A$ (Moffat, 1974; Bookchin et al., 1975; Goldberg et al., 1975; Table 4–1). X-ray crystallographic data of Wishner et al. (1975) (described below) indicate that only one of the two β chains has an intermolecular contact at β6.

Optical Studies

Perutz and Mitchison (1950) studied the absorption of sickled erythrocytes with polarized light. Their results, when interpreted in terms of the later x-ray structural information, indicated that the dyad axis of the hemoglobin tetramers in the sickle hemoglobin fiber lay perpendicular to the fiber axis. More recent optical data of Hofrichter et al. (1973) confirm this early conclusion. Their measurements further indicate that the long molecular axis of the tetramer (65 Å dimension) is within 22 degrees of the fiber axis. These results impose an important constraint on the orientation of the hemoglobin molecule within the fiber lattice.

Ultrastructural Studies

A number of investigators have studied the ultrastructure of deoxygenated sickle hemoglobin, both in intact red cells and in concentrated solutions (Stetson, 1966; Murayama, 1966; White, 1968; Bertles and Döbler, 1969; Edelstein et al., 1973; Finch et al., 1973; Josephs et al., 1976). Electron micrographs demonstrate bundles of long straight fibers whose axis is parallel to the long axis of the sickled erythrocyte. Ultrastructural examination of a gel of deoxyhemoglobin S revealed fibers that each have a diameter of approximately 170 Å, with spacing between fibers ranging between 180 and 240 Å (Finch et al., 1973). A representative electron micrograph is shown in Figure 4–1 (Finch et al., 1973).

From a consideration of the dimensions of the tetrameric hemoglobin molecule (65 × 55 × 50 Å), Murayama (1966) and others concluded that the hemoglobin fiber is a helical polymer consisting of six strands (i.e., six molecules per cross-sectional area) (Fig. 4–2*A*). The detailed structure of the helix, including the pitch and the orientation of the hemoglobin molecules within the helix, is not entirely clear. X-ray diffraction data of Magdoff-Fairchild and coworkers (1972) were interpreted to support a six-stranded helical structure. However, other preparations of hemoglobin S have yielded a different morphological appearance on electron microscopy. Recent data of Josephs et al. (1976) obtained on intact sickled cells indicate that most of the Hb S fibers have helical structures (200 Å diameter) consisting of eight strands, with adjacent strands staggered by half a molecule (Fig. 4–2*B*).

Wishner et al. (1975, 1976) have done *x-ray diffraction analyses* of crystals of deoxyhemoglobin S grown in 10 to 15 per cent polyethylene glycol. The unit cell consists of two tetrameric molecules with the dimensions 63 × 184 × 52 Å. At both 5 Å and 3 Å resolution, there were no significant differences between the crystals of deoxy Hb S and deoxy Hb A in the regions around the $\beta 6$ residues. As dis-

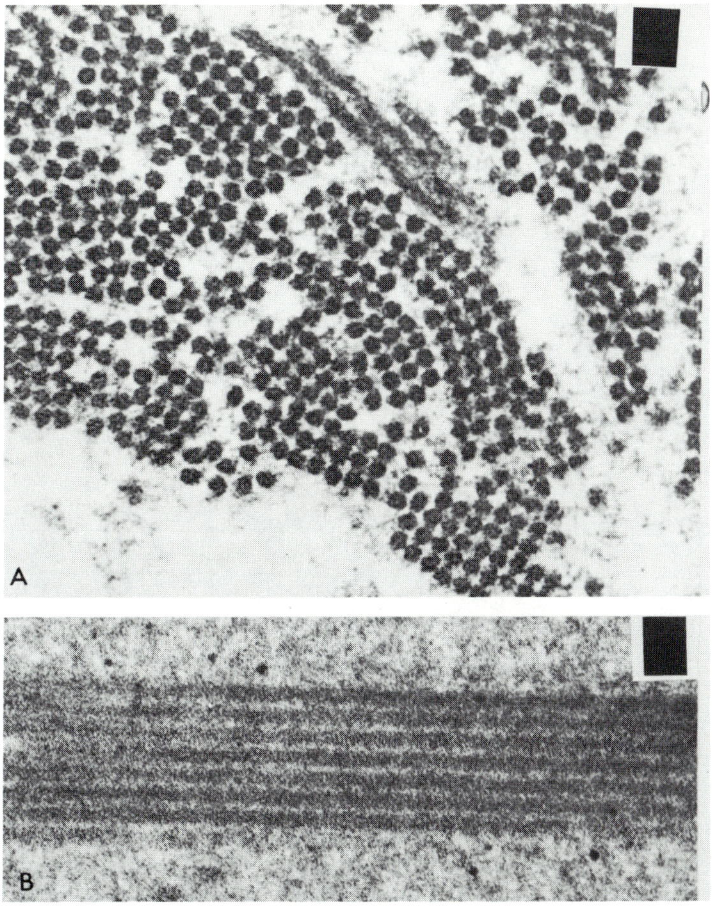

Figure 4–1. Electron micrographs of centrifuged pellet of deoxyhemoglobin S (× 325,000). *A*, Transverse section showing bundles of Hb S fibers. *B*, Longitudinal section showing parallel alignment of fibers. (From Finch, J. T., et al.: Proc. Natl. Acad. Sci. U.S.A. *70*:718, 1973.)

cussed in the section above on the interaction of sickle and nonsickle hemoglobins, a number of specific residues are known to affect the gelling behavior of sickle hemoglobin. These include β6 Val, β73 Asp, β121 Glu, and α23 Glu. The x-ray data of Wishner et al. indicate that these residues are all at sites of intermolecular contact, including interactions between molecules of the same strand and between molecules of adjacent strands. This is shown diagrammatically in Figure 4–3. Only one of the β6-valines is involved in an intermolecular interaction. These x-ray results indicate that adjacent interlocking strands are out of register by 32 Å (half the repeat distance) and rotated by half a turn. Such a structure does not fit the fiber model proposed by Finch et al. (1973) (Fig. 4–2A) but is compatible with the recent electron microscopic results of Josephs et al. (1976)

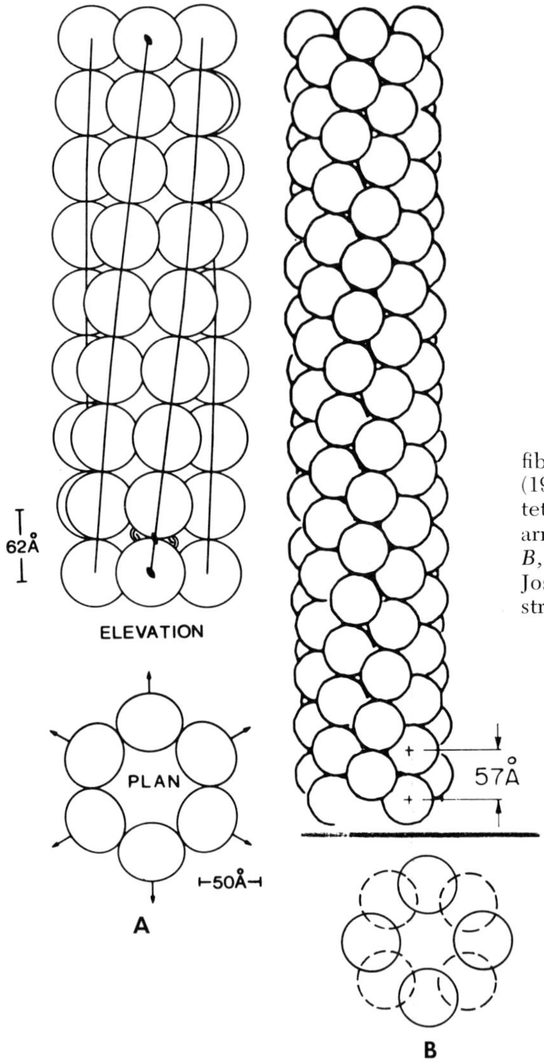

Figure 4–2 *A*, Model of Hb S fiber proposed by Finch et al. (1973) showing individual Hb S tetramers (represented as spheres) arranged in a six-stranded helix. *B*, Model of Hb S fiber proposed by Josephs et al. (1976) showing eight-stranded helix.

described above (Fig. 4–2*B*). It should be emphasized that the crystals analyzed by Wishner et al. (1975, 1976) were prepared under nonphysiological conditions and may not reflect the spatial orientation of molecules of deoxyhemoglobin S within the sickled red cell.

Participation of Small Molecules in the Sickling Phenomenon

In order to understand the sickling of red cells in vivo, it is necessary to determine how various intracellular mediators of hemoglobin function affect the polymerization of deoxy sickle hemoglobin.

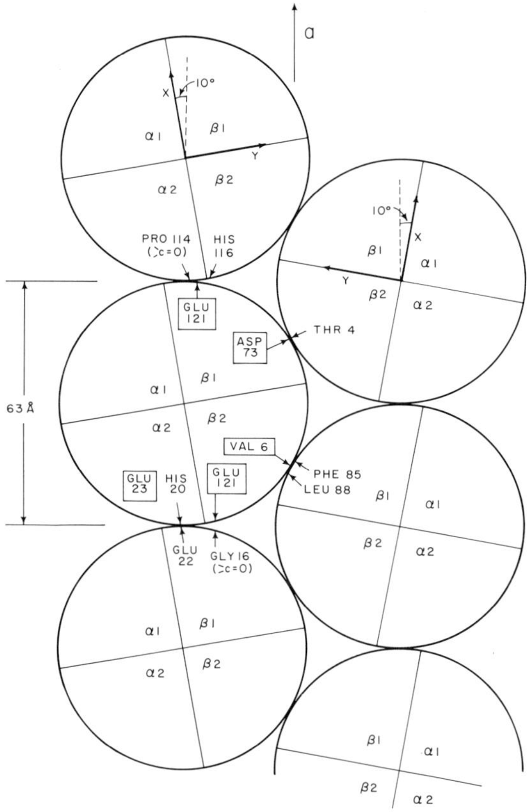

Figure 4–3. Intermolecular contacts between neighboring strands of Hb S. This model was constructed from x-ray crystallographic data of Wishner et al. (1975).

These factors include pH, ionic strength, organic phosphates (particularly 2,3-DPG), and PCO_2. The influence of these variables on sickling had not been studied until recently.

As pointed out in Chapter 1, 2,3-DPG is an important mediator of intracellular hemoglobin function. It has been demonstrated recently that 2,3-DPG facilitates the sickling phenomenon. Using analytical ultracentrifugation and viscosity measurements, Briehl and Ewert (1973) showed that the aggregation of deoxyhemoglobin S was enhanced by decreasing pH and increasing concentrations of 2,3-DPG. The promotion of sickling by 2,3-DPG has also been confirmed by measurements of viscosity (Paniker et al., 1972) and gelation (Nagel and Bookchin, 1974a) of Hb solutions and by intact cell preparations (Jensen et al., 1973a). X-ray diffraction data of Arnone (1972) indicate that there is a small, but significant, change in the three-dimensional structure of the N-terminal end of the β chain when 2,3-DPG is bound to hemoglobin. This alteration in the three-dimensional configuration may enhance sickling by an alteration at the primary binding site in the vicinity of β6-valine.

Water plays a complex role in the sickling phenomenon. Careful measurements of cell volumes indicate that, during sickling, the red cell loses osmotically active water (Masys et al., 1974). This phenomenon can be explained by a decrease in oncotic pressure due to hemoglobin polymerization. In addition, water molecules become incorporated into the fiber lattice. Transverse water proton relaxation times show a progressive increase in tumbling time for irrotationally bound water during the deoxygenation of sickle hemoglobin and its accompanying polymerization (Cottam et al., 1974; Chuang et al., 1975; Zipp et al., 1976).

Chemically Modified Sickle Hemoglobin

The gelation or polymerization of sickle hemoglobin has been studied following the chemical modification of the molecule at a number of sites. There has been a considerable amount of work done on the effects of cyanate on the sickling phenomenon both in vitro and in vivo following the introduction of sodium cyanate by Cerami and Manning (1971) as a potential form of therapy in sickle cell anemia. Nigen and his associates (1974) have shown that when sickle hemoglobin is selectively carbamylated at the N terminus of the α chain, there is little effect on minimum gelling concentration, whereas hemoglobin S carbamylated only on the β chain showed a decreased tendency to polymerize (Table 4–1). Recently, Benesch et al. (1974) reacted hemoglobin S selectively at the N terminus of the β chain with pyridoxal phosphate and found that this modification had a small effect on sickling. In contrast, they showed that selective blocking of the α-chain N-terminal amino group with pyridoxal sulfate caused a more marked increase in minimum gelling concentration (Table 4–1). These two sets of results seem to be in conflict. The effect of selective modifications at the N termini of α and β chains must be strongly dependent on the nature of the blocking groups. Recently, Roth and his associates (1974) found that nitrogen mustard, a potent alkylating agent, reacted specifically at β2-histidine (the second residue of the β chain) and caused a marked inhibition of sickling without a significant alteration in the functional properties of the molecule, such as oxygen affinity. Since this modification is close to the site of the primary amino acid substitution in sickle hemoglobin, it probably has a direct steric effect on the primary binding site. In contrast, selective chemical modification at the β93-sulfhydryl group appears not to have a profound effect on the polymerization of sickle hemoglobin (Yamaoka et al., 1974).

Effect of Conformation on Sickling

Since the early experiments of Hahn and Gillespie, it has been known that deoxygenation favors the sickling of red cells. Harris

(1950) subsequently demonstrated in cell-free solutions that the deoxy form of hemoglobin S was a prerequisite for the formation of liquid crystals (tactoids). Since hemoglobin undergoes a marked change in quaternary conformation upon deoxygenation, it has been assumed that this structural transition opens up one or more binding sites on the hemoglobin S molecule necessary for its aggregation. Bookchin and Nagel (1971) have found that the T quaternary conformation is not required for the participation of non-S hemoglobins in gelling. For example, mixtures of cyanmethemoglobin A (R structure) and deoxyhemoglobin S gel equally as readily as mixtures containing equivalent amounts of deoxyhemoglobin A and deoxyhemoglobin S. Further studies by Bookchin and Nagel (1973a) have been designed to assess the importance of the tertiary conformation of the subunits in the hemoglobin tetramers participating in aggregation. They examined hemoglobin hybrids in which either the α or the β chain of hemoglobin S was locked in the r tertiary structure by converting the heme to cyanmet. They observed that these hybrid hemoglobins, $\alpha_2{}^{CNMet}\beta_2{}^{S}$ and $\alpha_2\beta_2{}^{S\text{-}CNMet}$, both gelled at a hemoglobin concentration approximately 50 per cent higher than $\alpha_2\beta_2$ (see Table 4–1). These findings were unexpected because they implied that the tertiary conformation of the β^S chain was not essential in the sickling process. These studies are somewhat hard to interpret, since electron exchange probably occurs following preparation and incubation of these mixed liganded hemoglobin hybrids. This is a very difficult phenomenon to measure or to control. By this means, some of the hybrids would be converted into homogeneous tetramers, $\alpha_2\beta_2{}^S$ and $\alpha_2{}^{CNMet}\ \beta_2{}^{S\text{-}CNMet}$. Such a phenomenon would blunt any intrinsic difference in the sickling of the two hybrids.

Deoxyhemoglobin is not the only form of hemoglobin which is capable of undergoing a transition to the T quaternary structure. Perutz (1974) has found that methemoglobin, particularly at low pH and in the presence of organic phosphates, can assume a T-like structure. Briehl and Ewert (1974) have presented ultracentrifugation data showing that concentrated solutions of methemoglobin S can polymerize in the presence of organic phosphates. The binding of nitric oxide (NO) to the heme groups of hemoglobin also results in a species which is capable of assuming the T conformation (Salhany et al., 1974). Briehl and Salhany (1975) have also found that NO-hemoglobin S, under appropriate conditions, can polymerize into a gel. Both ultracentrifugation data and the demonstration of birefringence support this conclusion.

Sequence of Events in Sickling

Until recently the great majority of experimental studies on the polymerization of sickle hemoglobin have been assumed to be equilibrium measurements. However, the sickling phenomenon is markedly affected by kinetic considerations. The polymerization of deoxyhemoglobin S is very strongly concentration-dependent, so that above a critical concentration there is a concerted transition from hemoglobin sol to hemoglobin gel. This phenomenon was shown quite convincingly by ultracentrifugation studies (Williams, 1973; and Briehl and Ewert, 1973). Malfa and Steinhart (1974d), Harris and Bensusan (1975), and Hofrichter et al. (1974) have found that the polymerization of a solution of sickle hemoglobin can appear abruptly after a delay of up to several hours under appropriate incubation conditions. It has been estimated by Hofrichter and his associates (1974) that the rate of aggregation of sickle hemoglobin varies as the 30th power of hemoglobin concentration:

$$1/t_d = k(C/C_s)^n$$

where t_d = delay time, C = hemoglobin concentration, C_s = solubility (see below), and $n \cong 30$. Note that the delay time is markedly affected by small changes in hemoglobin concentration or solubility.

From their experimental observations, Hofrichter et al. (1973, 1974) proposed that sickling occurs in stages, as shown in Figure 4–4: nucleation followed by fiber growth and alignment of adjacent fibers. The last process is entropically driven and proceeds relatively slowly.

In some experimental systems, notably ultracentrifugation (Williams, 1973; Briehl and Ewert, 1973), no small aggregates are observed in solutions in equilibrium with the sickle gel. In contrast, Wilson et al. (1974) obtained quasi-elastic light scattering, data indicating demonstrable pregelation aggregation. Concerted gel formation implies an equilibrium between fibers or filaments and single

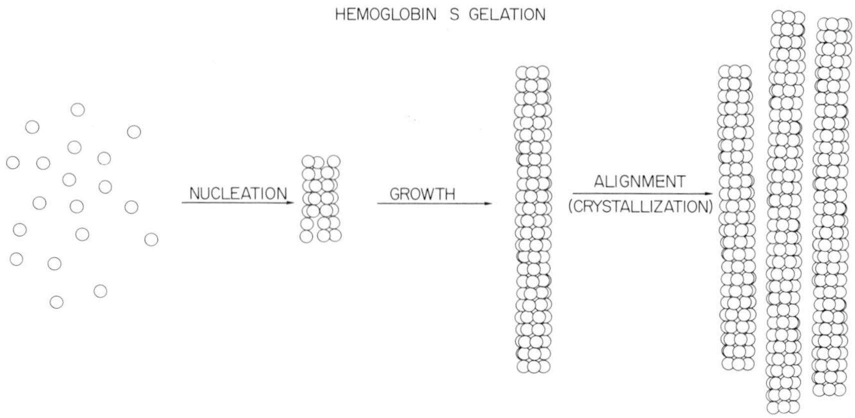

Figure 4–4. Model for the polymerization of deoxyhemoglobin S into aligned fibers. (From Hofrichter, J., et al.: Proc. Natl. Acad. Sci. U.S.A. *70*:3604, 1973.)

molecules of deoxyhemoglobin S, whereas the results of light-scattering experiments suggest that hemoglobin S molecules are bifunctional and that any size aggregate can combine with any other size aggregate in a linear array. Moffat and Gibson (1974), whose studies were based on changes in turbidity with temperature jump, favor a rate-limiting formation of nuclei containing a minimum of 15 deoxy Hb S molecules, followed by polymerization of the nuclei to one another or (more likely) by the addition of individual molecules to the nuclei. Aggregates of hemoglobin S adjacent to the membrane of the intact red cell may provide an initial site for nucleation. Sundin and Williams (1976) have shown that the addition of "inside out" red cell ghosts to concentrated solutions of deoxyhemoglobin S shortens the delay time. The lack of definitive information about the molecular structure of filaments of deoxyhemoglobin S and the different methods used to observe pregelation events make the detailed interpretation of the kinetic data uncertain.

Because of the complex kinetic factors discussed above, the commonly used determinations of sickling such as minimum gelling concentration and viscosity are not true equilibrium measurements. It is likely that at equilibrium there is a simple biphasic system consisting of sickle fiber (containing at least 30 molecules) and free tetramers. If so, sickling can be measured most precisely and directly by a determination of *solubility* (Hofrichter et al., 1976). This can be done by centrifugation, separating the dense gel from the sol. The hemoglobin concentration of the supernatant (sol phase) provides a measure of solubility. The slow transition from isotropic (randomly oriented) to anisotropic (aligned) fibers probably has little effect on solubility.

It is apparent that the sickling phenomenon in the intact red cell must be largely dependent upon kinetic considerations because the extent of deoxygenation during circulation through the capillary bed is strongly time-dependent. This subject is considered in detail in the next section and in a recent review by Eaton et al. (1975).

This large body of experimental information represents a considerable advance in the understanding of the molecular basis of the sickling phenomenon. However, the orientation of the individual sickle hemoglobin tetramers within the fiber is not yet established. Thus, the specific intermolecular contacts are not known. Such information would be useful in designing a suitable drug for the inhibition of sickling in vivo.

CELLULAR BASIS OF SICKLING

The growing body of information on the molecular basis of sickling, summarized in the previous section, provides only a partial understanding of the mechanisms underlying the clinical manifestations of sickle cell anemia. The *cellular* basis of sickling is dependent upon a number of additional factors such as the composition and concentration of the hemoglobin within the red cell, the age of the cell, the integrity of its membrane, the rate of extent of oxygen release as well as alterations or abnormalities in the microcirculation. In common with other types of hemolytic anemia, sickled red cells are unduly rigid and, as a result, have a shortened life span. In addition, plugging of the microvasculature by sickled red cells leads to tissue ischemia. All Hb S-containing cells will acquire the classic sickle-shape deformity upon deoxygenation because of the intracellular polymerization of hemoglobin (see Figures 4–5 and 4–6). This process is ordinarily reversible upon reoxygenation of the cell. However, repeated sickling induces sufficient membrane damage to certain susceptible cells that the rigidity and sickle shape persist, even after the cell has been reoxygenated. It is likely that both processes contribute to the various clinical findings encountered in the sickle syndromes.

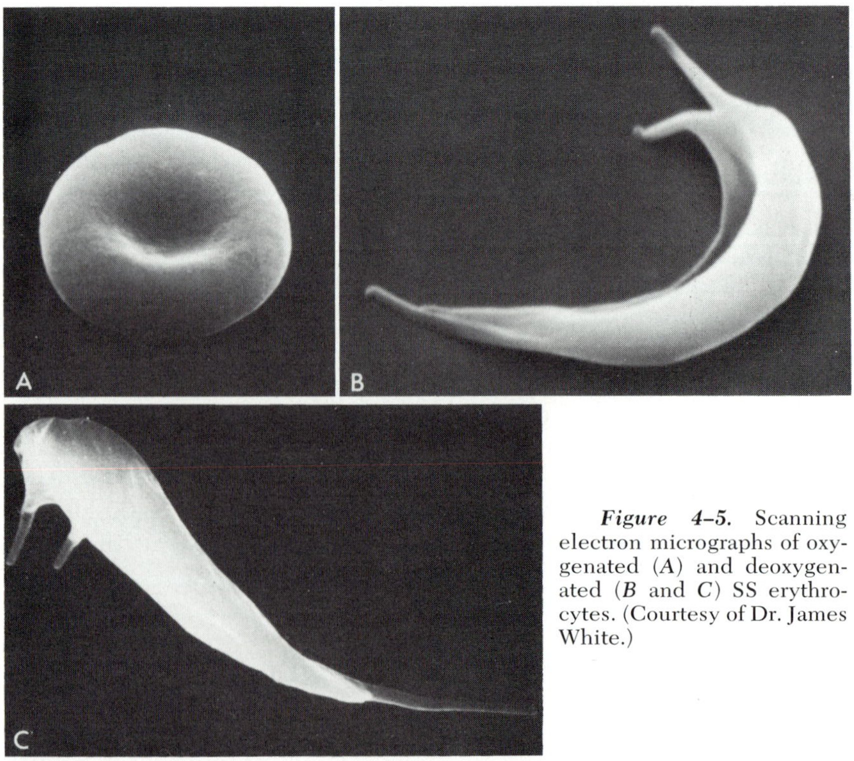

Figure 4–5. Scanning electron micrographs of oxygenated (*A*) and deoxygenated (*B* and *C*) SS erythrocytes. (Courtesy of Dr. James White.)

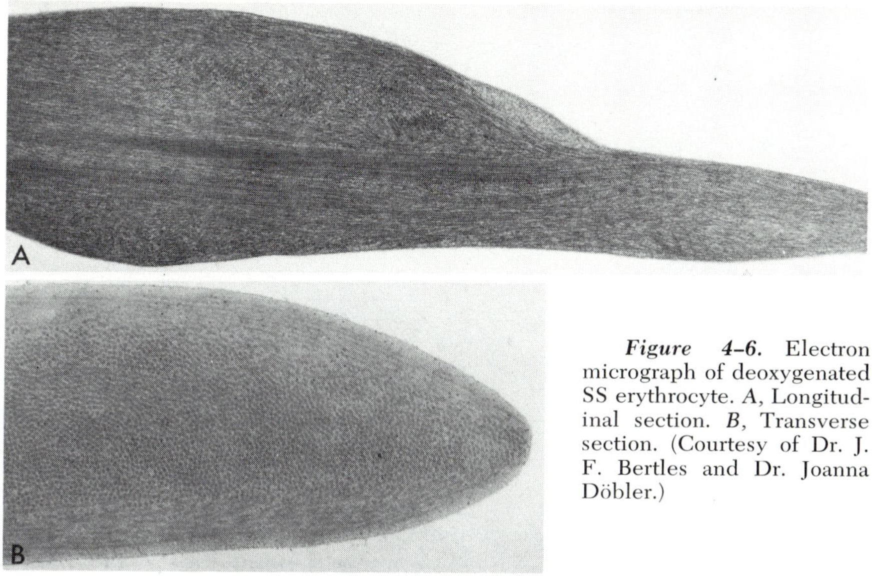

Figure 4–6. Electron micrograph of deoxygenated SS erythrocyte. *A*, Longitudinal section. *B*, Transverse section. (Courtesy of Dr. J. F. Bertles and Dr. Joanna Döbler.)

THE "SICKLE CYCLE"

When the oxygen tension of the Hb S-containing red cell is lowered to a critical point, intracellular polymerization of hemoglobin occurs, leading to the formation of the classic sickle shape (see Figure 4–5). This phenomenon can be monitored by direct morphological examination or by indirect measurements such as viscosity or filterability. The oxygen saturation at which a given cell sickles is determined by a number of factors. As Figure 4–7 shows, the presence of non-S hemoglobin has a profound effect on cellular sickling comparable to its influence on gelation of a cell-free solution (Table 4–1). Griggs and Harris (1956) showed that, under physiologic conditions, the sickling of red cells from homozygotes was first noted at O_2 saturations below 85 per cent. Sickling was nearly complete at 38 per cent O_2 saturation. A progressive increase in whole blood viscosity paralleled the appearance of sickled cells. In contrast, no sickling of AS red cells was observed until the O_2 saturation fell below 40 per cent. These in-vitro studies provide a crude assessment of the sickling phenomenon in vivo. SS homozygotes would be expected to have a significant amount of sickling at oxygen tensions normally encountered in the capillary and venous circulation. However, kinetic considerations discussed below make such predictions unreliable. The fact that AS heterozygotes rarely have clinical manifestations is not surprising in view of the severe and nonphysiologic degree of hypoxemia necessary to induce the sickling deformity.

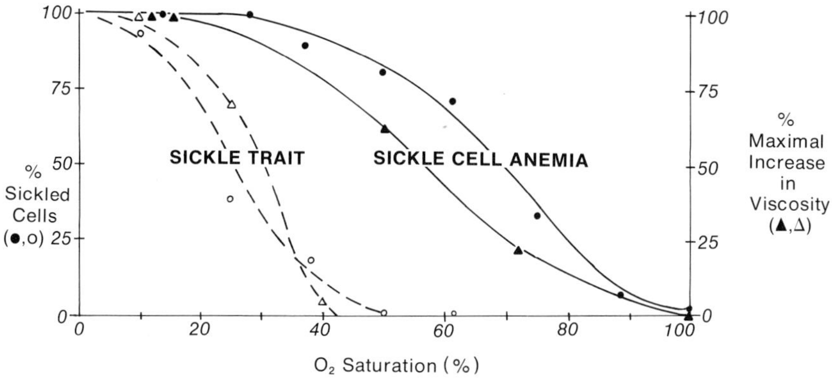

Figure 4–7. Measurement of viscosity and percentage of sickled forms in SS and AS red cell suspension at different oxygen saturations. (Figure prepared from data of Griggs and Harris [1956].)

The precise chain of events which initiates vaso-occlusive crises is not well understood. It is likely that rigid sickled cells (deformed by deoxygenation or irreversibly sickled) obstruct blood at the capillary level. The resulting stasis promotes local hypoxia, deoxygenation of red cells, and further sickling. In this way, the area of vaso-occlusion is amplified (Harris et al., 1956). Local anatomical and physiological factors such as distribution of blood vessels and rate of blood flow help to determine where and when this vicious cycle will occur. Of equal importance is the relationship between the rate of sickling of a partially deoxygenated red cell and the duration of its flow through the microcirculation. In the past few years, a variety of elegant techniques have been applied to this problem. If oxygen is rapidly and exhaustively removed by chemical means, such as addition of dithionite, sickling is very rapid. Zarkowsky and Hochmuth (1975) observed the characteristic deformities of SS red cells within 2 seconds of deoxygenation. However, the rate of sickling of partially deoxygenated cells is a more physiologically relevant consideration (Allison, 1956; Charache and Conley, 1964).

A number of investigators have noted an intermediate phase prior to the assumption of the classic "holly leaf" sickle shape. Padilla et al. (1973) observed a loss of the flicker phenomenon, indicating an increase in cell rigidity that preceded the shape change. Messer and Harris (1970) documented this intermediate phase of cell rigidity by filtration measurements of rapidly deoxygenated SS red cells. Rampling and Sirs (1973) also noted nonspecific abnormalities that preceded true sickling. Recently, Messer et al. (1975) have correlated the rheological properties of deoxygenated SS red cells with serial electron micrographs. They found that during the intermediate phase in which increased rigidity was first detected, there was no ultrastructural evidence of aligned fibers. In contrast, the formation of the classic elongated sickle shape was accompanied by the presence of parallel fibers similar to those shown in Figure 4–5. This intermediate cellular phase of sickling may be closely analogous to the intermediate phase of gelation mentioned above, in which the sickle fibers are randomly oriented.

The mean in-vivo capillary circulation time varies widely from one tissue to another but it ranges between 0.5 and 2.0 seconds. Most SS cells will not have enough time to assume the sickle shape during their rapid passage through capillaries. Jensen et al. (1960) and Serjeant et al. (1973) found that the percentage of sickled forms in venous blood from various sites correlated inversely with the oxygen saturation of the blood sample. However, most if not all of this sickling probably occurred following the transit of blood through capillaries. Beyond that point, the rigid cell should pose no threat to the perfusion of the tissue. The fact that sickle infarcts rarely occur in the myocardium despite its very large oxygen extraction is probably due to rapid circulation through this tissue. Because of these kinetic considerations it is unlikely that the transformation of red cells into sickled forms is the initial event that triggers a vaso-occlusive crisis. However, it is plausible that red cells in the intermediate phase of sickling are sufficiently rigid that they could impede blood flow and initiate the "vicious sickle cycle."

Irreversibly Sickled Cells

Upon examination of peripheral blood films of patients with sickle cell anemia, anywhere from 2 to 30 per cent of the red cells have the characteristic elongated sickle deformity (see Figure 3–5). The presence of such cells is surprising, since the red cells in a peripheral blood smear are fully oxygenated and therefore would not be expected to sickle. Electron microscopy of such cells fails to reveal any aligned sickle fibers so characteristic of deoxygenated sickle cells (Bertles and Döbler, 1969). Thus, these cells have a permanently sickled shape even in the absence of any intracellular polymerization of hemoglobin. These observations indicate that such cells have a damaged membrane which is no longer capable of assuming the normal biconcave disc shape upon reoxygenation.

Irreversibly sickled cells (ISC's) are unduly rigid. Indeed, the presence of these cells explains why oxygenated SS blood has a higher viscosity than normal blood having a comparable packed cell volume (Chien et al., 1970). As mentioned above, these cells may be responsible in part for the plugging of capillaries and, perhaps, the initiation of vaso-occlusive crises. Because of their rigidity, ISC's have a markedly shortened life span (Bertles and Milner, 1968) and contribute significantly to the hemolytic anemia of patients with SS disease. The percentage of ISC's in the peripheral blood provides no insight concerning the *turnover* of these cells. Because of their high MCHC, these cells are dense and can readily be separated from other red cells by centrifugation. Bertles and Milner (1968) have shown that these cells have a relatively low content of Hb F. It is likely that cells that are not well endowed with Hb F are at a distinct disadvantage from the time they emerge from the bone marrow. Without the protection provided by Hb F, these cells have a high probability of repeated sickling and within a few days become ISC's.

Shen et al. (1949) were able to generate ISC's in vitro by prolonged incubation of deoxygenated blood from a patient with sickle cell anemia. Tosteson et al. (1956) showed that such treatment induces a membrane lesion, with enhanced leakage of potassium ion from the cell. Deoxygenation of SS red cells also results in a significant loss of cell water (Masys et al., 1974). In addition to changes in cation permeability, sickling also causes disruption in the anatomical integrity of the red cell membrane. With the use of phase-optic cinematography, Padilla et al. (1973) showed that repetitive sickling can lead to fragmentation and loss of small segments of membrane (microspherules) in excess of hemoglobin. This phenomenon may explain why a small population of SS red cells has increased osmotic fragility, even though the majority of cells are less fragile than normal (Harris et al., 1956). Repeated injury to the red cell membrane eventually leads to the formation of an irreversibly sickled cell.

Recently, a number of investigators have attempted to unravel the physico-chemical factors which put the ISC membrane into rigor mortis. Normal red cells lose their pliability and become rigid echinocytes when depleted of ATP (Weed et al., 1969). Furthermore, stiffening of red cell ghosts is also correlated with accumulation of membrane-bound calcium. Weed et al. (1969) proposed that red cell ATP may serve to chelate calcium, thereby preserving the pliability of the membrane. Jensen et al. (1973c) observed a similar relationship when ISC's were artificially generated during in-vitro incubations. They found a close relationship between the decline of red cell ATP and the generation of ISC's. Furthermore, the formation of ISC's was markedly inhibited by omission or chelation of Ca^{++} during the incubation. Subsequently, low levels of ATP (Glader et al., 1976) and high levels of membrane-bound calcium (Eaton et al., 1973; Palek, 1973) were demonstrated in naturally occurring ISC's. Upon deoxygenation, the influx of extracellular Ca^{++} into SS red cells was markedly enhanced, while deoxygenation had no effect on calcium leak into normal red cells (Eaton et al., 1973).

The precise role of calcium in the pathogenesis of ISC's is controversial. The fact that a calcium ionophore can induce a temporary retention of the sickled shape after reoxygenation (Eaton et al., 1975) implies that Ca^{++} may be directly responsible for the generation of

ISC's. However, Palek et al. (1975) found that the rate of transformation of SS red cells into ISC's was not influenced by either intracellular ATP or extracellular calcium. They have pointed out the difficulties in distinguishing between Ca^{++}-loaded stiff echinocytes and naturally formed ISC's. It is likely that the primary membrane lesion in ISC's is induced by intracellular polymerization of hemoglobin and that enhanced Ca^{++} influx, like K^+ efflux, is a secondary phenomenon. In support of this conclusion, Clark and Shohet (1976) have found that normal red cell ghosts reconstituted with Hb S were able to form irreversibly sickled forms even in the absence of calcium.

The direct interaction of Hb with the inner surface of the red cell membrane may also affect the rheology of SS red cells. Red cell membranes are capable of binding more Hb S than Hb A (Fischer et al., 1975). Furthermore, in AS reticulocytes, newly synthesized β^S chains are more adherent to red cell stroma than are β^A chains (Bank et al., 1974) and, in some cases, have a faster turnover rate compatible with membrane binding (DeSimone et al., 1974a; Shaeffer et al., 1976). These phenomena may account for the presence of dense precipitates of hemoglobin adherent to the membranes of both SS and AS red cells which have been observed by dark-field and phase microscopy (Schneider et al., 1972). The inclusions from AS red cells were found to contain more Hb S than Hb A.

Irrespective of the sequence of steps leading to its formation, the ISC's owe their increased rigidity to a permanently altered membrane protein lattice. Lux and John (1975) observed that the sickled shape of ISC's was preserved even after hemoglobin-free ghosts had been extracted with triton, which removed membrane lipid and the majority of membrane protein. The remaining protein was shown to be composed primarily of spectrin and red cell actin.

Oxygenation of Sickle Blood

Since the sickling phenomenon depends on the formation of deoxyhemoglobin S, it is important to define the oxygen binding properties of sickle red cells. As mentioned above, Hb S in dilute solution has normal oxygen equilibria. However, SS blood has markedly decreased oxygen affinity (Bromberg and Jensen, 1967b). Like patients with other types of anemia, SS homozygotes have elevated red cell 2,3-DPG (Charache et al., 1970). However, P_{50} values of SS blood are higher than would be predicted from red cell 2,3-DPG values, and there is not a significant correlation between P_{50} and red cell 2,3-DPG (Seakens et al., 1973). In view of the intracellular polymerization of deoxyhemoglobin S, Allen and Wyman (1954) predicted, from thermodynamic principles, that high concentrations of Hb S would have low oxygen affinity, but they did not have adequate methods to test their prediction. Recently, May and Huehns (1972b) showed that the P_{50} of SS red cells suspended in artificial media rose sharply when the MCHC was increased from 10 g/100 ml to 30 g/100 ml, while the oxygen affinity of AA red cells was nearly unaffected. Seakens et al. (1973) found that SS red cells having the highest MCHC (irreversibly sickled cells) had the highest P_{50} values. As Rossi-Bernardi et al. (1975) have pointed out, the decreased oxygen affinity of SS red cells is a two-edged sword. On the one hand, the right-shifted curve greatly facilitates oxygen unloading (see Chapter 1) and helps to explain why SS homozygotes tolerate severe degrees of anemia surprisingly well when they are free of crises or infection. On the other hand, decreased oxygen affinity promotes the formation of deoxyhemoglobin and, as a result, promotes sickling.

EPIDEMIOLOGY OF SICKLING

Sickle cell syndromes are found among Africans, Greeks, Italians, Saudis, Israeli Arabs, and the Veddoids of Southern India. Most of the sickle cell anemia found in the New World is of African origin, but sickle cell thalassemia is far commoner in Americans of Greek or Italian origin than is sickle cell anemia.

The sickle cell gene is found largely in the tropical parts of Africa in which malaria parasites flourished over past centuries. Prevalence of sickle trait is as high as 30 per cent in some areas of Africa. During the early surveys of sickling in Africa, it was stated that sickle cell anemia was rare or absent despite the high frequencies of sickle cell trait. The laboratory evaluations which formed the basis for these statements were incomplete: in populations affected with hookworm and with malaria, anemia and splenomegaly were frequent, and the diagnosis of sickling was based solely on sickle cell preparations. Presumably the severely affected sicklers died in childhood, and the laboratory methods used did not permit the identification of mild sicklers. A large loss of Hb S genes from the gene pool due to the loss of homozygotes would be expected in populations with high gene frequency for Hb S. The maintenance of such high gene frequencies implies a selective advantage for heterozygotes for hemoglobin S. Allison (1954, 1957a) suggested that a balanced polymorphism was based upon a selective advantage possessed by individuals heterozygous for hemoglobin S, as compared with normal individuals, with respect to infections with falciparum malaria. The protection conferred by sickle cell trait appears to reduce the mortality rate of children with cerebral malaria. Parasitemia can be demonstrated in sickle cell trait or anemia with falciparum malarial infections but the degree of parasitemia appears to be somewhat lower in sickle cell trait than in individuals with normal hemoglobin. In-vitro studies by Luzzato et al. (1970) provide information on the mechanism by which sickle trait provides protection against malaria. Once an AS cell is parasitized, it is more likely to sickle. This rigid cell is then removed from the circulation and destroyed. Power's (1975) detailed analysis of this model offers an explanation for the restriction of this protection to children with falciparum malaria. With the declining incidence of malaria, the selective advantage of heterozygotes in resistance to infection no longer affects gene frequencies.

SICKLE CELL TRAIT

Sickle cell trait is found in high incidence in many populations of African ancestry; about 8 per cent of American blacks and up to 30 per cent of certain African populations are affected.

Clinical Features

The presence of sickle cell trait is rarely associated with clinical manifestations. While spontaneous hematuria or splenic infarction at high altitudes occurs in AS individuals, such an association should not be regarded as unequivocal evidence of the pathogenicity of sickle cell trait under ordinary circumstances. The occurrence of spontaneous hematuria in sickle cell trait is so rare that the coexistence of another condition, such as an anomaly in the renal microcirculation, in affected individuals is very likely. Diminished vasa recta in the renal medulla have been reported (Statius van Eps et al., 1970). Most individuals with sickle cell trait have an impairment in the ability to make concentrated urine (Schlitt and Keitel, 1960) due to small medullary infarcts. However, renal acidification is normal (Oster et al., 1976).

Reports of sudden death following severe muscular exercise in individuals with sickle cell trait have lacked pertinent information concerning other potential but undetected illnesses in the patients. Observation that sickle cell trait is found with the expected frequency among black professional football players suggests that the tolerance of individuals with sickle cell trait for severe muscular exertion is not impaired (Murphy, 1973). Flying at high altitudes in unpressurized aircraft has apparently resulted in splenic infarctions in a few individuals with sickle trait. Nearly all the vaso-occlusive phenomena seen in SS disease have been described in individuals with sickle trait. (For references see Harris and Kellemeyer, 1970.) However, the significance of these anecdotal reports is difficult to assess in view of the very large group of AS individuals at risk. It is safe to conclude that vaso-occlusive complications are extremely rare in those with sickle trait. Nevertheless, it would seem prudent for individuals with sickle cell trait to avoid exposure to potentially low ambient oxygen, e.g., high altitude flying without pressurization[2] or scuba diving. If general anesthesia is properly administered, AS individuals are not subject to any added risk (Searle, 1972). However, there may be increased morbidity in the application of a tourniquet to an injured extremity of an individual with sickle trait (Stein and Urbaniak, 1975). Data are now being accumulated about the relationship between sickle cell trait and a variety of other diseases (Heller, 1974). It is not possible to make firm statements on the basis of evidence at hand. Certainly, the denial of employment or of life insurance to individuals with sickle cell trait on the grounds of increased risk of illness or of early death is not justified.

Diagnosis

Individuals with sickle trait have normal blood counts. Red cell morphology is usually normal, although some AS individuals may have occasional target cells. The diagnosis of sickle trait is established by the combination of a positive test for sickling (such as the metabisulfite slide test or solubility test [Sickledex]) and a characteristic pattern on hemoglobin electrophoresis. If performed properly, the metabisulfite test is highly reliable, but since it requires a microscope and a skilled observer it is not suitable for large-scale screening or field studies. Several solubility tests are commercially available in kit form. They are easy to perform and quite reliable, but occasional false positives have been noted in individuals with unstable hemoglobins (Fairbanks and Pettit, 1972). Hemoglobin electrophoresis reveals about 60 per cent Hb A, 35 per cent Hb S, and normal amounts of Hb A_2. The proportion of Hb S in AS individuals may be diminished in the presence of folic acid deficiency (Heller et al., 1963b), iron deficiency (Levere et al., 1964), or α thalassemia (De Simone et al., 1974b; Steinberg et al., 1974).

Screening Programs

The advisability of screening programs has become a controversial issue. Certainly the appropriate tests should be available to all individuals who want to know if they or their children have a sickling disorder. Occasionally screening clinics detect individuals with clinically significant disorders such as SS, SC, or S/thalassemia.

---

[2]Even pressurized cabins in commercial airplanes flying at high altitudes (40,000 ft) have a relatively low atmospheric PO_2 (120 mm Hg) corresponding to an alveolar PO_2 of 66 mm Hg (normal = 107 mm Hg) (Liebman et al., 1976).

Few people derive any obvious benefit from the knowledge that they have sickle trait unless they are engaged in occupations that may confer increased risk. In addition, establishing the diagnosis of sickle trait may be useful to some individuals who are planning families. If screening programs are employed, it is very important that confidentiality be preserved and that affected individuals have the benefit of adequate education and counseling. Such services are now being provided in a number of Sickle Centers in various urban areas in the United States.

SICKLE CELL DISEASE

The term sickle cell disease generally includes the symptomatic forms of sickling: sickle cell anemia (SS disease, homozygosity for Hb S), sickle cell–hemoglobin D disease (SD disease/$\alpha_2^A\beta^S\beta^{121\ Gln}$), sickle cell–hemoglobin O disease (SO disease/$\alpha_2^A\beta^S\beta^{121\ Lys}$), sickle cell–hemoglobin C disease (SC disease), and sickle cell–β thalassemia of either the S/β^0 or S/β^+ type. Other rarer forms of sickle cell disease may also be found. The approximate order of decreasing severity is SS, SD, SO, SC; the variable severity of sickle β thalassemia probably reflects the type of thalassemia present. Since β thalassemia is itself so heterogeneous in its clinical severity, the wide spectrum of clinical expression of S/β thalassemia might be expected: the disorder may be as severe as sickle cell anemia or nearly asymptomatic, detected in the course of hospitalization for other illnesses. However, the possibility remains that other factors, e.g., altered primary structure of Hb S, or different hemoglobin-membrane interactions, might influence the manifestations of sickle β thalassemia in different individuals. The presence of α thalassemia probably ameliorates sickle cell anemia (Van Enk et al., 1972).

While some clinical features of the genetic variants of sickling may differ from those of sickle cell anemia (e.g., the frequency of severe retinal lesions of SC disease), in general the differences in symptoms between sickle cell anemia and the genetic variants of sickling are in the severity and frequency of the manifestations of sickling. Powars (1975) has emphasized the observation that the deaths in young children associated with infection are nearly confined to patients with sickle cell anemia.

The manifestations of sickle cell disease may be considered in four major groups:

(1) Chronic hemolytic anemia.

(2) Systemic manifestations, including impairment of growth and development and increased susceptibility to infections.

(3) Vaso-occlusive or painful "crises"–episodes of pain of varying severity which come on over a few minutes or hours and last for a

few hours or several days. The pain may involve one or more sites; pleural, abdominal, and bone or muscular pain are common. The pain is attributed to the occlusion of small vessels by sickled cells with release of kinins and, in many instances, microinfarctions.

(4) Organ damage which is the consequence of multiple microvaso-occlusive events and of chronic anemia. Organ damage is to some extent cumulative, and adults with severe sickle cell anemia have greater or lesser impairment of a number of different organ systems; cardiac, pulmonary, renal, skeletal, cerebral, and hepatic damage may all be evident.

Anemia of Sickle Cell Disease

The anemia of sickle cell disease is due to accelerated red cell destruction, which is independent of red cell age. The populations of red cells which have the greatest proportions of fetal hemoglobin do, however, appear to survive longer than do the red cells which contain little or no fetal hemoglobin (Bertles and Milner, 1968). Patients with sickle cell anemia are usually jaundiced, but this finding is not a constant feature of the other sickling disorders.

The marked shortening of red cell survival places a high demand on erythropoiesis. Temporary decline in erythropoiesis consequent to infection results in a more severe anemia. If the initial clinical observations on the patient are made as the infection is subsiding, a remarkable reticulocytosis (up to 50 per cent) may be observed. This recovery phase from temporary bone marrow suppression is probably more common than a true hyperhemolytic crisis, although the latter may be observed, particularly in children. Glucose-6-phosphate dehydrogenase (G-6-PD) deficiency is found in the expected frequency in patients with sickle cell anemia, and some examples of hyperhemolytic crises have been associated with this deficiency (Smits et al., 1969). In other patients an increasingly severe anemia probably represents an episode of acute splenic sequestration.

The greatly increased erythropoiesis of sickle cell anemia leads to a significant increase in requirements for folic acid, and evidence of folate deficiency is sometimes encountered. In patients who have a good dietary intake, it is doubtful whether supplemental folic acid is necessary, but in the presence of infection or when dietary intake is poor, the administration of 1 or 2 mg per day of folic acid is often recommended. The high folic acid content of milk usually prevents folic acid deficiency in children. Iron deficiency is occasionally and unexpectedly encountered in sicklers (Peterson et al., 1974a). Medicinal iron should not be given, however, unless the diagnosis of iron deficiency is firmly established, since iron overload may develop in later life.

Systemic Manifestations of Sickle Cell Disease

The two outstanding manifestations which might be classed as systemic are (a) increased susceptibility to infections, particularly bacterial infections, and (b) impaired growth and development.

Powars (1975) has recently described the clinical findings of sickle cell disease in a series of 422 patients who resided in the Los Angeles area during the preceding 20 years. The diagnosis was well established in this large group of patients. Firm distinctions between sickle cell disease and sickle β^0 thalassemia can be made with the usual laboratory tests on the blood of the affected child (excluding tests of in-vitro synthesis of β polypeptide chains) when the patient is above 6 months of age. Studies of the parents may of course permit earlier diagnosis.

Susceptibility to Infection

The clinical manifestations during the early years, particularly the first year of life, deserve particular attention. Evidence of accelerated red cell destruction is apparent by age 3 months, but growth and development are usually normal in infancy. Powars (1975) and others (Jenkins et al., 1960; Pearson, 1974) have called attention to the frequency of sudden death in infants with sickle cell anemia and the relationship of sudden deaths to infections, particularly pneumococcal sepsis (Seeler et al., 1972). Sudden death in early childhood in patients with sickle cell anemia is probably most frequently caused by bacterial infection (Seeler et al., 1972): the concomitant intravascular sickling may be less impressive on autopsy examination than is intravascular sickling in adults who have died in sickle cell crises. Nearly all the patients in whom sudden death has been related to pneumococcal sepsis have had SS disease, rather than the other sickling disorders.

The relationship of recognizable bacterial infection to mortality in sickle cell disease is also reflected in the morbidity. *Diplococcus pneumoniae* is much more frequently isolated in young children with pulmonary symptoms and fever (Barrett-Connor, 1971; Powars, 1975) than in adult SS homozygotes with the same symptoms.

Both Powars (1975) and Pearson (1974) have called attention to the frequency of pneumococcal infections, including sepsis and meningitis in American children with sickle cell disease, an association noted earlier by Janet Watson (Robinson and Watson, 1966). In her detailed survey of infections in Dade County, Florida, Barrett-Connor (1971) reported a greatly increased incidence of bacterial infections, including pneumococcal meningitis and *Haemophilus influenzae* meningitis, in children with sickle cell anemia as compared with the black population of that county; Salmonella, Shigella, and tuberculous infections were also more frequent but their incidence was less striking than that of pneumococcal infections. Ward and Smith (1976) also noted a high incidence of *H. influenzae* sepsis in children with SS disease. In another series (Robinson and Halpern, 1974; Robinson, 1974), *Escherichia coli* constituted the second most frequently encountered pathogen in children with sickle cell disease, many of whom had urinary tract infections. In Ghana, the increased susceptibility to infection is reflected in malaria and typhoid rather than pneumococcal infections (Ringelhann, 1973).

The pathophysiological basis for the increased susceptibility to infection of infants with sickle cell anemia has recently been reviewed by Johnston (1974). This phenomenon is at least partially related to altered reticuloendothelial function, particularly in the spleen. Pearson and O'Brien (1974) have shown that at age 9 to 12 months, a time when the spleen is regularly palpable in infants with sickle cell anemia, the phagocytic function of the spleen as measured by uptake of isotopes is impaired. The presence of Howell-Jolly bodies also attests to the presence of functional asplenia. As a result of successive infarctions, the spleen slowly decreases in size and is usually not palpable in children with sickle cell anemia after the age of 7. Children with sickle cell anemia are prone to the same kinds of life-threatening bacterial infections as other asplenic children. In young children the spleen appears to play a major role in host defense, a role that appears to diminish with advancing age. Alternatively, decreasing incidence of infections with age may reflect immunity induced by previous infection. While repeated infections occurred in several children in the series of Barrett-Connor (1971) and Ward and Smith (1976), recurrences were nearly absent in Powars' group (1975).

The basis of the increased susceptibility of young children with sickle cell anemia to infection is probably related in part to the reticuloendothelial blockage by sickled cells and cell fragments. The role of the spleen as a site of synthesis of proteins important in host defenses in young children has not been fully evaluated. A functioning spleen may be necessary for the formation of antibodies to particulate antigens. Schwartz and Pearson (1972) found that SS children failed to develop a normal rise in heterophil antibody titer following the intravenous injection of sheep red cells. A deficiency of pneumococcal serum opsonizing activity found in some children with sickle cell disease (Winkelstein and Drachman, 1968) appears to be related to an abnormality in the properdin pathway with impaired fixation of the third component of complement (C_3) to the pneumococci (Johnston et al., 1973).

A defect in neutrophil kinetics and delayed chemotaxis has also been demonstrated by Boggs et al. (1973).

Improved clinical care has resulted in longer survival for patients with sickle cell anemia in Africa (Konotey-Ahulu, 1973, 1974) as well as in America. The greatest risk for severe bacterial infection appears to be in children 7 years of age or younger. In Powars' study (1975) the peak morbidity occurred between the second and third year of life, and except for hospital admissions for pregnancy and complications thereof, morbidity as measured by hospital admissions was essentially the same between ages 7 and 30. Children who appear to constitute an exception are those who have had cerebrovascular accidents: many have repeated episodes and resulting neurological impairment. Powars (1975) found the death rate during the first decade of life to be 10 per cent, with a rate of 5 per cent or less during any of the subsequent decades.

Patients with SC disease do not appear to share the susceptibility to bacterial infections in childhood, but patients with either SC or S/β thalassemia have crises, particularly the chest syndrome, and bone infarcts in childhood.

Growth and Development

Impairment of growth and development correlates fairly well with the severity of the anemia and symptoms of sickle cell disease. No abnormalities in growth are encountered until late infancy. Thereafter, growth is probably slower in many patients with SS disease, but delayed puberty allows for continuing growth. Consequently, most adult patients with SS disease do not differ appreciably from their siblings in height or appearance. A few patients with severe sickle cell anemia form "a subset," with severely retarded growth and delayed puberty. The "tower skull" of chronic hemolytic anemia is occasionally seen; Konotey-Ahulu (1974) has called attention to gnathopathy, an overgrowth of the maxillary portion of the skull which occurs frequently in Ghanian patients with sickle cell anemia but is not commonly encountered in America.

Coagulation in Sickle Cell Disease

Among other "systemic" manifestations of sickle cell disease are abnormalities in coagulation. This topic has been reviewed by Rickles and O'Leary (1974). Haut et al. (1973) demonstrated a significant, although transient, shortening of platelet survival in three patients during sickle crises. A modest fall in platelet count has also been observed during painful crises (Gordon et al., 1974). Freedman and Karpatkin (1975) have reported elevated platelet counts in patients with SS disease with significant decline in numbers of circulatory platelets during vaso-occlusive crises. There are conflicting reports on platelet function during crises. Although fibrinogen levels are often elevated, particularly during crisis (Gordon et al., 1974), fibrinogen turnover is enhanced (Mattii et al., 1973). Furthermore, the presence of increased amounts of plasma high molecular weight fibrinogen complexes in SS patients may reflect enhanced rates of in vivo fibrin formation (Alkjaersig et al., 1976). The levels of these complexes decreased toward normal after patients were treated with antiplatelet drugs (aspirin and dipyridamole).

Sickle Cell Crisis

While sickle cell crisis in young children is often associated with evident bacterial or presumed viral infections, clear evidence for infection is frequently absent in older children or adults. Overall, about one-third of acute painful crises in adults are probably associated with a concurrent or preceding infection. A shortening in survival of SS red cells has been noted for a few days after the induction of pyrexia (Basu and Woodruff, 1963). An associated enhancement of sickling may be responsible for precipitating a vaso-occlusive crisis.

The frequency and severity of painful crises vary considerably among patients and even in a given patient. Crises may occur rather infrequently in some patients, while in others recurrent episodes of painful crises interfere with schooling or steady employment. Common experience is documented by Powars' (1975) observation that in any group of sicklers, a few patients account for most of the hospital admissions. While cerebral thrombosis carries grave implications for recurrence with continuing or progressive disability, particularly in children, and recurrent bone infarctions may lead to bone changes by x-ray (which are generally asymptomatic except in the hips), the organ damage of adult patients does not correlate very well with the observed frequency or severity of sickle crises in childhood.

The effects of recurrent episodes of severely painful crises on the mental state of the affected patient and on the structure of the family are variable in the extreme. Some patients with little chronic disability are psychologically incapacitated and others with similar histories of painful crises have succeeded in attending school and have had permanent employment thereafter. That such contrasts can be observed in two affected siblings reflects some unknown variation in the disease or in the reactions of affected individuals.

Chest Crises

The "chest syndrome" is one of the frequent manifestations of sickling vaso-occlusive crises. Since the pathogenesis of the symptoms is not entirely clear, we have retained the designation "chest syndrome." Affected patients have sudden onset of pleural pain with fever. X-ray findings may be absent initially or evanescent, or areas of possible infarction or infection may be demonstrated. The obvious problem is the difficulty in distinguishing pulmonary infection, infarction due to sickling in situ, or pulmonary embolism.

The susceptibility of young children with sickle cell anemia to bacterial infections, particularly to pneumococcal infections, has been referred to earlier. Barrett-Connor (1973) has called attention to the prolonged course of bacteriologically proven pneumococcal pneumonia in patients with sickle cell disease. In addition, severe bouts of Mycoplasma pneumonia are frequently encountered in these patients (Shulman et al., 1972). Etiological agents are less frequently identified in adults with pulmonary symptoms, but in all age groups the "chest syndrome" appears to be the commonest diagnosis for sicklers admitted to the hospital. Pulmonary vascular occlusion has been demonstrated in sickle cell anemia as well as in its genetic variants. While vascular occlusion may occasionally be caused by marrow or fat emboli from infarcted bone, it is generally believed to represent thrombosis of sickled cells in situ rather than embolization of blood or marrow clots (Moser and Shea, 1957; Diggs, 1969). Infection and infarction of the lung in these patients share so many clinical features (fever, leukocytosis, pleurisy with or without pleural effusion) that it may be difficult to distinguish firmly between the two pathological processes (Barrett-Connor, 1973). Since infection may be accompanied by microinfarctions, and thrombosis by superimposed infection, the distinction in clinically severe examples of the chest syndrome may be somewhat academic. The frequency of episodes of chest pain in the last trimester of pregnancy in patients with SC disease has been noted by many hematologists, and chronic pulmonary occlusion with pulmonary hypertension and cor pulmonale has been noted in SS and SC patients. It may be that the viscosity of the higher hematocrit plus sickling carries an increased risk in SC patients for pulmonary as well as for ocular (see below) disability. Anticoagulation has been of no demonstrated value in the chest syndrome.

Musculoskeletal Crises

Musculoskeletal crises occur in all age groups. An erroneous diagnosis of acute rheumatic fever is occasionally made at the time of the initial crisis. The frequency of objective findings such as swelling and tenderness appears to be higher in children. Dactylitis may be the initial symptom of SS disease in infants. It is characterized by the rather sudden onset over hours to a day or two of painful swelling of the dorsum of both hands and feet. Usually at least two

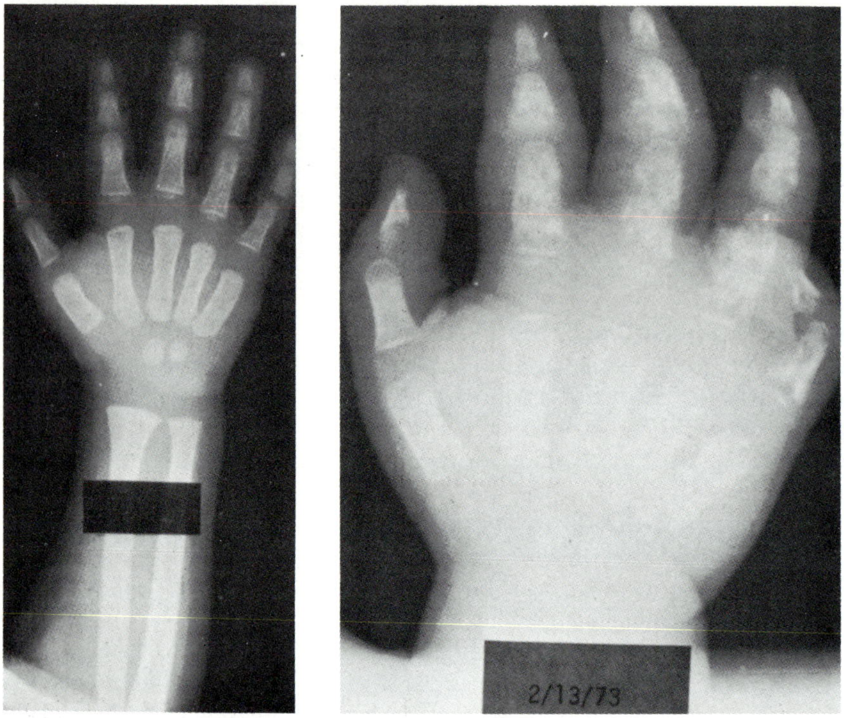

Figure 4–8. X-ray of child's hand during (left) and two weeks following (right) an attack of dactylitis. Note the development of destructive bony lesions (From Nathan, D. G., and Oski, F. A.: Hematology of Infancy and Childhood, W. B. Saunders Co., 1974.)

and frequently all four extremities are involved. Dactylitis may occur before the first year of age and generally does not occur after the age of 5. Children with dactylitis usually have fever and, as might be expected, irritability. A single episode may last for one to two weeks and may recur one or more times during the next several months or years. X-rays may show no abnormalities, but evidence of cortical thinning and marked bone destruction with healing may be seen (Fig. 4–8). Most episodes subside without sequelae, but deformity of hands due to infarction and destruction of the carpal or metacarpal bones may rarely occur. A shortened digit secondary to infarcted bone has been reported (Serjeant and Ashcroft, 1971).

The age predilection of dactylitis is thought to result from the rapid growth of bone which has a limited blood supply. The occlusion of a vessel by sickled cells may not be easily compensated for by a collateral blood supply in bone. The regular features of symmetrical local swelling and involvement of more than one extremity are admittedly not so readily explained. The growing bones appear to be a site at which sickling is particularly likely to occur once the proportion of sickle hemoglobin in the infant has greatly exceeded that of Hb F. The absence of dactylitis in older children or adults may be due either to lower growth rate of bones after the age of 5 or to greater osseous vascularity.

Powars (1975) has found that patients who have had skeletal crises as children are more likely to have bone deformities as adults. The painful crises with localization of pain to a small area of bone may be difficult to distinguish from osteomyelitis, particularly if the patient has fever and leukocytosis. Bone infarctions can sometimes be demonstrated by aspiration (Charache and Page, 1967) or by x-ray (Reynolds, 1965) but not until several days have elapsed after onset of pain. Recently, ^{99m}Tc-sulfur colloid scans have been used to localize bone infarction due to sickling (Alavi et al., 1974), but similar abnormalities are seen in osteomyelitis. In known sicklers, it is usually advisable to wait for a day or two to observe the progress of symptoms of sudden onset isolated to a single bony site rather than to undertake a long course of probably unnecessary antibiotic therapy for osteomyelitis.

Occasional musculoskeletal vaso-occlusive crises begin suddenly with back pain, which is followed by pain in other areas of the body. Such a sequence of symptoms may reflect an initial infarct in the spine, particularly in the lumbosacral spine, followed by fat embolization. Fat emboli have been described in a few patients, but it is not known how often such emboli occur in nonfatal crises.

Sometimes, a sickle crisis may present as an acute monarticular or polyarticular arthritis. The elbows and knees are most often involved. The presence of signs of inflammation and joint effusion may mimic rheumatoid arthritis, gout, or acute septic arthritis (Schumacher et al., 1973). Examination of the joint fluid is helpful in this differential diagnosis. If the effusion is due to sickling, the synovial fluid will be clear and yellow with normal viscosity. Microscopic examination reveals a low white cell count ($\sim$100 to 1000/mm^3) with a predominance of mononuclear cells and an absence of bacteria or uric acid crystals. Synovial biopsy may show sickled erythrocytes in the lumen of small vessels. SS patients have a higher incidence of gout than normal individuals (Ball and Sorenson, 1970), although this complication is less common than sickle arthropathy.

Splenic Sequestration Crises

The frequent "autosplenectomy" which results in the absence of splenic function in older children and adults with sickle cell anemia was referred to earlier. Only a few patients with sickle cell anemia retain splenomegaly. In contrast, over half the patients with SC disease and S/β thalassemia have enlarged spleens. Splenic calcifications are sometimes visualized roentgenographically in a few SS patients with splenomegaly.

Rarely, again usually in children, the presence of continuing splenomegaly seems to predispose to life-threatening episodes of so-called "sequestration crises" (Pearson, 1969; Seeler and Schwiaki, 1972). In such crises, the already enlarged spleen rapidly enlarges over several hours as the child becomes progressively more anemic. A child with splenic sequestration is usually admitted to the hospital with impending or actual shock, grossly enlarged spleen, and severe anemia. The sequence of events suggests that blood has collected in the spleen. Prompt transfusion and supportive measures are necessary. There is some uncertainty as to whether a single episode of splenic sequestration is an indication for splenectomy when the patient's condition has stabilized. A history of a single episode of sequestration implies an increased risk for a second episode.

Abdominal Crises

When the sole manifestations of sickle cell crises are abdominal symptoms and signs, the differential diagnosis may include many causes of the acute abdomen. Gallstones occur with increased frequency in sickle cell disease (Barrett-Connor, 1968) and causes of acute abdominal pain other than crises must be considered. Patients with sickle crises may have classic rebound tenderness. The presence of bowel sounds favors the diagnosis of sickle crisis rather than an acute process requiring surgical intervention. The white count and differential and the leukocyte alkaline phosphatase levels are not helpful in making this differential diagnosis. Because of these uncertainties, SS patients have often undergone unnecessary abdominal surgery. After the age of 10, many patients have similar pain patterns with recurrent crises, and the perceptive patient's assessment of his or her pain is frequently helpful. The hepatobiliary manifestations of sickle cell disease are discussed below.

Crises with Neurological Manifestations

Occlusion of vessels in the brain by sickle cells may be manifest either by seizures or by sudden onset of neurological deficits, including hemiplegia. Such occlusive events, although not common, occur in young individuals; dramatic improvement in the initial symptoms may be seen over the course of days or weeks, although Powars (1975) has pointed out that affected children may have continuing or recurring neurological deficits. Recent studies which suggest that exchange transfusion should be employed in the treatment of neurological manifestations need to be verified with larger numbers of patients in both treated and control groups (Russell et al., 1974, 1976; see pp. 168 and 169).

Sudden Death

Death of patients with sickle cell anemia is frequently sudden, occurring within minutes or hours following symptoms of crisis. The information that the patient died suddenly at home or on the way to the hospital is frequently obtained when efforts are made to secure information about patients who have failed to keep appointments with physicians. Sometimes the historical sequence of events suggests that the patient had an infection followed by occlusion of cardiac or cerebral vessels. Autopsy findings of massive occlusion of vessels by sickled cells are difficult to interpret, since post-mortem sickling will lead to similar findings. Probably in most of these patients, particularly in young children, pneumococcal sepsis or other infection is the commonest precipitating cause of the fatal outcome.

Chronic Organ Damage in Sickle Cell Disease

Manifestations of specific organ damage appear in SS patients after mid-childhood and constitute significant aspects of the illness of adult sicklers. Many different organs may be affected; the heart, lungs, kidneys, liver, skin, and skeletal, ocular, and central nervous systems all bear the scars of the disease (Diggs, 1973).

Cardiovascular Manifestations

The cardiovascular manifestations of sickle cell anemia are generally related to anemia, with a hyperdynamic state, and to the pulmonary abnormalities which follow occlusion of pulmonary vessels by sickled cells. Klinefelter (1942), in an attempt to distinguish sickle crisis with musculoskeletal symptoms from acute rheumatic fever, concluded that the auscultatory findings in sickle cell disease might indeed closely mimic those of rheumatic heart disease. The degree of anemia in children with sickle cell anemia would be expected to result in a sustained increase in cardiac output (Varat et al., 1972; Lindsay et al., 1974), which increases even further on exercise. Arterial hypoxemia, related in part to pulmonary disease, probably causes a further demand on the heart in older patients. The pulmonary disease (see below) is only slowly cumulative, but pulmonary hypertension is occasionally found. The chronicity and severity of sickle cell anemia find few counterparts in other diseases and most of the findings are probably related to the long-standing anemia. Hemosiderosis of remarkable degree is more common in thalassemia and indeed is likely to be more significant, in the authors' experience, in sickle thalassemia than in sickle cell anemia.

The symptoms of cardiac origin are those of dyspnea on exertion and, in a few patients, symptoms of overt congestive heart failure. An enlarged, hyperactive heart, with a loud systolic murmur, is commonly encountered, and in perhaps a third of the cases a diastolic murmur is heard. Structural mitral stenosis may be distinguished by echocardiography. While it was originally believed that rheumatic heart disease was very uncommon in sickle cell disease, there have been numerous examples of the coexistence of rheumatic valvular disease (as well as congenital heart disease) and sickle cell anemia. There is no evidence for the existence of a sickle cell cardiomyopathy. In view of the very low O_2 tensions in the coronary sinus, which might in theory favor sickling, clinical evidence of coronary artery insufficiency is strikingly absent.

Pulmonary Involvement

Since sickling occurs in deoxygenated red cells containing hemoglobin S, the development of impaired pulmonary function is particularly troublesome in patients with sickle cell disease. In adults with sickle cell disease, gas exchange is frequently abnormal even during the stable noncrisis state (Bromberg, 1974). Resting arterial PO_2 is usually decreased in adult patients with sickle cell anemia, S thalassemia, and SC disease, although it is seldom at dangerously low levels. Since the oxygen affinity of the blood in sickle cell anemia is shifted to the right, the reduction in arterial PO_2 usually produces lowered oxygen saturation of the arterial blood. Most patients with sickle cell disease have arterial unsaturation (Sproule et al., 1958). In compensation for the anemia, larger volumes of oxygen per red cell must be delivered to the tissues than is the case in nonanemic individuals. Curiously, the values for pulmonary arterial oxygen saturation have been found to be higher than would be expected from systemic arterial PO_2 values in SS patients, suggesting peripheral arteriovenous shunting (Sproule et al., 1958).

The calculated alveolar-arterial (A-a) PO_2 differences in these patients, which may range upward of 20 mm Hg, resemble or exceed those in patients with comparable degrees of anemia of other cause (Bromberg and Jensen, 1967a). The widened alveolar-arterial PO_2 difference apparently reflects a large contribution of intrapulmonary shunting, since such gradients were observed in patients breathing 100 per cent oxygen (Sproule et al., 1958). Inequality in ventilation and perfusion appears to play a significant role in some of the patients. Decreased oxygen diffusion does not appear to be a major factor in the etiology of the oxygen unsaturation, although some impairment in gas diffusion can usually be demonstrated. (Reduction of diffusing capacity as measured by CO methods is generally demonstrable in anemia of any cause; the observed reduction is attributed to the reduction of the numbers of red cells in capillaries.) In most patients with sickle cell disease, tissue oxygen supply on exercise is limited by cardiac output rather than by impaired pulmonary function. Cor pulmonale is distinctly unusual in sickle cell disease, and pulmonary vascular resistance is generally normal.

Despite the absence of evidence for remarkable pulmonary abnormalities in most patients with sickle cell disease, it appears logical to consider the observed arterial oxygen unsaturation a significant factor in the morbidity of sickle cell disease. Hypoxemia may well promote the formation of irreversibly sickled cells (ISC) and the sequence of microthrombi that may be initiated by the trapping of ISC's.

Hepatobiliary Involvement

The chronic jaundice of patients with sickle cell anemia reflects accelerated red cell destruction. Hepatic injury in sickle cell disease frequently occurs as a result of transfusion-induced hepatitis. In addition, these patients may develop hepatic infarcts, which occasionally become infected, resulting in hepatic abscess (Brittain et al., 1966). If a significant portion of hepatic parenchyma becomes infarcted, fibrosis and deterioration of liver function may result (Green, 1953).

Like patients with other types of congenital hemolytic anemia, patients with sickle cell disease have a high incidence of cholelithiasis (Barrett-Connor, 1968). Although about one-third of these patients have gallstones, only 10 per cent develop symptoms that can be attributed to biliary disease. On occasion, sicklers are subject to attacks of cholestatic jaundice in which very high serum bilirubin and alkaline phosphatase levels suggest choledocholithiasis (Klion et al., 1964). However, such episodes are difficult to distinguish from hepatic crises due to sickling. Both usually resolve uneventfully. The decision to recommend cholecystectomy in sickle cell disease must be individualized: the existence of asymptomatic gallstones in a severely anemic patient is probably of no great moment, while significant symptoms of gallbladder disease (e.g., recurring attacks of cholecystitis) would constitute a strong indication for surgical intervention.

Genitourinary Manifestations

The involvement of the kidney in sickle cell disease is rather constant if the loss of the ability to produce a concentrated urine is considered renal involvement. The impairment in renal concentrating capacity appears in childhood in sickle cell trait. Since the concentrating defect in children is reversed following transfusions of normal blood, the pathogenic mechanism must be secondary to the abnormal red blood cells (Keitel et al., 1958; Statius van Eps et al., 1967). In the hypertonic environment of the renal medulla, red cells sickle even with normal O_2 tensions (Perillie and Epstein, 1963). A disorder of the countercurrent distributor in the medullary circulation has been proposed as the etiological factor for the concentrating defect. However, as Buckalew and Someren (1974) have pointed out, the mechanism by which the decreased medullary blood flow would produce the isosthenuria is not clear. By injection at autopsy of kidneys of patients with sickle cell disease Statius van Eps et al. (1970) demonstrated decreased filling of medullary vasa recta, dilated capillaries, and extravasation of contrast material from ruptured capillaries. The renal concentrating defect of sicklers is unusual because tubular reabsorption of free water appears to be normal or decreased only slightly (Heinemann and Cheung, 1957). Lief et al. (1969) have shown in rats after papillectomy that tubular reabsorption of free water is normal in spite of a marked defect in maximum urine osmolality. Buckalew and Someren (1974) have suggested that the concentrating defect is due to decreased perfusion of nephrons with long loops of Henle extending into the papillae. The preservation of tubular reabsorption of free water reflects normal function of the shorter ascending loops of Henle in the outer medulla which are not affected by the damage to papillae.

HEMATURIA. Hematuria occurs in patients with sickle cell anemia and in those with the genetic variants of sickling, including some patients with sickle cell trait. Diggs (1973) indicated that the anatomical lesion is a papillary necrosis with formation of a papillary ulcer. Peritubular extravasation of blood in kidneys surgically removed for hematuria has also been observed. Again, the evidence suggests a papillary lesion secondary to impaired blood supply as in the concentrating defect. While, in the authors' experience, hematuria has been rather common in patients with sickle cell/Hb C disease, it is distinctly uncommon in sickle cell trait when one considers the number of individuals at risk in each of the two groups. The possibility of causes of painless hematuria other than sickling should be carefully evaluated in such patients. In some sicklers with hematuria, blood loss continuing over many weeks may lead to iron deficiency anemia. The therapeutic maneuver of oral iron administration should not be overlooked in the frustration of both physician and patient concerning the prolonged hematuria. The use of diuretic agents to decrease medullary hypertonicity has been recommended and should be used in the attempt to stop prolonged hematuria. Occasionally renal bleeding has been so extensive and prolonged that nephrectomy was performed (Mostofi et al., 1957; Lucas and Bullock, 1960). However, nephrectomy has largely been abandoned because, in many patients, bleeding has occurred on separate occasions from each kidney. Epsilon-aminocaproic acid (EACA) may be useful (Bilinski et al., 1969); however, it should be used with caution, since it may prevent the dissolution of clots in the renal pelvis.

RENAL FAILURE AND THE NEPHROTIC SYNDROME. Morphological renal changes are found in patients with sickle cell anemia in the absence of clinical signs of renal disease. The glomerular capillaries, afferent arterioles, interlobular arteries, and small medullary vessels are distended with erythrocytes, some of which appear sickled (Buckalew and Someren, 1974). Enlarged glomeruli (Bernstein and Whitten, 1960) may have electron-dense material in the mesangial cytoplasm (Pitcock et al., 1970). Similar changes were found on electron microscopy by McCoy (1969) and Antonovych (1971) in renal sections of patients with sickle cell anemia and the nephrotic syndrome. It was suggested by McCoy (1969) that the electron-dense deposits represent some form of iron which remains from phagocytosis of red cells or hemoglobin by mesangial cells. Since iron is frequently found in renal tissues in patients with hemolytic anemia (primarily in proximal tubular cells), it is difficult to attribute renal insufficiency to the presence of the metal. Pardo et al. (1975) have proposed that the glomerular lesion in SS disease is due to an immune complex composed of renal tubular epithelial antigen and antibody directed toward that antigen.

Frank renal failure, sometimes following the nephrotic syndrome, occurs in a relatively small number of patients with sickle cell anemia. Patients who become uremic develop an increased transfusion requirement which can be reduced by hemodialysis (Friedman et al., 1974). In patients with sickle cell anemia who have survived to the fourth and fifth decades, mild nitrogen retention is common. Some of the patients have elevated levels of uric acid due to increased purine turnover (Walker and Alexander, 1971; Diamond et al., 1976); but uric acid stones are rare. It is likely that renal insufficiency of variable degree will be encountered more frequently as longer average life span leads to an older population with sickle cell anemia.

PRIAPISM. Male patients with sickle cell disease occasionally develop spontaneous and painful engorgement of the penis. This distressing symptom accounted for 3 to 5 per cent of admissions of male SS patients in two series from the southern United States (Campbell and Cummins, 1951; Hasen and Raines, 1962). Priapism occurs with about equal frequency in prepubertal and postpubertal patients, although the latter are more difficult to treat and may develop impotence following the acute episode. While a number of approaches to therapy have been employed, conservative management is recommended (Karayalcin et al., 1972). As with other types of sickle crises, the patient should be given sedation, analgesia, and adequate intravenous fluids. Seeler (1973) has treated 6 boys with packed red cell transfusion. Twenty-four hours after doubling the hematocrit, a marked decrease in pain was noted, followed by a resolution of priapism over the next several days. Surgical intervention such as incision and drainage or irrigation is only indicated when conservative measures fail. It is uncertain whether surgery decreases (Grace and Winter, 1968) or increases (Karayalcin et al., 1972) the likelihood of impotence.

Ocular Abnormalities

Impressive changes in the eyes may accompany sickle cell anemia and its genetic variants. These changes were reviewed recently by Armaly (1974). Condon and Serjeant (1972a and 1972b) compared the incidence of a variety of ocular manifestations in 70 patients with SC disease and 76 patients with SS disease. Whitened peripheral retina (88 per cent), peripheral vessel disease (96 per cent), tortuosity of vessels (11 per cent), and peripheral arteriovenous anomalies (28 per cent) were found in about equal frequency in SS and SC disease, but the ocular lesions leading to the greatest disability are found primarily in SC disease. In SC disease the following lesions were found: vitreous hemorrhages (16 per cent) and retinitis proliferans (33 per cent). Retinal detachment occurs more frequently in patients with SC disease. The reason for the higher incidence of major ocular disability in SC disease than in SS disease is not understood; since lesions follow vessel occlusion by sickled cells, it may be that the higher packed cell volume in SC disease plus sickling leads to large changes in viscosity, with capillary plugging in the microvasculature of the eye. The early diagnosis of retinal lesions in SS and SC disease is important, since retinal detachment may be prevented by laser beam therapy (Ryan and Goldberg, 1971).

Musculoskeletal Manifestations

The great variety of bony changes that result from infarctions of bone and from the marrow hyperplasia consequent to accelerated red cell destruction have been described in the monograph by Reynolds (1965). Calvarial thickening is frequent, but the “hair-on-end” appearance so often encountered in thalassemia is uncommon in sickle cell disease. X-rays of the spine may reveal sclerosis consequent to old infarcts as well as the nearly pathognomonic biconcave deformity of the vertebrae, called “fishmouth vertebrae” (Fig. 4–9). This abnormality is generally encountered in older patients with sickle cell disease and is distinguished from a similar nonspecific deformity of a number of skeletal disorders by the flat “floor” or “roof” on the depressed area, sparing the peripheral bone, and by the coarse bony trabeculae of sickle cell disease. Bony changes may be seen in any of the long bones but the most symptomatic changes occur in the hip,

Figure 4–9. *A*, X-ray of lumbosacral spine of patient with SS anemia. Note classic fishmouth deformity. (Courtesy of Dr. Charles Peterson.) *B*, Pathogenesis of fishmouth deformity. The central depression of the vertebral end plates is caused by local inhibition of bone growth from ischemia. The central portion of the growth plate suffers ischemic damage owing to impaired circulation through the main vertebral artery. In contrast, the ring epiphyses and outer portion of the vertebral plates are spared because of numerous perforating apophyseal arteries.

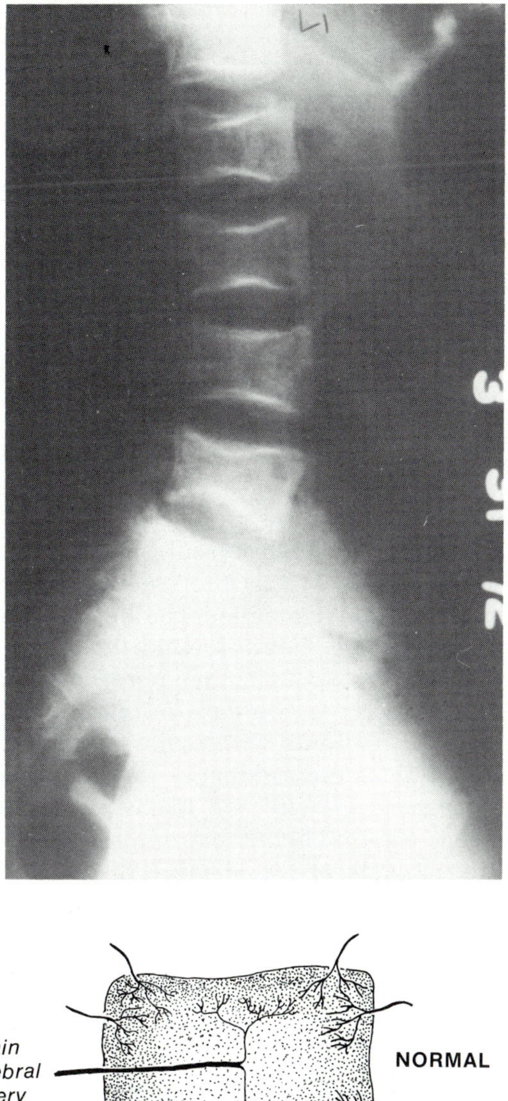

A

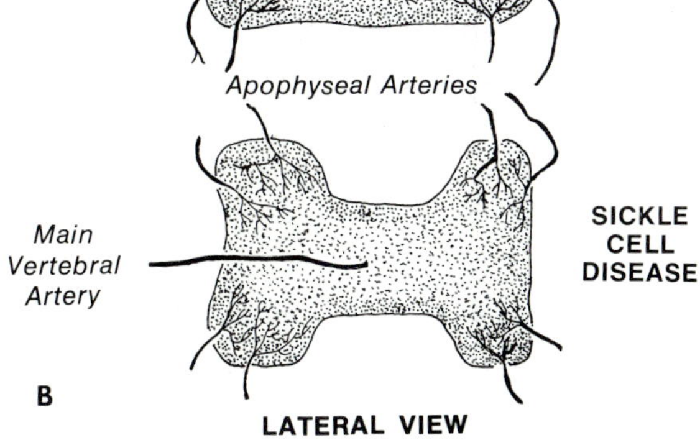

B

where avascular necrosis of the femoral head may lead to disability, requiring surgical correction. Some patients may require a total hip prosthesis. Aseptic necrosis of the femoral head occurs both in SS disease and in the genetic variants. The suggested higher incidence in patients with the genetic variants is not convincing when patients of similar age are compared.

Osteomyelitis has been found in sickle cell disease of all types. Staphylococcus is the commonest etiological agent. In addition, SS and S/β thalassemia patients have a peculiar susceptibility to develop Salmonella osteomyelitis. Chronic osteomyelitis in sickle cell disease appears to be less common than formerly, probably because of the administration of effective antibiotics earlier in the course of the disease. The infection probably begins in a nidus of infarcted bone.

Skin Ulcers

One of the most troublesome problems of many patients with sickle cell disease is the recurrent chronic skin ulcers of the lower extremities. This subject has been reviewed by Serjeant (1974). The lesions usually begin around the ankle and may become very large. The ulcers appear to be more common in the patients with more severe anemia. Similar lesions have been described, admittedly rarely, in patients with thalassemia and in other types of congenital hemolytic anemia. Most of the leg ulcers are found in patients with SS disease or with S/β thalassemia. The finding of scars of healed ulcers on the lower extremities of young black patients strongly suggests one of the sickling diseases. Unfortunately, the ulcers are very slow to heal, and healing is not infrequently followed by the appearance of another ulcer months or years thereafter. Leg ulcers may be more frequent in tropical areas, but both the frequency and the chronicity may reflect difficulty in keeping the ulcer clean.

Some ulcers heal fairly well with frequent simple clean dressing changes or with weekly application of supportive paste (Unna) boots. If these measures are ineffective, transfusions may be added to the regimen to reduce the circulating Hb S to less than 50 per cent. Rarely, skin grafting is necessary. Skin grafting should be undertaken only after conservative measures (including transfusion) have failed, since both prolonged elevation and transfusions are usually used as adjuncts to grafting, and the simpler measures make the graft unnecessary. The oral administration of zinc sulfate may hasten the healing of leg ulcers (Serjeant et al., 1970).

Neurological Complications of Sickle Cell Disease

There is a significant incidence of neurological complications in sickle cell disease, but the actual incidence is not known because of the paucity of prospective studies. Portnoy and Herion (1972) found that 26 per cent of 89 patients with sickle cell disease had neurological complications; the commonest manifestation, hemiplegia, occurred in 17 per cent of patients with sickle cell anemia. Coma, convulsions, and visual disturbances were the next most common symptoms. A few of these patients (3 of the 23 in the series of Portnoy and Herion) had recurrent cerebrovascular incidents with spastic quadriplegia and disability. Two additional patients died promptly after the onset of hemiplegia. The potentially ominous significance of neurological manifestations is also noted by Powars (1975). However, in 15 of the episodes of hemiplegia, improvement occurred, while 6 showed little neurological improvement.

In the series of Portnoy and Herion, convulsions occurred in 11 of the patients (12 per cent) and constituted an isolated manifestation in 7 patients. Coma occurred as an isolated finding or associated with other non-neurological findings, e.g., sepsis.

Thrombosis, hemorrhage, and berry aneurysms have been described in sickle cell disease. Thrombosis appears to be the more common lesion. In 6 of 7 patients with neurological manifestations on whom angiograms were done (Russell et al., 1974), 3 had complete occlusion of vessels, and 2 had small aneurysms. Three of the patients who were transfused for one year had improved or stable angiograms, while in two who were not transfused the vascular lesions appeared to progress over the same period. This study suggests the need for further data on the potential benefit of transfusions in children with neurological manifestations.

Differential Diagnosis

The diagnosis of moderate or severe forms of sickle cell anemia is usually quite straightforward. Such patients will have recurrent painful crises, marked anemia, fixed sickle forms on peripheral smear, and >80 per cent Hb S on routine hemoglobin electrophoresis. However, as Table 4–2 shows, these findings may also be present in patients with S/D-Punjab. Agar-gel electrophoresis at low pH is required to separate these two variants. Severe cases of S/β thalassemia may present the same clinical findings, but microcytosis is evident on blood smears in this genetic variant.

In patients who have milder clinical manifestations, other forms of the "sickle syndrome" must be considered. Some of these entities are listed in Table 4–2 and are discussed at the end of the chapter. If the diagnosis remains in doubt after the routine hematological evaluation is completed, it may be necessary to perform structural analysis of the patient's hemoglobin. In addition, studies of family members can provide important additional information which may prove vital in establishing the diagnosis.

TABLE 4–2. *Differential Diagnosis of SS Disease*

Diagnosis	Clinical Severity	Hematocrit	RBC Morphology	Electrophoresis	Distribution of Hb F
SS	Marked	18 to 30	Targets; 2 to 30% ISC's	80 to 95% S 2 to 20% F 2 to 4% A_2	Uneven
S/D-Punjab	Moderate to Marked	20 to 30	Targets; frequent ISC's	~50% S ~50% D*	
S/β^0 Thal	Moderate to Marked	20 to 35	Hypochronic; microcytic; targets; rare ISC's	50 to 85% S 10 to 30% F 3 to 6% A_2	Uneven
S/β^+ Thal	Mild to Moderate	25 to 40	Slightly microcytic; targets; rare ISC's	55 to 75% S 15 to 30% A 5 to 20% F 3 to 6% A_2	Uneven
S/HPFH	Mild	38 to 48	Targets	70 to 80% S 20 to 30% F 1 to 3% A_2	Even

*Agar-gel electrophoresis.

TREATMENT OF SICKLE CELL DISEASE

The improved prognosis in sickle cell disease which has attended better living conditions, nutrition, and medical care (including antibiotics) has been observed not only in the United States (Powars, 1975) but also in some parts of Africa (Konotey-Ahulu, 1973). The serious acute complications mostly occur in the youngest age group: the life-threatening infections, sepsis and meningitis, the sequestration crises, and the sudden collapse and death which may also be related to infection occur with diminishing frequency in older patients.

Supportive Therapy

Infections

Since patients with sickle cell disease have increased susceptibility, antibiotics should be administered at the earliest sign of infection, particularly to children, in whom bacterial infections constitute a major hazard. In some centers, children are given prophylactic penicillin. Antimalarial prophylaxis is indicated in endemic areas.

In the vaso-occlusive crisis—the most common reason for hospital admission of adults—evidence of bacterial infection is frequently absent. However, the slow resolution of the chest syndrome following the administration of antibiotics cannot constitute evidence against bacterial infection.

Anemia

Patients with sickle cell anemia usually tolerate anemia quite well. Worsening of anemia because of folic acid deficiency is readily prevented by administering a daily supplement of this vitamin. Androgen treatment results in a significant increase in red cell mass (Lundh and Gardner, 1970; Alexanian and Nadell, 1975) and may be indicated in selected patients who appear to be symptomatic because of severe anemia. The rise in red cell 2,3-DPG and decrease in oxygen affinity during androgen therapy (Chapter 1) would theoretically enhance sickling. However, treatment had no significant effect on red cell survival (Lundh and Gardner, 1970; Alexanian and Nadell, 1975). The possible benefits from long-term oral androgen therapy must be weighed against adverse effects, chief among which is hepatotoxicity. Furthermore, male sicklers have a tendency to develop priapism during treatment (Lundh and Gardner, 1970).

Blood transfusions are seldom indicated in the treatment of the anemia of sickle cell disease. However, vaso-occlusive complications can be prevented by exchange transfusions. Charache (1974c) has described this procedure in detail. In order to be effective, at least 50 per cent of the patient's red cells should be of donor origin. This clinical impression is supported by whole blood viscosity measurements by Charache and Conley (1975). Exchange transfusion should not be undertaken lightly, since it entails a considerable commitment of time and resources as well as the familiar risks of hepatitis, red cell sensitization, and iron overload. Nevertheless, such a program may be indicated in selected patients, particularly if they are going through a period of increased risk such as major surgery or pregnancy. It is important to match the patient's blood carefully, particularly for red cell antigens which have a relatively low frequency in blacks.

Painful Crises

The management of the painful vaso-occlusive crisis is best achieved by vigorous hydration, analgesics, and appropriate antibiotics if there is any evidence of infection. Because of their inability to produce concentrated urine, SS patients have an increased fluid requirement and are prone to dehydration. Careful attention should also be paid to the patient's acid-base status. Acidosis should be promptly corrected, since it can trigger a painful crisis (Greenberg and Kass, 1958). However, alkali therapy does not appear to be effective either in the treatment of acute painful crises (Cooperative Urea Trials Group, 1974) or in their prevention (Mann and Stuart, 1974). Oxygen is usually administered during acute painful crises but its efficacy is doubtful unless the patient has a significant ventilatory hypoxia. In contrast, hyperbaric oxygen may be an effective albeit cumbersome form of treatment (Reynolds, 1971). Prompt and adequate relief of pain is of prime importance. Unfortunately, many patients who have frequent painful crises become dependent upon, if not addicted to, a variety of narcotics and analgesics. Nevertheless, such an individual deserves the benefit of the doubt. Blood transfusion has been recommended in the management of acute painful crises (Brody, 1970) but the efficacy of this treatment is doubtful. In contrast, exchange transfusion is effective in the prevention of painful crises.

Surgery

Since patients with sickle cell disease may not tolerate major surgery very well, hematologists are conservative in recommending surgical procedures. Close attention should be paid to maintenance of adequate hydration and acid-base balance as well as to optimal oxygenation before, during, and after surgery (Flye and Silver, 1973;

Searle, 1972). If extensive surgery is planned on an elective basis, such as a total hip replacement, it is reasonable to prepare the patient with exchange transfusion.

Pregnancy

The management of sickle cell disease in pregnancy has been the subject of considerable discussion. There is an increased risk of fetal wastage, but with appropriate management the maternal risk is probably not greatly increased. This statement does not apply in patients who do not receive antenatal care; such patients have a much higher risk of serious complications. (Diggs [1973] cites a maternal mortality of 6 per cent and fetal mortality of 50 per cent for these patients.) In the antenatal period, folic acid should be administered daily. A superimposed physiologic anemia of pregnancy may appear to increase the anemia. Most of the serious complications occur in the last trimester, and in some clinics regular transfusions of normal red cells are given during the last three months. Regular prophylactic exchange transfusion is not usually necessary, but the occurrence of serious complications just before or after delivery is not predictable. Pritchard et al. (1971) has found that this treatment resulted in a lower incidence of fetal wastage. Transfusions should be given in any pregnant patient with sickle cell disease in whom markedly increased anemia or crises have occurred in the final trimester. Whether to interrupt an early pregnancy is ultimately dependent on the patient's informed decision. The risks should be defined as clearly as our limited knowledge makes possible.

Anti-Sickling Agents

During the past 20 years, a variety of agents have been proposed for the treatment of sickle cell anemia. Many of these are listed in Table 4–3. Usually, an initial wave of enthusiasm has been followed by the sober realization that the drug was either ineffective or in some cases unsafe. Currently, none of the anti-sickling agents appear to be of clinical value.

Present-day knowledge of the molecular bases of sickling should enable the design of specific anti-sickling agents. The ligand-dependent polymerization of molecules of sickle hemoglobin suggests that agents which would (1) shift the oxygen dissociation curve to the left (i.e., increase the oxygen affinity), thereby favoring the oxy conformation of the tetramer, or (2) interfere with the intermolecular contacts involved in polymerization of deoxyhemoglobin S would be beneficial in sickle cell disease. Cyanate, which carbamylates the N-terminal residues of proteins, was extensively investigated by Cerami

TABLE 4–3. *Agents Which Have Been Proposed for the Treatment of Sickle Cell Anemia*

Agents	Proposed	Efficacy Contested
Priscoline	Smith (1953)	
Cobalt	Gross et al. (1955)	
Met Hb	Beutler (1961)	
Anticoagulants		Salvaggio et al. (1963)
CO	Sirs (1963) Beutler (1975)	Perruganan and McElfresh (1964)
Alkali		Schwartz and McElfresh (1964)
Dextran	Watson and Williams (1963) Barnes et al. (1965)	Oski et al. (1965)
Carbonic Anhydrase Inhibitors	Hilkowitz (1957)	dosSantos and Lehmann (1959) Finney and Hatch (1965)
Phenothiazines	Hatborn and Lewis (1966)	Pearson and Noyes (1967) Oski et al. (1968)
Androgens	Isaacs, Hayhoe (1967)	Raper et al. (1970)
Urea	Nalbandian (1970)	Cooperative Urea Trials Group (1974)
Cyanate	Gilette et al. (1974)	Harkness and Roth (1975)

and his associates (Gillette et al., 1973; Peterson et al., 1974b). Patients treated with cyanate in low doses generally exhibited prolongation of the red cell life span and a higher circulating hemoglobin with increased oxygen affinity. Unfortunately, the appearance of reversible peripheral neuropathy in patients treated with cyanate made it impossible to evaluate the effects of higher doses of this carbamylating agent on incidence of crises or on the long-term course of sickle cell disease in a large number of patients (Peterson et al., 1974c; Charache et al., 1975c). It is likely that orally administered sodium cyanate has a low therapeutic index. In a double-blind crossover study, Harkness and Roth (1975) found that patients on oral cyanate for six months had the same incidence of painful crises as when they received a placebo. Extracorporeal carbamylation of the patient's blood may be a reasonable alternative. This approach permits more extensive chemical modification of the hemoglobin without risk of toxic side effects. Diederich et al. (1976) found that a small number of patients derived considerable clinical benefit from extracorporeal carbamylation. Such an approach may be potentially useful for the administration of other anti-sickling agents, such as nitrogen mustard (Roth et al., 1972), that cannot be administered systemically.

A number of other anti-sickling drugs are now being investigated, and a safe pharmacological approach to sickle cell disease may emerge in the next decade. Some agents, such as zinc (Brewer and Oelschlegel, 1974) and procaine (Baker et al., 1974), appear to prevent sickling by interacting with the red cell membrane. Other agents, such as alkyl ureas (Roth et al., 1974), dimethyladipimidate (Lubin et al., 1975), and dichloromethane (Milosz and Settle, 1975), penetrate through the membrane and interfere with the polymerization of sickle hemoglobin.

PROGNOSIS

In many of the early reviews on sickle cell anemia the assessment of prognosis has been unduly pessimistic. This has been due in part to case selection. Only patients with relatively severe disease tend to require frequent emergency room visits and hospital admissions. There is a surprisingly large group of SS homozygotes who remain relatively symptom-free and who do not solicit medical attention. Furthermore, during the past 30 years there has been a marked improvement in the care of patients with sickle cell anemia. Infections are treated more promptly with increasingly effective antibiotics. More careful attention is devoted to the maintenance of fluid balance and the prevention of dehydration, and blood transfusions are used for more severe anemia secondary to complications of sickling. It also appears that maternal mortality of SS patients has decreased in recent years. In underdeveloped nations, the mortality in sickle cell anemia remains high. A recent survey from Nigeria reports an alarmingly high death rate, particularly in children from rural areas (Attah and Ekere, 1975).

No single factor is a consistent predictor of prognosis in SS disease. The section on molecular pathogenesis of sickling discusses the impairment of the polymerization of deoxyhemoglobin S by hemoglobin F. One might expect that those SS homozygotes who have relatively high levels of hemoglobin F should have a decreased tendency to sickle and milder clinical manifestations. Although this relationship appears to be true when a large group of patients are analyzed statistically (Jackson et al., 1961), the level of hemoglobin F is not of prognostic value in any given patient. Steinberg et al. (1973) have reported a mean Hb F of 5.4 per cent in a group of 21 patients with relatively mild disease (compared to a mean value of 3.2 per cent in 12 patients with severe sickle cell disease). The group with mild disease did have significantly higher hematocrits. The percentage of irreversibly sickled cells in blood smears is also not useful as an indicator of prognosis.

Considerable variation in the severity of sickle cell disease has been reported among different ethnic and geographical groups. Patients from Jamaica were initially considered to have relatively mild disease (Serjeant et al., 1968). However, it is now conceded that the spectrum of clinical severity in Jamaica does not differ significantly from that in the United States. In contrast to the United States, virtually every SS homozygote in Jamaica is registered and followed by physicians who have an interest and expertise in sickle cell disease. In the United States, mild cases would often escape attention.

There are small ethnic groups of SS homozygotes who appear to have a genuinely milder form of the disease. A group of Shi Arabs from Saudi Arabia have been found to have a very benign form of

TABLE 4–4. *Sickling Disorders**

	Genotype Adult Hb	Hemoglobins Present	Clinical Expression
Group I. Homozygous for Hb S			
A. Without other Hb abnormality (sickle cell anemia)	$\alpha\alpha\beta^S\beta^S$	S, F(1-20%), A_2	Severe anemia, vaso-occlusive crises and complications
B. With α thalassemia	$\alpha^{Thal^1}, \alpha^{Thal^2}\beta^S\beta^S$	S, F(43%), Bart's, A_2	Mild anemia in childhood
	$\alpha^{Thal}\alpha\beta^S\beta^S$	S, F(27%), A_2	Doubtful
C. With α-chain structural varient			
1. With Hb Memphis	$\alpha\alpha^{23\ Gln}\beta^S\beta^S$	S, F, A_2, Memphis/S	Mild course, with hemolytic anemia and few crises
2. With Hb G-Philadelphia	$\alpha\alpha^{68\ Lys}\beta^S\beta^S$	S, G/S, F, A_2, G_2	Like severe sickle cell anemia
3. With Hb Stanleyville-II	$\alpha\alpha^{76\ Lys}\beta^S\beta^S$	S, Stanleyville/S F, A_2, $Stanleyville_2$	Like severe sickle cell anemia
Group II. Heterozygous for Hb S			
A. Without other Hb abnormality	$\alpha\alpha\beta^A\beta^S$	A, S, A_2	Asymptomatic; rare complications
B. With α thalassemia	$\alpha\alpha^{Thal}\beta^A\beta^S$	A, S(<30%), A_2	Asymptomatic; RBC microcytic, hypochromic
C. With β thalassemia (1)	$\alpha\alpha\beta^S\beta^{Thal^0}$	S, F, A_2(increased)	Moderate to severe anemia and crises; RBC microcytic; may be mistaken for SS
(2)	$\alpha\alpha\beta^S\beta^{Thal+}$	A(6-25%), S, F, A_2 (increased)	Ranges from mild to severe
(3)	$\alpha\alpha\beta^s(\delta\beta)^{Thal}$	S, F (10-25%) A_2(decreased)	Mild anemia without crises

D. With hereditary persistence of Hb F	$\alpha\alpha\beta^S$ –	S, F(18–25%), A_2 (decreased)	Hb F homogeneously distributed in RBC
E. With β-chain structural variants			
1. Hb C**	$\alpha\alpha\beta^S\beta^{6\ Lys}$	C, S, A_2**	Moderate anemia, occasional crises
2. Hb G-San Jose†	$\alpha\alpha\beta^S\beta^{7\ Gly}$	G†, S, A_2	Asymptomatic
3. Hb J-Baltimore	$\alpha\alpha\beta^S\beta^{16\ Asp}$	J, S, A_2	Asymptomatic
4. Hb E**	$\alpha\alpha\beta^S\beta^{26\ Lys}$	S, E, A_2**	Moderate to severe anemia
5. Hb K-Ibadan	$\alpha\alpha\beta^S\beta^{46\ Glu}$	K, S, A_2	Asymptomatic
6. Hb Osu-Christianborg†	$\alpha\alpha\beta^S\beta^{52\ Asn}$	Osu-Christianborg†, S, A_2	Asymptomatic
7. Hb Ocho-Rios†	$\alpha\alpha\beta^S\beta^{52\ Ala}$	Ocho-Rios†, S, A_2	Asymptomatic
8. Hb Korle-Bu†	$\alpha\alpha\beta^S\beta^{73\ Asn}$	Korle-Bu†, S, A_2	Asymptomatic
9. Hb D-Ibadan†	$\alpha\alpha\beta^S\beta^{87\ Lys}$	D†, S, A_2	Asymptomatic
10. Hb Richmond	$\alpha\alpha\beta^S\beta^{102\ Lys}$	Richmond, S, A_2	Asymptomatic
11. Hb D-Punjab†	$\alpha\alpha\beta^S\beta^{121\ Gln}$	D†, S, A_2	Moderate anemia, crises
12. Hb O-Arab**	$\alpha\alpha\beta^S\beta^{121\ Lys}$	O, S, A_2**	Moderate to severe anemia, crises
13. Hb K-Woolwich	$\alpha\alpha\beta^S\beta^{132\ Gln}$	K, S, A_2	Asymptomatic
14. Hb Lepore†	$\alpha\alpha\beta^S\beta^{\delta\times\beta}$	S, F, Lepore†, A_2	Mild to severe anemia
15. Hb C-Harlem	$\alpha\alpha\beta^S\beta^{6\ Val,\ 73\ Asn}$	S, C-Harlem	Moderate to severe anemia crises

*Modified from Milner, 1974.
**Hb C, Hb O Arab, and Hb E are not separated from Hb A_2 on routine alkaline electrophoresis.
†Not separated from Hb S on routine alkaline electrophoresis.

sickle cell disease (Brown et al., 1972). Appropriate genetic and laboratory studies have documented that these individuals are SS homozygotes. This group has very high levels of hemoglobin F (15 to 30 per cent). It is not surprising that these patients have a much lower incidence of cholelithiasis than those with more severe sickle cell disease (Perrine, 1973). A similar form of SS disease with elevated hemoglobin F encountered among the Veddoids of India has recently been studied by Brittenham and his associates (1974).

Associated genetic factors may be important determinants of the overall clinical severity of sickle cell anemia. The coexistence of α thalassemia may result in a significantly lower mean corpuscular hemoglobin concentration and, consequently, a decreased tendency to sickle (Van Enk et al., 1972). Piomelli and his colleagues (1972) reported that glucose-6-phosphate dehydrogenase deficiency was more common in SS homozygotes than in the general Afro-American population. Such an association could be interpreted to mean that this enzyme deficiency might improve the fitness and survival rate of patients with SS disease. However, two subsequent studies have failed to confirm this finding (Beutler et al., 1974a; Steinberg and Dreiling, 1974).

Prevention

Genetic counseling can play an important role in the prevention of sickle cell anemia. If both marital partners are known to be AS heterozygotes, they may elect not to have children, knowing that there is a 25 per cent chance that their offspring will be homozygous.

The antenatal diagnosis of sickle cell anemia can now be made early in the second trimester of pregnancy by the testing of a very small sample of fetal blood obtained from the placenta (Kan et al., 1976b; Alter et al., 1976a). If it is established that the fetus is an SS homozygote, the parents may decide to interrupt the pregnancy. Antenatal diagnosis is discussed in detail on page 85.

SICKLING DISORDERS OTHER THAN SICKLE CELL ANEMIA

As might be expected of a gene with the high frequency of Hb S, sickle cell hemoglobin is frequently encountered in association with other genetically determined abnormalities of the α or β polypeptide chains (Table 4–4).

Hemoglobin SC Disease

Hemoglobin C trait is found in about 3 per cent of Afro-Americans (Motulsky, 1973), and hemoglobin SC disease is the commonest of the genetic variants of sickling in populations of African ancestry. Indeed, in older adults, patients with Hb SC disease probably outnumber SS homozygotes since SC disease is milder and leads to fewer lethal complications in the younger age groups. Typically, patients with Hb SC disease have infrequent crises and a hemolytic anemia of a milder degree than that usually found in sickle cell anemia (McCurdy et al., 1975). Examination of the peripheral blood reveals numerous target cells and occasional plump sickled cells (see Figure 3–5). Sometimes intracellular crystals can be seen (Diggs and Bell, 1965). Most of the complications described under sickle cell anemia may be seen in Hb SC disease, and a few manifestations seem to be at least as common in SC as in SS disease: (1) serious eye lesions (Condon and Serjeant, 1972a and b; see above); (2) hematuria, presumably from renal papillary lesions; (3) avascular necrosis of the heads of the femora; and (4) acute "chest syndromes," particularly in the last trimester of pregnancy. The increased viscosity of the venous blood in Hb SC disease (as compared to SS blood) results from the presence not only of deoxygenated sickle cells but also of a higher packed red cell volume than in sickle cell anemia. Sickle cell hemoglobin C disease is quite variable in its clinical manifestations, and many patients are first detected in adult life. The most common complaint in childhood is generally musculoskeletal or growing pains. Splenomegaly is present in about 60 per cent of patients (Milner, 1974).

Sickle Cell Thalassemia

Sickle cell thalassemia is next in frequency to Hb SC disease among the genetic variants of sickling. Since β thalassemia is common in Greece and in Italy, and sickle cell trait is found generally in lower incidence in some of these populations, the genetic variant, sickle cell–β thalassemia, is the most common form of the sickle syndrome in individuals of Mediterranean ancestry. Beta thalassemia is also found in Africans, and the expression of S/β thalassemia in Africans is generally milder than in the Mediterranean populations. (This difference probably reflects the observed clinical differences in thalassemia in the two groups: thalassemia major generally is an incapacitating disease in Greeks and Italians, and while severe thalassemia has been described in Africans, the usual manifestations of homozygosity for thalassemia in the latter group are considerably milder—sometimes designated thalassemia intermedia [see Chapter 2].)

It is sometimes difficult to distinguish between sickle cell anemia and S/β thalassemia (Table 4–2). The finding of an enlarged spleen in an older patient may be useful in the differential diagnosis. Splenomegaly is much more likely to be encountered in patients (>6

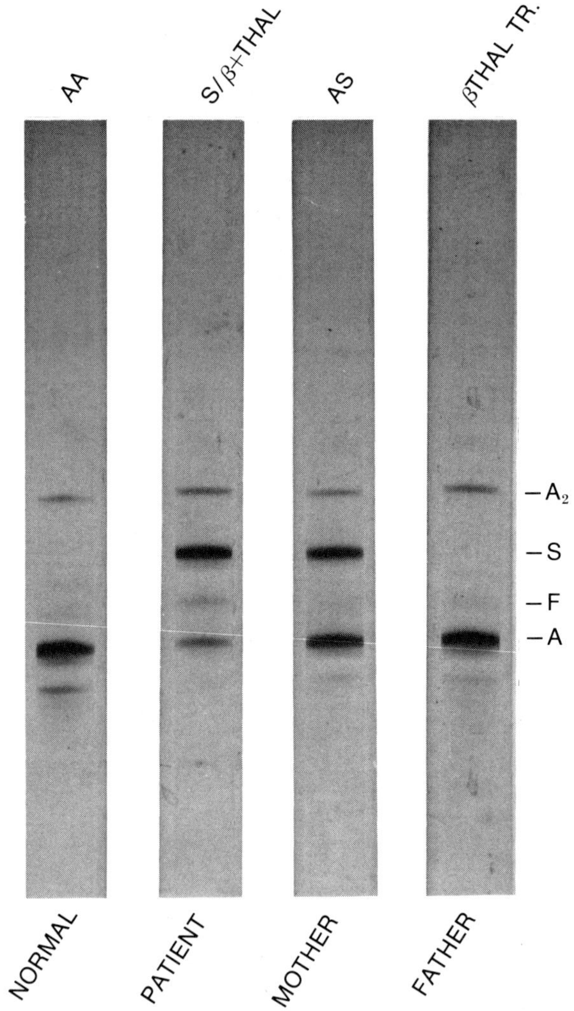

Figure 4–10. Hemoglobin electrophoresis of patient with sickle/β^+ thalassemia and his parents. The mother has sickle trait (AS) and the father has β-thalassemia trait. Note that both the patient and his father have elevated Hb A_2. In addition, the patient has elevated Hb F. The presence of Hb A in the patient's hemolysate indicates that he has S/β^+ thal rather than S/β^0 thal. Hemolysates were analyzed by electrofocusing on polyacrylamide gels.

years) with sickle/β thalassemia than in homozygous sicklers. The hypochromia and microcytosis of the erythrocytes of patients with sickle/β thalassemia is usually established by the age of one year. Hemoglobin electrophoresis provides important independent evidence. If the proportion of Hb A_2 is remarkably increased, e.g., 6 per cent, the diagnosis of sickle/β thalassemia is suggested. Of course, the presence of 10 to 20 per cent hemoglobin A in a patient who has not been transfused, together with Hb S, strongly suggests the presence of S/β^+ thalassemia (Fig. 4–10). The differential between SS and S/β^0 thalassemia is more difficult, since the elevation in hemoglobin A_2 may not be accurately measured, and in either disorder, the sum of Hb S and Hb F accounts for nearly all the hemoglobin. Sometimes family studies are used to establish the diagnosis (Fig. 4–10). The diagnosis of S/β thalassemia can also be made by measuring the biosynthesis of α and β subunits in blood reticulocytes. In S/β thalassemia the β^S/α ratio is 0.5, while it is 1.0 in SS disease. Alpha thalassemia in association with sickle cell anemia is uncommon; the abnormal red cell indices suggest the diagnosis.

Sickle cell thalassemia varies in its severity and outlook; the degree of anemia may be as marked as in sickle cell anemia, or the hemoglobin concentration may be nearly normal. As shown in Table 4–2, S/β^0 thalassemia tends to be more severe than S/β^+ thalassemia. Ocular and bony manifestations may be present, and splenic sequestration crises have been described.

Sickle Cell/Hb D Disease

Sickle cell/Hb D disease is usually due to the presence of Hb S and Hb D-Punjab (in which the glutamic acid residue at β^{121} is replaced by glutamine). The combination of sickle and D-Punjab hemoglobins has been encountered in a number of patients of African origin who have had occasional crises and moderate hemolytic anemia. The electrophoretic pattern of SD disease at alkaline pH is identical with that of SS disease. Hemoglobins S and D-Punjab can be separated by electrophoresis at pH 6.2 in citrate agar. In this acid medium, Hb D migrates like hemoglobin A and is distinct from Hb S.

At least nine hemoglobins with the electrophoretic properties of Hb D (or S) have been found in association with Hb S (McCurdy et al., 1974) (Table 4–4). Of these, only two—Hb D-Punjab and Hb Lepore—each in association with Hb S, have given rise to symptomatic sickle cell disease. Another 12 variants have the same electrophoretic mobility as Hb S but have not thus far been found in association with sickling. The definitive diagnosis of each of these hemoglobins with the electrophoretic properties of Hb D can be made only with detailed structural analysis, since they migrate similarly (like Hb D-Punjab or A, unlike Hb S) on citrate-agar electrophoresis.

Inheritance of Hb S with Other Hemoglobin Variants

Hemoglobin Lepore/S (or Pylos/S) is manifest by the presence of a sickle cell disease of moderate severity, with a thalassemia-like blood picture. The proportion of the nonsickling hemoglobin is lower than in the other β variants.

Hemoglobin S/O-Arab has been described in a number of patients who were previously thought to have Hb SC disease (Milner et al., 1970). Hemoglobin S/O-Arab is generally somewhat more severe than Hb SC disease. A presumptive diagnosis of Hb S/O-Arab disease can be made from the electrophoretic properties at alkaline and acid (pH 6.2) pH: at alkaline pH, Hb O-Arab migrates like Hb C and at pH 6.2 like Hb S (rather than C).

Recently, a patient was found to be doubly heterozygous for hemoglobin S and hemoglobin C-Harlem (Moo-Penn et al., 1975). The hemoglobin electrophoretic patterns resembled that of SC or S/O-Arab. In this disorder, all the β chains have the β6 Glu $\rightarrow$ Val substitutions and half of the β chains have an additional substitution: β73 Asp $\rightarrow$ Asn. The patient suffered numerous crises as a child and became less symptomatic as she approached adulthood. The clinical manifestations of hemoglobin S/C-Harlem disease resemble those of SS disease.

The combination of structural α-chain abnormalities with heterozygosity for Hb S has not resulted in sickle cell disease. These combinations can generally be recognized by the appearance of multiple major components ($\alpha_2^A\beta_2^A$, $\alpha_2^X\beta_2^A$, $\alpha_2^X\beta_2^S$, $\alpha_2^A\beta_2^S$) as well as two minor components ($\alpha_2^A\delta_2 \cdot \alpha_2^X\delta_2$) on electrophoresis. Depending upon the charge of the α-chain variant, three or four major bands may be visualized on electrophoresis in alkaline media. (See Figure 3–2.)

Since sickle cell trait is itself asymptomatic, it is perhaps not surprising that amelioration of sickling by the presence of a structural variant has not generally been recognized. However, Hb Memphis ($\alpha_2{}^{23\ \mathrm{Gln}}\ \beta_2^S$) has been observed in association with homozygosity for Hb S. These patients have very mild symptoms of sickling (Kraus et al., 1966; Cooper et al., 1973). In vitro, impaired gelling of Hb S has been demonstrated in the presence of Hb Korle-Bu ($\alpha_2^A\beta_2^{73\ \mathrm{Asn}}$) and Hb F. As might be expected, gelling of Hb S in vitro is favored by the presence of variants which are associated with sickle cell disease—hemoglobins C, D-Punjab, and O-Arab (see Table 4–1).

HEMOGLOBIN S/HPFH

As explained in Chapter 2, the gene for hereditary persistence of fetal hemoglobin (HPFH) is encountered in approximately 0.1 per cent of blacks (Motulsky, 1973). Thus, it is not surprising that occasional individuals have been encountered who are doubly heterozygous for Hb S and HPFH (Bradley et al., 1961). Affected individuals have about 70 per cent Hb S, 20 to 30 per cent Hb F, low Hb A_2, and no Hb A. Peripheral blood counts are usually normal with no evidence of anemia or hemolysis. Red cells are normochromic and normocytic. The peripheral blood film reveals target cells but no fixed sickle forms. Although the sickle preparation and sickle solubility tests are positive, there is rarely clinical evidence of sickling. The mild expression of S/HPFH is due to the fact that the fetal hemoglobin is evenly distributed, thereby protecting all red cells from sickling. This can be demonstrated by differential staining of red cells by acid elution (Kleihauer-Betke stain) or by the use of fluorescently labeled anti-Hb F antibody (Stamatoyannopoulos et al., 1975).

In the great majority of cases the HPFH gene is either allelic or very closely linked to the β-chain structural chain. However, a much less common type of HPFH can be transmitted in cis to the β-chain structural gene (Martinez and Colombo, 1974; Huisman et al., 1975; Stamatoyannopoulos et al., 1975; Friedman and Schwartz, 1976) (see Chapter 2). Stamatoyannopoulos et al. (1975) have reported a patient with homozygous sickle cell disease and HPFH. The increased level of Hb F (20 per cent) and its nearly uniform distribution among red cells probably explain the patient's benign clinical course. This diagnosis should be considered in other patients with mild SS disease and elevated levels of fetal hemoglobin.

Chapter 5

UNSTABLE HEMOGLOBIN VARIANTS—CONGENITAL HEINZ BODY HEMOLYTIC ANEMIA

INTRODUCTION

As mentioned in Chapter 3, most human hemoglobin variants are not associated with detectable clinical manifestations. Many are discovered by chance or during the screening of large populations. However, a growing number of variants are known to have an enhanced propensity to denature, and the denatured hemoglobin precipitates in the red cell. As a result, the abnormal hemoglobin tends to aggregate within the red cell, forming an amorphous mass which has the morphological appearance of a Heinz body. These patients have a disorder of varying clinical severity which is generally called congenital Heinz body hemolytic anemia (CHBA).

In 1952 Cathie described a child with congenital nonspherocytic hemolytic anemia. At 10 months of age the patient had anemia, jaundice, splenomegaly, and pigmenturia. Splenectomy, performed six months later, resulted in no significant clinical improvement. Subsequently, large Heinz bodies were demonstrated in the patient's red cells. Following this report, a number of similar cases have been encountered throughout the world. In most of these cases, a defect in hemoglobin structure and function was suggested by the demonstration of a copious precipitate upon heating the patient's hemolysate (for details, see below). Nearly all these patients have been shown to have a hemoglobin variant. Cathie's patient was found to have Hb

Text continued on page 188.

TABLE 5–1. *Unstable Hemoglobin Variants*

Name	Structure	Helical Site	Inclusion Bodies	Heat Labile	Dark Urine	Hb g/100 ml	Reticulocytes (%)	Per Cent Abnormal Hb	Oxygen Affinity	Comments
I. β-Chain Variants										
Leiden	$\alpha_2\beta_2^{6 \text{ or } 7\ Glu\to 0}$	A3 or A4	?			11-13	3-6	30	Decreased	Mild; one residue deletion
Sögn	$\alpha_2\beta_2^{14\ Leu\to Arg}$	A11				12-13	0.4	30		No clinical abnormality
Saki	$\alpha_2\beta_2^{14\ Leu\to Pro}$	A11								
Belfast	$\alpha_2\beta_2^{15\ Trp\to Arg}$	A12	+			11-13	4	28	Slightly increased	
Lyon	$\alpha_2\beta_2^{17,18\ Lys,Val\to 0}$	A14,15	+			14.5	4	37	Increased	
Freiburg	$\alpha_2\beta_2^{23\ Val\to 0}$	B5		+		13	9	30	Increased	Cyanosis; ↑ methemoglobin, one residue deletion
Riverdale-Bronx	$\alpha_2\beta_2^{24\ Gly\to Arg}$	B6		+	0	11-12	10	30		
Savannah	$\alpha_2\beta_2^{24\ Gly\to Val}$	B6	+	+		4→6*	50	15-30		Severe
Moscva	$\alpha_2\beta_2^{24\ Gly\to Asp}$	B6	+	+				17	Slightly decreased	Patient also had leukemia
St. Louis	$\alpha_2\beta_2^{28\ Leu\to Gln}$	B10	+			12	10	29	Increased	15% methemoglobin
Genova	$\alpha_2\beta_2^{28\ Leu\to Pro}$	B10	+	+	±	8→14*	10-50	10-25	Increased	
Tacoma	$\alpha_2\beta_2^{30\ Arg\to Ser}$	B12	0	+	0	13	4		Increased	No clinical abnormality
Perth	$\alpha_2\beta_2^{32\ Leu\to Pro}$	B14	+	+	+	8→11*	27	≃38	Normal	
Philly	$\alpha_2\beta_2^{35\ Tyr\to Phe}$	C1	+	+	?	12-14	2-8			
Mequon	$\alpha_2\beta_2^{42\ Phe\to Tyr}$	C7								Hemolysis during infection
Hammersmith	$\alpha_2\beta_2^{42\ Phe\to Ser}$	CD1	+	+	+	6→7*	20-50	30	Decreased	Severe
Louisville	$\alpha_2\beta_2^{42\ Phe\to Leu}$	CD1	+	+		11-13	7-9	30-35	Decreased	
Okaloosa	$\alpha_2\beta_2^{48\ Leu\to Arg}$	CD7							Decreased	
Duarte	$\alpha_2\beta_2^{62\ Ala\to Pro}$	E6	+	+		15	10	~100	Increased	Heterozygous with β thalassemia

Table continued on following page.

TABLE 5–1. *Unstable Hemoglobin Variants*–Continued.

Name	Structure	Helical Site	Inclusion Bodies	Heat Labile	Dark Urine	Hb g/100 ml	Reticulocytes (%)	Per Cent Abnormal Hb	Oxygen Affinity	Comments
Zürich	$\alpha_2\beta_2^{63\ His\rightarrow Arg}$	E7	+	+	+	11-12	5-6	25	Increased	Mild; drug-sensitive
Toulouse	$\alpha_2\beta_2^{66\ Lys\rightarrow Glu}$	E10	0	+	0	12-15	1-4	40	Normal	No clinical
Sydney	$\alpha_2\beta_2^{67\ Val\rightarrow Ala}$	E11	+	+	+	12	8	30		
Bristol	$\alpha_2\beta_2^{67\ Val\rightarrow Asp}$	E11	+	+		7→7*	37	36	Decreased	Severe hemolysis
Seattle	$\alpha_2\beta_2^{70\ Ala\rightarrow Asp}$	E14	+	+	+	9-10	3	40	Decreased	
Christchurch	$\alpha_2\beta_2^{71\ Phe\rightarrow Ser}$	E15	+	+						
Shepherds Bush	$\alpha_2\beta_2^{74\ Gly\rightarrow Asp}$	E18				12-13	5-8		Increased	Impaired reactivity of Hb with 2,3-DPG
Bushwick	$\alpha_2\beta_2^{74\ Gly\rightarrow Val}$	E18					1-2			Mild; drug-sensitive
St. Antoine	$\alpha_2\beta_2^{74,75\ Gly,Leu\rightarrow 0}$	E18,19	+	+	0	11	8	25	Normal	
Buenos Aires	$\alpha_2\beta_2^{85\ Phe\rightarrow Ser}$	F1	+	0	0	12-14	8-15		Increased	Compensated hemolysis
Tours	$\alpha_2\beta_2^{87\ Thr\rightarrow 0}$	F3	+	+	0	13-14*	9	20	Increased	
Boräs	$\alpha_2\beta_2^{88\ Leu\rightarrow Arg}$	F4	+	+		8-12*		10		
Santa Ana	$\alpha_2\beta_2^{88\ Leu\rightarrow Pro}$	F4	+	+	+	8-13*	6-28	10		Two hemes per molecule
Gun Hill	$\alpha_2\beta_2^{91\text{-}95\rightarrow 0}$	F + FG	0	+	0	13.5	4-10	30	Increased	Five residue deletion; two hemes per molecule
Sabine	$\alpha_2\beta_2^{91\ Leu\rightarrow Pro}$	F7	+	+		8-10*	35-65	8		Two hemes per molecule
Istanbul	$\alpha_2\beta_2^{92\ His\rightarrow Gln}$	F8	+	+		9-13*	4	12-15	Increased	Two hemes per molecule
Köln	$\alpha_2\beta_2^{98\ Val\rightarrow Met}$	FG5	+	+	+	11-13	5-16	10	Increased	Commonest of unstable hemoglobins
Nottingham	$\alpha_2\beta_2^{98\ Val\rightarrow Gly}$	FG5	+	+	0	6.7	50		Increased	

Rush	$\alpha_2\beta_2^{101\ Glu \to Gln}$	G3		+		11-12	3-7	34	Normal	
Casper	$\alpha_2\beta_2^{106\ Leu \to Pro}$	G8	+	+		4-7→13*	20-90		Increased	Severe hemolysis
Peterborough	$\alpha_2\beta_2^{111\ Val \to Phe}$	G13	0	+		12	3.5		Decreased	Mild
Madrid	$\alpha_2\beta_2^{115\ Ala \to Pro}$	G17	+	+	+	9.7	33	23		Severe hemolysis
Khartoum	$\alpha_2\beta_2^{124\ Pro \to Arg}$	H2	0	+						Very mild
Wien	$\alpha_2\beta_2^{130\ Tyr \to Asp}$	H8	+	+		10*	43			
Leslie	$\alpha_2\beta_2^{131\ Gln \to 0}$	H9								
Hope	$\alpha_2\beta_2^{136\ Gly \to Asp}$	H14							Decreased	
Olmsted	$\alpha_2\beta_2^{141\ Leu \to Arg}$	H19				5-6*	3-8			
Cranston	$\alpha_2\beta_2^{144 \to 157}$	C terminus	+	0	0	14	6-8	35	Increased	Elongated β chain
II. α-Chain Variants										
Torino	$\alpha_2^{43\ Phe \to Val}\beta_2$	CE1	+	+	?	8→12*	6-16	8	Decreased	Moderately severe; aggravated by drugs
L-Ferrara	$\alpha_2^{47\ Asp \to Gly}\beta_2$	CE5					9	14-20	Normal	Mild
Hasharon	$\alpha_2^{47\ Asp \to His}\beta_2$	CE5	0	±	0	Normal	1-5	14-19	Normal	Mild
Russ	$\alpha_2^{51\ Gly \to Arg}\beta_2$	CE9								
Ann Arbor	$\alpha_2^{80\ Leu \to Arg}\beta_2$	F1				12	10	2-12		Mild
Etobicoke	$\alpha_2^{84\ Ser \to Arg}\beta_2$	F5		+		11-14	1-3	15	Increased	Mild
Setif	$\alpha_2^{94\ Asp \to Tyr}\beta_2$	G1		+	0			15	Slightly low	
Bibba	$\alpha_2^{136\ Leu \to Pro}\beta_2$	H19	+	+		6-7.5	6-16	5-11		Severe
III. γ-Chain Variant										
F-Poole	$\alpha_2\gamma_2^{130\ Trp \to Gly}$	H8	+	+						Hemolysis in newborn

*After splenectomy.

Bristol ($\alpha_2\beta_2{}^{67\ Val \rightarrow Asp}$) (Steadman et al., 1970). At present about 47 structurally different unstable hemoglobin variants have been reported (Table 5–1). Some, such as Hb Köln, have been encountered repeatedly in unrelated families from widely scattered parts of the world. Thus, CHBA represents an important type of congenital hemolytic disease. In this chapter we will review its pathogenesis at the cellular and molecular levels, its clinical manifestations, and finally its laboratory diagnosis and treatment.

PATHOGENESIS

The understanding of the mechanism underlying the hemolysis in CHBA was considerably enhanced when Grimes and his associates (Grimes and Meisler, 1962; Grimes et al., 1964) showed that hemolysates from these patients, when incubated at 50° C, formed flocculent precipitates. Such precipitation in stroma-free hemoglobin solutions indicated that an abnormality in soluble cell constituents, probably hemoglobin, was responsible for Heinz body formation. Subsequently, it was shown that heat-labile hemoglobin could be synthesized by reticulocytes (Grimes et al., 1964). Hence its presence was not related to some type of aberrant catabolism or denaturation of aged normal hemoglobin. Hb Zürich was the first unstable variant to be analyzed structurally. Muller and Kingma (1961) demonstrated that at β63(E7), histidine was replaced by arginine. The intimate steric relationship between this residue and the heme group was not known at this time (see Chapter 1). Subsequently, many other patients with CHBA and heat-labile hemoglobin were shown to have electrophoretically abnormal hemoglobins. It became apparent that the great majority of patients whose clinical and laboratory findings suggest the diagnosis of CHBA have structurally abnormal hemoglobin variants. In other patients with the clinical findings of CHBA, current methods may not permit the delineation of structural changes in hemoglobin.

A list of the unstable hemoglobin variants appears in Table 5–1.[1] It is apparent that there are about four times as many β-chain as α-chain variants. The relatively large number of unstable β-chain variants can be best explained by the strong likelihood that there are four α-chain genes but only two β-chain genes (see Chapter 2). Accordingly, a structural mutation of an α-chain gene would result in the synthesis of only 25 per cent of abnormal α chains. There may

[1]The preparation of Table 5–1 was greatly facilitated by information provided by Dr. Dominique Labie, Dr. Titus Huisman, and Professor Hermann Lehmann and by recent comprehensive reviews by White and Dacie (1971) and White (1974).

be a relatively high incidence of unstable α-chain variants which escape clinical recognition because they make up only a small proportion of the total hemoglobin in the red cell and therefore result in less significant hemolysis. Indeed, most of the α-chain variants listed in Table 5–1 are associated with mild clinical manifestations. It is noteworthy that of the 14-odd *stable* hemoglobin variants associated with increased O_2 affinity and familial polycythemia, all but two are β-chain variants (see Chapter 6).

Molecular Basis of Instability

As discussed in Chapters 1 and 2, considerable knowledge has been amassed on the three-dimensional structure of normal human hemoglobin, allowing rather precise structural-functional interpretations. Thus, the properties of a number of human hemoglobin variants have been explained in terms of the stereochemical consequences arising from an amino acid substitution (or deletion) at a specific site in a globulin subunit (Perutz and Lehmann, 1968; Morimoto et al., 1971). The instability of most of the variants listed in Table 5–1 can be attributed to one of the following five mechanisms:

1. *Amino Acid Substitution in the Vicinity of the Heme Pocket.* The binding of heme to globin involves a very specific stereochemical fit which helps to stabilize the tertiary conformation of the subunit (see Chapter 1). The heme is inserted into a hydrophobic cleft on the surface of the subunit. The porphyrin interacts with certain nonpolar amino acids in the CD, E, F, and FG regions of the subunits. Most of these nonpolar amino acids are invariant residues. Thus, it is not surprising that substitutions of these residues may result in a decrease in the stability of the heme-globin linkage and, secondarily, of the entire subunit. Figure 5–1 shows a three-dimensional diagram of a β chain. Unstable hemoglobin variants in the vicinity of the heme pocket have been marked by arrows. A number of the unstable hemoglobins have substitutions or deletions in the heme pocket. In some, such as hemoglobins Hammersmith, Zürich, Köln (Jacob et al., 1968; Jacob et al., 1968a), and Sabine (Schneider et al., 1969), experimental evidence supports the prediction that heme binding is impaired. Four of these variants (Bristol, Boräs, Olmsted, and Shepherds Bush) involve the substitution of a polar for a nonpolar residue. Such substitutions may allow the entrance of water into the normally hydrophobic heme pocket and thereby weaken heme-globin linkage. The consequences of displacement of heme from its normal binding site will be discussed below in further detail.

2. *Disruption of Secondary Structure.* The primary amino acid sequence of a protein determines how much of it will be ordered into some form of secondary structure such as the α helix or β pleated

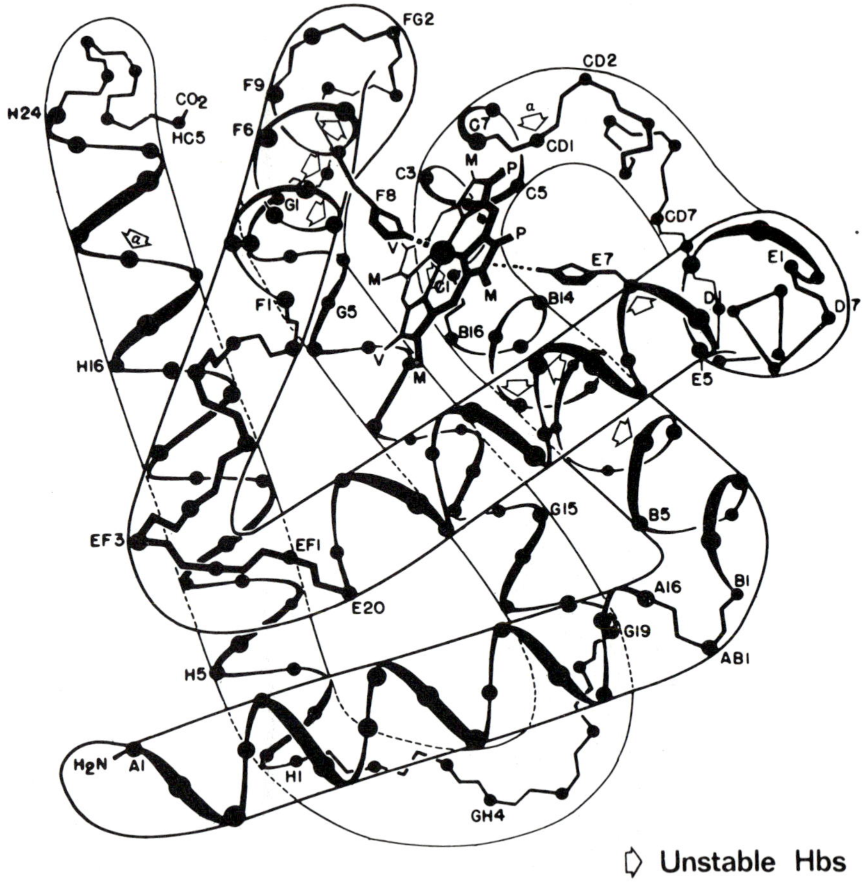

Figure 5–1. Three-dimensional representation of β chain. Arrows indicate sites of substitutions in a number of unstable hemoglobins. Note their proximity to the heme group. (This figure was constructed by Dr. Helen Ranney, using a three-dimensional diagram of myoglobin published by Dickerson, R. E. in Neurath, H. (ed.): The Proteins: Composition, Structure and Function, Vol. II. 2nd ed. New York, Academic Press, 1964, pp. 603–778.)

sheet. As mentioned in Chapter 1, native hemoglobin is about 75 per cent in the form of α helix. The remaining segments of the chains are in random coil. Certain residues have a higher probability of forming an α helix than others. Thus, an analysis of primary structure can give a good prediction of secondary structure (Chou and Fasman, 1974). Certain amino acid substitutions could shift the equilibrium between α helix and random coil in a given segment of the subunit. This would have a marked effect on tertiary structure and the overall stability of the subunit. Proline cannot participate in an α helix except as one of the initial three residues. Eight of the unstable variants are substitutions of proline for leucine. In addition, Hb Duarte and Hb Madrid involve a substitution of proline for alanine. In each case, the substitution involves a residue beyond the third place in the helix. Among the 101 stable hemoglobin variants associated with no clinical manifestations, only one involves a proline substitution at the C-terminal residue of the α chain (Hb Singapore $\alpha^{141\ Arg \rightarrow Pro}$). Thus, the disruption of the α helix probably accounts for the instability of the ten variants mentioned above.

3. Substitution in the Interior of the Subunit. As mentioned in Chapter 1, the globin subunits are folded in such a way that all the charged amino acids such as lysine, arginine, glutamic acid, and aspartic acid are situated on the surface of the molecule, allowing their ionized groups to be in contact with solvent water. In contrast, the residues oriented toward the interior of the molecule have nonpolar side groups. The interior of the molecule is thus stabilized by hydrophobic interactions. A number of unstable variants involve the substitution of a polar for a nonpolar residue. These include hemoglobins Sögn, Riverdale-Bronx, Bristol, Shepherds Bush, Boräs, Olmsted, Russ, Ann Arbor, and Wien. As mentioned above, four of these (Bristol, Boräs, Shepherds Bush, and Olmsted) are near the heme pocket. Polar for nonpolar substitutions could result in significant alterations in tertiary structure if water is allowed access to the hydrophobic interior of the subunit. In addition, a variant having a neutral amino acid substitution may owe its instability to an alteration of the stereochemical fit of the residue's side group. This is difficult to predict without very precise atomic coordinates. Nevertheless, it is interesting that 17 out of 46 unstable variants (35 per cent) involve the substitution of one noncharged residue for another (including the 6 Leu→Pro substitutions), whereas only 3 out of 110 functionally normal and clinically silent variants encountered to date involve such a substitution (3 per cent). As mentioned in Chapter 1, hemoglobin readily dissociates symmetrically into $\alpha\beta$ dimers: $\alpha_2\beta_2 \rightleftharpoons 2\alpha\beta$. The subunits cleave at the interface between the α_1 and β_2 subunits. In contrast, the bonding between the α_1 and β_1 subunits is considerably stronger. In normal Hb A, the dissociation of the subunits at this interface ($\alpha_1\beta_1 \rightarrow \alpha + \beta$) is observed only under extremes of pH or ionic strength or in solutions which favor disruption of secondary and tertiary structure, such as concentrated urea. A few hemoglobin variants owe their instability to substitutions at the $\alpha_1\beta_1$ interface, which permits the dissociation of the $\alpha\beta$ dimer into monomers and allows hidden sulfhydryl groups to become reactive. Hb Philly is one of the best studied of this type of unstable variant (Rieder et al., 1969).

4. Amino Acid Deletion(s). Nine hemoglobin variants have been reported to date to have deletions from one to five residues in sequence: Leiden, Lyon, Freiburg, Leslie (Deaconess), St. Antoine, Tours, Niteroi, Tochigi, and Gun Hill. All of these are unstable variants (Table 5–1). Variants having multiple deletions have only been encountered at or near interhelical corners. Such an alteration in structure can have a marked effect on the overall conformation of the molecule involving intra- and inter-subunit interactions. Distortion of structure is particularly marked in Hb Gun Hill, in which no heme binding to the β chain is possible because of the deletion of five residues in the F–FG region. Despite this, individuals with Hb Gun Hill have relatively mild hemolysis (Bradley and Rieder, 1966; Bradley et al., 1967).

5. *Elongation of Subunit.* A few hemoglobin variants have elongated subunits, owing either to an error in chain termination or to nonhomologous crossover (see Chapter 3). Most of these are present in only small amounts. Hb Cranston is found in association with a compensated hemolytic state (Bunn et al., 1975b). The instability of this variant is probably due to a hydrophobic segment attached to the C-terminal end of the β chain. The stability of the other elongated β chain variant, Hb Tak, has not yet been determined.

HEINZ BODY FORMATION

The mechanisms underlying the formation of intracellular inclusions in CHBA have been studied extensively, particularly by Jacob and his associates (1968a, 1968b; Jacob and Winterhalter, 1970a, 1970b), Rachmilewitz (Rachmilewitz and Harari, 1972; Rachmilewitz and White, 1973; Rachmilewitz, 1974), and Winterbourn and Carrell (1972, 1973, 1974). Their experiments were done on selected variants, but the results are likely to be relevant to many of the other unstable hemoglobins. The following phenomena have been demonstrated.

Displacement of the Heme Group in the Abnormal Subunit

The stability of the heme-globin linkage is dependent on the precise stereochemical fit conferred by the surrounding residues in the heme pocket (see Chapter 1). As mentioned above, this fit is perturbed in a number of the unstable variants because of amino acid substitutions or deletions in this region. Furthermore, the oxidation state of the heme iron has an important influence on the stability of the heme-globin linkage. In normal oxyhemoglobin and deoxyhemoglobin, the ferrous heme group remains tightly bound to globin. In contrast, the ferriheme group in methemoglobin has a much lower affinity for globin (Bunn and Jandl, 1968). Jacob and his coworkers (1968b) showed that ferriheme dissociated more readily from methemoglobin Köln than from methemoglobin A. During incubation of hemolysates at 50° C, those containing unstable hemoglobin variants (Köln, Zürich, Hammersmith) showed a rapid decrease in the ratio of absorptions at 540 nm and 280 nm (Jacob and Winterhalter, 1970a, 1970b). These results do not necessarily mean "heme loss." Free hematin is very insoluble at neutral pH and binds avidly and non-specifically to a number of proteins. It is likely that in many cases the heme group is displaced from its normal position in the subunit during the incubation, and as a result its absorption in the visible spectrum is significantly altered.

Hemichrome Formation

Recent observations by Rachmilewitz and his associates (Rachmilewitz and Harari, 1972; Rachmilewitz and White, 1973; Rachmilewitz, 1974) indicate that hemichromes are a common intermediate in various types of hemoglobin denaturation. They are characterized by a specific absorption in the visible spectrum (Fig. 5–2). The incubation of methemoglobin can lead to hemichromes, particularly under circumstances in which hemoglobin lacks its normal stabilizing interactions. For example, isolated hemoglobin subunits (α or β chains), certain chemically modified hemoglobins, and a number of unstable hemoglobin variants have been shown to form hemichromes readily (Rachmilewitz et al., 1971). Electron paramagnetic (spin) resonance (EPR) has proved a very useful physical measurement in the further characterization of these intermediates (Rachmile-

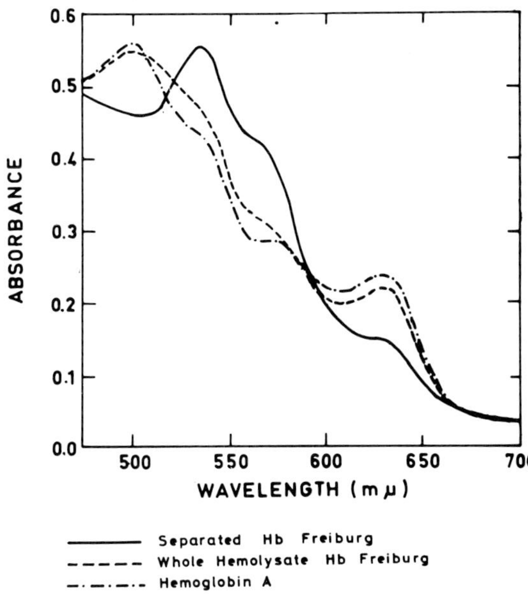

Figure 5–2. Absorption spectra of whole hemolysate and purified hemoglobins from a patient with Hb Freiburg (β23 Val→0), 48 hours after oxidation with ferricyanide (0.05 M phosphate, pH 7.0, 4° C). Purified Hb A (—·—·—·) has an absorption spectrum indicating methemoglobin. Purified Hb Freiburg (———) has an absorption spectrum of a hemichrome. (With permission of Dr. E. A. Rachmilewitz.)

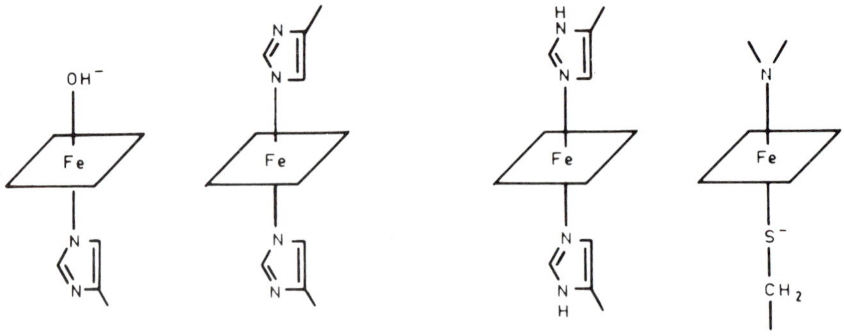

Reversible Hemichromes Irreversible Hemichromes

Figure 5–3. Diagrammatic structure of hemichromes showing proximal histidine below the plane of the porphyrin ring and distal histidine above the plane. (From Rachmilewitz, E. A.: Sem. Hemat. *11*:441, 1974.)

witz et al., 1971). The bonding of the distal (E7) histidine imidazole to the oxidized heme results in the transition from high spin to low spin state having a characteristic EPR signal (Fig. 5–3). This type of hemichrome has been shown to be reversible (hemichrome 1 in Figure 5–5). Upon reduction of the heme iron to the ferrous state, deoxyhemoglobin is formed. Further distortion of the subunit's conformation allows other groups to form an internal ligand with the heme, resulting in the formation of irreversible hemichromes which have distinguishing EPR spectra (hemichrome 2 in Figure 5–5). The formation of irreversible hemichromes is accompanied by precipitation of the hemoglobin.

A number of unstable hemoglobin variants have been shown to form hemichromes, particularly following incubation of the oxidized (methemoglobin) form. These include hemoglobins Köln, β98 Val→Met (Rachmilewitz and Harari, 1972); Louisville (Bucuresti), β42 Phe→Leu (Rachmilewitz, 1974); Freiburg, β23 Val→0 (Rachmilewitz and Harari, 1972); Riverdale-Bronx, β24 Gly→Arg (Rachmilewitz and Harari, 1972); Hammersmith, β42 Phe→Ser (Wajcman et al., 1973b); Seattle, β70 Ala→Asp (Rachmilewitz, 1974); Sydney, β67 Val→Ala (Winterbourn and Carrell, 1974); and Christchurch, β71 Phe→Ser (Winterbourn and Carrell, 1974). It is likely that such hemichromes are formed during the denaturation of other unstable variants. The amino acid substitution apparently causes sufficient disruption in the tertiary structure of the subunit to permit the opposition of the iron atom of the ferriheme group to certain nearby groups of the globin chain. The formation of hemichromes involves a marked reduction in absorption at 540 nm and probably contributes to the decreased ratio of optical density observed for several unstable variants (OD-540/OD-280) (Jacob and Winterhalter, 1970a, 1970b).

Enhanced Reactivity of the β93 Sulfhydryl Groups

Jacob et al. (1968a, 1968b) showed that Hb Köln had an increased rate of reaction with labeled glutathione to form the mixed disulfide. Red cell glutathione has been found to be decreased in a few patients with CHBA (Fairbanks et al., 1969; White and Dacie, 1971; Honig et al., 1973), although normal or elevated in others (Fairbanks et al., 1969; White and Dacie, 1972). The enhanced sulfhydryl reactivity of some of the unstable variants may explain their tendency to become highly labeled with radioactive chromium. White and Dacie (1971) incubated intact CHBA red cells with ^{51}Cr-labeled sodium chromate and then separated the globin peptide chains by column chromatography. The variant β chains (Köln, Hammersmith, and Shepherds Bush) had two- to sixfold higher specific activity than the β^A chains. Jacob and his coworkers (1968a, 1968b) have suggested that in patients with Hb Köln, Heinz bodies may be attached to the inner surface of the red cell membrane by a disulfide bond between hemoglobin and a membrane protein. The inclusions could be released from erythrocyte ghosts by the addition of mercaptoethanol, a reagent capable of reducing disulfide bonds (Jacob et al., 1968a).

Recent studies by Winterbourn and Carrell (1973, 1974) have raised some doubt about the importance of sulfhydryl oxidation in the pathogenesis of CHBA. Experiments on three unstable variants (Köln, Sydney, Christchurch) revealed no blocked cysteines and no protection by reduced glutathione. Although precipitation of the oxy and carboxy forms of these hemoglobins was accompanied by the formation of intermolecular disulfide bonds, there was no evidence that this phenomenon affected the rate of precipitation. Furthermore, these authors examined red cells containing inclusions of Hb Christchurch and failed to demonstrate the presence of any covalent linkage (such as disulfide bonds) between globin and membrane protein. They concluded that the adherence of the Heinz body to the inner surface of the red cell membrane is due to hydrophobic bonding (Winterbourn and Carrell, 1973).

The two phenomena—dissociation of heme and enhanced sulfhydryl reactivity—may be linked according to the following scheme:

$$
\begin{array}{ccccc}
\text{Globin—Fe}^{3+}\text{heme} & \underset{K_1}{\rightleftharpoons} & \text{Globin} & + & \text{Fe}^{3+}\text{heme} \\
| & & | & & \\
\text{SH} & & \text{SH} & & \\
K_2 \downarrow\uparrow +\text{RSH} & & K_4 \downarrow\uparrow +\text{RSH} & & \\
\text{Globin—Fe}^{3+}\text{heme} & \underset{K_3}{\rightleftharpoons} & \text{Globin} & + & \text{Fe}^{3+}\text{heme} \\
| & & | & & \\
\text{SR} & & \text{SR} & &
\end{array}
$$

The following observations support such a relationship: (1) the dissociation of ferriheme from normal methemoglobin A is enhanced when the $\beta 93$ sulfhydryl group is blocked by N-ethylmaleimide ($K_3 > K_1$) (Bunn and Jandl, 1968); (2) hemoglobin lacking heme groups on the β chains ($\alpha_2\beta_2^0$) has markedly enhanced sulfhydryl reactivity ($K_4 > K_2$) (Jacob and Winterhalter, 1970a; and (3) in several of the unstable variants both of these reactions are favored. From these considerations it is not surprising that the rate of denaturation of the unstable hemoglobins can be enhanced by sulfhydryl blockade (Jacob et al., 1968, 1968a) and that it can be reduced by the addition of a heme ligand such as cyanide (Jacob and Winterhalter, 1970a; Rieder, 1970) which stabilizes the heme-globin linkage (Bunn and Jandl, 1968) (see Figure 5–4). Rieder (1970) has shown that cyanide also inhibits the denaturation of normal hemoglobin.

The unstable hemoglobins have properties very similar to the artificial Hb $\alpha_2\beta_2^0$ (Jacob and Winterhalter, 1970a). As mentioned above, both have enhanced sulfhydryl reactivity. Both form a flocculent precipitate when incubated at 50° C. This denaturation is inhibited by the addition of ligands such as cyanide or hemin. Both $\alpha_2\beta_2^0$ and many of the unstable variants have an increased degree of dissocia-

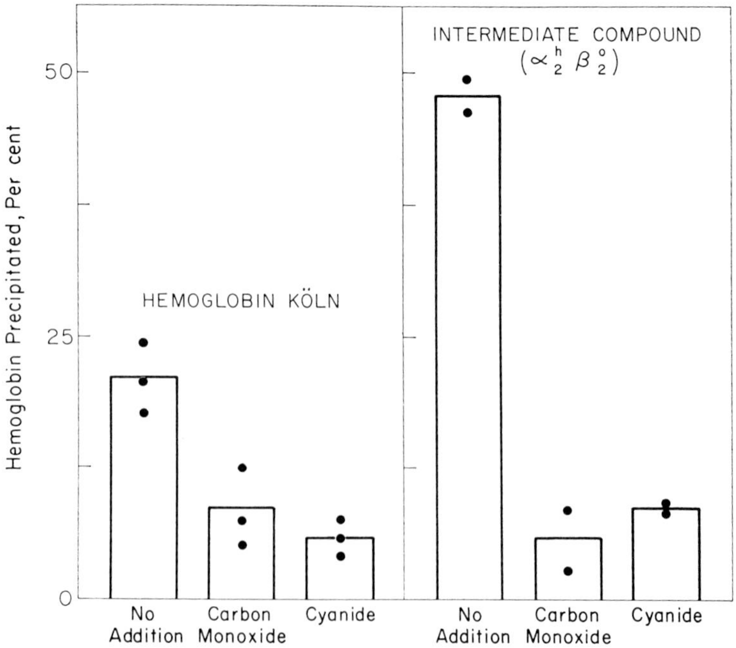

Figure 5–4. Inhibition of heat precipitation of hemoglobin Köln (left) and $\alpha_2^{heme}\beta_2^0$ (right) by cyanide or carbon monoxide. Both heme proteins copiously precipitate when heated at 50° C for 2 hours unless the heme ligands, cyanide or carbon monoxide, are present. (From Jacob, H. S., and Winterhalter, K. H.: J. Clin. Invest. *49*:2008, 1970a.)

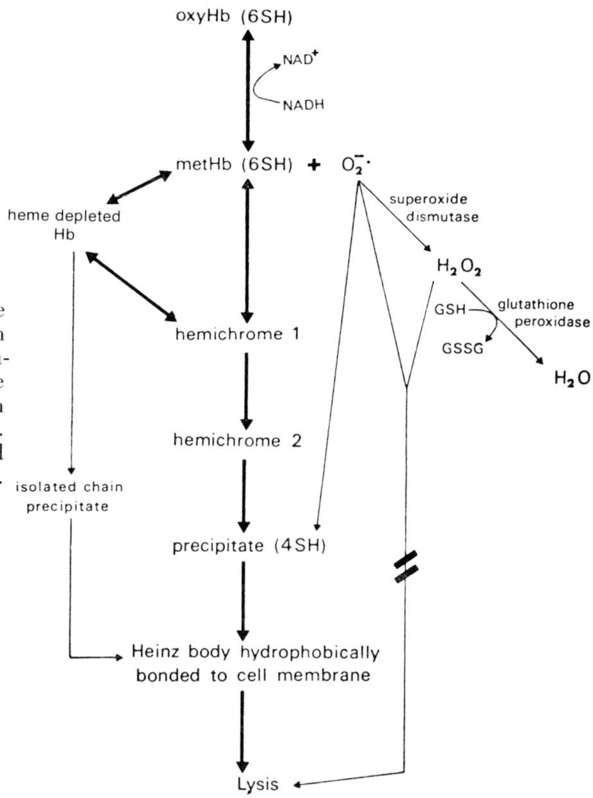

***Figure* 5–5.** Scheme proposed by Winterbourn and Carrell for the intracellular denaturation of unstable hemoglobins resulting in Heinz bodies and hemolysis. (From Winterbourn, C., and Carrell, R. W.: J. Clin. Invest. *54*:678, 1974.)

tion from tetramer to dimer: $\alpha_2\beta_2 \rightarrow 2\alpha\beta$ (Winterhalter, 1972; Waks et al., 1973).

During the circulation of the CHBA red cell in vivo or the incubation of the hemolysate in vitro, the three-dimensional structure of the hemoglobin variant is altered sufficiently so that its solubility decreases and it forms a precipitate. It seems unnecessary to postulate (Rachmilewitz and Harari, 1972; Rachmilewitz, 1974) that the hemoglobin tetramer dissociates into individual subunits prior to the precipitation of the abnormal chain. Winterbourn and Carrell (1972) have performed amino acid analyses and peptide mapping of precipitates of several variants, including Christchurch, Sydney, Köln, and Hammersmith, and have demonstrated the presence of equal amounts of α and β chains. Furthermore, some α chain polymerized with β chain by means of disulfide bond formation. The precipitates of hemoglobins Christchurch and Sydney contained a full complement of heme, whereas Hb Köln appeared to be depleted of half the heme. Thus, the precipitation of most unstable variants probably involves the entire molecule rather than selective heme loss with subsequent aggregation of the denatured globin subunits (Jacob et al., 1968a, 1968b).

The scheme proposed by Winterbourn and Carrell (1974) for the denaturation of unstable hemoglobins is depicted in Figure 5–5. Oxyhemoglobin is converted to methemoglobin. The release of superoxide anion (O_2^-) or its product, H_2O_2, may result in oxidant damage to globin thiols and to the membrane. As yet there is no experimental evidence on this point. Because of its structural abnormality, the unstable methemoglobin is converted first to a reversible hemichrome intermediate and then to an irreversible hemichrome (hemichrome 2). Precipitation of this latter species may be hastened by the formation of disulfide bonds between globin subunits.

Mechanism of Hemolysis in CHBA

There is both morphological (Rifkind, 1965; Schnitzer et al., 1971) and experimental (Jacob et al., 1968a) evidence that in CHBA, Heinz bodies become adherent to the inner surface of the red cell membrane. As mentioned above, this attachment is probably due to hydrophobic rather than covalent interactions (Winterbourn and Carrell, 1973; Chan and Desforges, 1974). The membrane-bound inclusions cause crater-like indentations on the surface of the cell (Schnitzer et al., 1971). Red cells containing Heinz bodies have been shown to have decreased pliability and filterability (Jandl et al., 1961; Miller et al., 1971). It is not surprising that they have difficulty negotiating the microcirculation. Rifkind (1965) has presented convincing morphological evidence that Heinz body red cells get hung up in transit between the cords and sinuses of the spleen. The membrane-bound Heinz body may be ensnared during this passage. The remainder of the red cell then reseals its membrane after it has been relieved of this excess baggage. These considerations help to explain why the number of Heinz bodies increases markedly after patients with CHBA have undergone splenectomy.

The metabolism of CHBA red cells has been studied by a number of investigators. In general, specific enzyme activities have either been normal or increased in keeping with a young population of red cells. In some cases, glucose consumption is increased in conjunction with decreased levels of ATP (Miller et al., 1971; White and Dacie, 1971). Indeed, one case of CHBA-(Schneider et al., 1969) was initially reported as a defect in red cell metabolism (Mills et al., 1968). Red cell 2,3-DPG is usually found to be normal. The enhanced potassium efflux (Jacob et al., 1968a; Miller et al., 1971) found in erythrocytes from certain patients with CHBA has been attributed to the adherence of Heinz bodies to the inner surface of the red cell membrane. However, this increased potassium efflux is rather nonspecific and has been reported in a diverse group of hemolytic states, including sickle cell anemia, pyruvate kinase deficiency, hereditary stomatocytosis, and red cells treated with amphotericin B. To the extent that CHBA red cells leak potassium, the energy-dependent Na-K pump is stimulated in order to maintain osmotic equilibrium, thereby increasing the rate of glycolysis and decreasing ATP concentrations. Osmotic fragility is generally normal in CHBA.

The activity of the hexose monophosphate shunt has been increased in some cases of CHBA. Nevertheless, red cell glutathione is more often normal or increased than decreased (White and Dacie, 1971) and does not have an enhanced turnover rate (White and Dacie, 1971) (see above).

Biosynthesis of Unstable Variants

As Table 5–1 shows, the unstable hemoglobin variant usually makes up only a minority of the total hemoglobin. The remainder is Hb A, A_2, and perhaps some F. Furthermore, in some hemolysates of individuals with unstable β-chain variants, a very small amount of free α chains is observed on electrophoresis (Grimes et al., 1964; Sansone and Pik, 1965; Raik et al., 1967; Monn et al., 1968; Rieder and Bradley, 1968; Jacob and Winterhalter, 1970a; Rieder et al., 1975). The presence of free α chains can be explained by either decreased synthesis or enhanced destruction of the unstable β subunit. As the previous discussion on the pathogenesis of CHBA implies, the latter mechanism predominates.

The biosynthesis of a number of unstable variants has been studied. As Table 5–2 shows, the rate of synthesis of normal and variant chains is equal in most cases. Exceptions include hemoglobins Riverdale-Bronx, Boräs, Abraham Lincoln, and Ann Arbor. In all cases, the specific activity of the abnormal β chain greatly exceeded that of β^A because of the selective loss of the unstable variant as CHBA red cells circulate through the RE system (see previous section). It is likely that in red cells containing very unstable variants, a small pool of free α chains exchanges readily with the α chains of the variant. Rieder's (1971) observations on Hb Gun Hill provide a striking illustration of this point. Following incubation of the reticulocyte-rich blood with ^{14}C leucine, hemoglobins A and Gun Hill were separated by electrophoresis. The α chains of the purified hemoglobin A had virtually no radioactivity, while the α chains of Gun Hill were highly labeled. Thus, the newly synthesized α chains appeared to be diluted by a pre-existing pool of unlabeled α chains, thereby lowering α^A radioactivity. The high activity of the α chains must have been due to exchange of the partially labeled free α chain pool with the α chains of the unlabeled (but labile) Gun Hill. A similar phenomenon has been noted for hemoglobins Hammersmith (White and

TABLE 5–2. *Synthesis of Globin Chains of Unstable Hemoglobin Variants*

Hb	Per Cent Abnormal Hb	Subunit Specific Activity var/A	Rate of Synthesis of Variant Chain*	Total $\alpha:\beta$ Synthesis	Reference†
Gun Hill β91–95 deleted	32	2.4	120	1.0	Adams et al., 1972†
Köln β98 Val→Met	12	7.4	100	1.2–1.4	White and Brain, 1970; Huehns, 1970†
Hammersmith β42 Phe→Ser	40	1.5	100	1.1	White and Dacie, 1970†
Bristol β67 Val→Asp	36	1.4	98		Steadman et al., 1970†
Riverdale-Bronx β24 Gly→Arg	28	1.4–1.5	56–59	~1.2	Bank et al., 1970, and Zulsky et al., 1970†
Boräs β88 Leu→Arg	10		33		White, 1971†
Shepherds Bush β74 Gly→Asp	25		100		White and Dacie, 1971†
Abraham Lincoln β32 Leu→Pro	18	2.5	50	1.18	Honig et al., 1974
Zürich β63 His→Arg	32		110		Rieder et al., 1965
Leiden β6,7→0	24	1.5	100	1.8	Rieder and James, 1974
Cranston β Elongated chain	30	1.4	100	1.0	Shaeffer et al., in preparation
Bushwick β74 Gly→Val	1–2	20–60	~100	1.0	Rieder et al., 1975
Sabine β91 Leu→Pro	12	~1.5–3	~100		Shaeffer, 1973
Ann Arbor α80 Leu→Arg	2–15	2.5	20	4.0	Adams, 1974

*Expressed as percentage of the rate of synthesis of normal subunit.
†Unless stated otherwise, data have been taken from paper of Honig et al., 1974.

Dacie, 1970), Köln (White and Brain, 1970), Shepherds Bush (White and Dacie, 1971), Riverdale-Bronx (Zalusky et al., 1970), Sabine (Shaeffer, 1973), and Abraham Lincoln (Honig et al., 1974). Because of this exchange of α chains, the ratio of the total radioactivity of the normal and variant hemoglobins is not a reliable indication of the relative synthetic rates. It is curious that despite the marked distortion of primary structure of Hb Gun Hill, which has a deletion of the 5 residue segment at the proximal heme binding site, the rate of translation of $\beta^{\text{Gun Hill}}$ was equal to that of β^{A} (Rieder, 1971). Thus, if heme normally binds to the nascent polypeptide chain, it has no apparent effect on the rate of synthesis. As Table 5–2 shows, in most of the synthesis studies done on reticulocytes containing unstable hemoglobins, total α and β chain production is balanced. However, Hb Leiden is an interesting exception (Rieder and James, 1974). The overall β/α synthetic ratio was found to be 0.47 to 0.63 in peripheral blood and 0.82 in marrow. These values are similar to what has been encountered in individuals with β thalassemia. The mechanism for this imbalance in subunit synthesis is not known.

CLINICAL MANIFESTATIONS

Inheritance

Congenital Heinz body hemolytic anemia exhibits an autosomal dominant pattern of inheritance. Thus, affected individuals are heterozygotes. Because the spleen selectively removes the Heinz bodies, the unstable hemoglobin makes up only a minority (10 to 30 per cent) of the total. As expected in the heterozygous state, the remainder is predominantly normal hemoglobin A. An interesting exception is the recent report of Hb Duarte (Beutler et al., 1974b). This unstable β-chain variant was inherited in conjunction with β thalassemia. Accordingly, the production of normal β^{A} chains was markedly suppressed and, therefore, most of the patient's hemoglobin was Duarte. Fortunately, the variant was only mildly unstable, so that the individual survived into adulthood with a well compensated hemolytic state. Because of the low gene frequency for unstable variants, homozygosity would be very rare (except in offspring of consanguineous marriages) and most often incompatible with life. Such genetic considerations also apply to erythrocytosis accompanying hemoglobin variants with abnormally high oxygen affinity. A sizable minority of cases of CHBA appear to have arisen because of a spontaneous mutation, both parents being unaffected. Viewed another way, of the 20 instances of apparent spontaneous mutations among hemoglobin variants reported up until 1973, 17 involved patients with CHBA (Table 5–3). This is not surprising, since most

***TABLE 5–3.** Apparent Spontaneous Mutations Among Hemoglobin Variants*

Hemoglobin	Structure	Clinical Status	Blood Antigens Tested	RNA Base Change
Hammersmith*	$\alpha_2\beta_2{}^{42\ \mathrm{Phe \to Ser}}$	Hemolysis	No	U → C
Köln†	$\alpha_2\beta_2{}^{98\ \mathrm{Val \to Met}}$	Hemolysis	Yes (36)	G → A
Santa Ana†	$\alpha_2\beta_2{}^{88\ \mathrm{Leu \to Pro}}$	Hemolysis	No	U → C
Olmsted	$\alpha_2\beta_2{}^{141\ \mathrm{Leu \to Arg}}$	Hemolysis	No	U → G
Freiburg	$\alpha_2\beta_2{}^{23\ \mathrm{Val \to 0}}$	Hemolysis	No	
Sabine	$\alpha_2\beta_2{}^{91\ \mathrm{Leu \to Pro}}$	Hemolysis	Yes	U → C
Savannah	$\alpha_2\beta_2{}^{24\ \mathrm{Gly \to Val}}$	Hemolysis	No	G → U
Toulouse	$\alpha_2\beta_2{}^{66\ \mathrm{Lys \to Glu}}$	Hemolysis	No	A → G
Bristol	$\alpha_2\beta_2{}^{67\ \mathrm{Val \to Asp}}$	Hemolysis	No	U → A
Bryn Mawr	$\alpha_2\beta_2{}^{85\ \mathrm{Phe \to Ser}}$	Hemolysis	No	U → C
Casper†	$\alpha_2\beta_2{}^{106\ \mathrm{Leu \to Pro}}$	Hemolysis	Yes	U → C
M-Saskatoon†	$\alpha_2\beta_2{}^{63\ \mathrm{His \to Tyr}}$	Cyanosis	Yes	C → U
M-Hyde Park	$\alpha_2\beta_2{}^{92\ \mathrm{His \to Tyr}}$	Cyanosis	Yes	C → U
M-Boston	$\alpha_2\beta_2{}^{58\ \mathrm{His \to Tyr}}$	Cyanosis	No	C → U
Bethesda	$\alpha_2\beta_2{}^{145\ \mathrm{Tyr \to His}}$	Erythrocytosis	Yes	U → C
Abraham Lincoln	$\alpha_2\beta_2{}^{32\ \mathrm{Leu \to Pro}}$	Hemolysis	Yes	U → C

*Three instances.
†Two instances.

cases are sufficiently severe that medical attention and evaluation are sought. In contrast, the chances are very remote of finding an asymptomatic individual with a hemoglobin variant due to a spontaneous mutation. Furthermore, the reproductive potential of patients with severe CHBA may be decreased.

Presentation

Congenital Heinz body hemolytic anemia varies widely in clinical severity (Table 5–1). The variability depends primarily on the structural differences among the unstable variants. A given variant tends to produce similar clinical sequelae in affected individuals whether they are within the same family or are unrelated. Thus far, Hb Köln has been the most frequently encountered unstable variant. At least seven unrelated kindred or sporadic cases from various parts of the world have been reported to have Hb Köln. These patients all have a moderate hemolytic state that is well compensated, particularly following splenectomy.

Patients with severe CHBA may present with anemia in early childhood.[2] These include hemoglobins Bristol and Hammersmith. These β-chain variants emerge at approximately 6 months of age when the transition from γ to β chain production is complete. More commonly, patients present at different ages with unexplained hemolytic anemia. In many cases patients come to a physician's attention during an "aplastic" crisis, in which erythropoiesis has been temporarily suppressed by either infection or folic acid deficiency. Like other patients with chronic hemolysis, individuals with CHBA have an increased tendency to develop pigmented gallstones.

In some patients hemolysis may be aggravated by viral or bacterial infections or following the exposure to an oxidant agent such as sulfonamides. Hb Zürich has been encountered in three unrelated families (Frick et al., 1962; Rieder et al., 1965; Dickerman et al., 1973a). Affected individuals have normal hematocrits and absent or minimal hemolysis unless they are exposed to an oxidant stress. A few days of treatment with a sulfa drug can result in a hemolytic crisis with a 50 per cent drop in hematocrit, the emergence of Heinz bodies, and marked hyperbilirubinemia. The anemia remits promptly upon withdrawal of the drug. Those affected family members who have not been exposed to oxidant drugs have no history of hemolysis. Sulfonamides have also been found to exacerbate hemolysis in individuals with hemoglobins Torino (Beretta et al., 1968; Prato et al., 1970), Shepherds Bush (White et al., 1970), and Peterborough (King et al., 1972). Oxidant drugs do not affect hemolysis in patients with Hb Köln (Miller et al., 1971).

A significant proportion of patients with CHBA give a history of passing dark urine. In the absence of liver disease, patients with hemolytic anemia do not have bilirubinuria. Indeed, an outmoded term for hemolytic anemia is "acholuric jaundice." Furthermore, patients with CHBA do not have enough intravascular hemolysis to produce hemoglobinuria. It turns out that the pigmenturia in such patients with CHBA is probably due to dipyrrolmethenes of the mesobilifuscin group (Schmid et al., 1959). The structure of this pigment

---

[2]An unstable γ-chain variant (Hb F-Poole, $\alpha_2{}^G\gamma_2{}^{130\ Trp\rightarrow Gly}$) has been reported to cause hemolytic disease in the newborn (Lee-Potter et al., 1975). The hemolysis disappeared when Hb F switched to Hb A in the first few months of life.

is not yet definitely established. Pigmenturia is an inconsistent finding in CHBA. As shown in Table 5–1, pigmenturia is not well correlated with the severity of hemolysis. Dipyrroluria has also been encountered in β thalassemia (major) (Kreimer-Birnbaum et al., 1966a, b), another disorder associated with Heinz body production (see Chapter 2). It is likely that the urinary pigment is a reflection of aberrant heme catabolism, perhaps via a pathway that bypasses heme oxygenase, an enzyme responsible for the physiological catabolism of heme (Tenhunen et al., 1968). Goldstein et al. (1968) have found that experimentally induced Heinz bodies are also broken down aberrantly with decreased conversion of heme to bilirubin and the formation of a urinary pigment having properties indicative of dipyrroles. It may be that during the auto-oxidation of the unstable hemoglobin in vivo, sufficient superoxide anion or peroxide is generated that heme (or its porphyrin) is oxidized in a nonspecific, nonenzymatic fashion leading to these abnormal products.

A number of the unstable hemoglobin variants are unassociated with any clinical manifestations and have been discovered fortuitously or during surveys of large populations. The frequency of finding these mild unstable variants is increasing because of the development of more sensitive and specific methods for detection (see below).

Physical Findings

The physical findings of patients with CHBA are variable and depend primarily upon the severity of the disease. Those with moderate or severe hemolysis have jaundice and splenomegaly. Some patients may have hypersplenism with significant thrombocytopenia (Hutchison et al., 1964; Pederson et al., 1973). Severe hypersplenic hemolysis has been observed in newborns with Hb Hasharon (Tatsis et al., 1972). A few patients with CHBA may be mildly cyanotic, owing either to the presence of methemoglobinemia (as encountered in Hb Freiburg) (Jones et al., 1966) or to decreased oxygen affinity leading to deoxygenation of the peripheral blood (Hb Hammersmith). Some patients with CHBA have been reported to have leg ulcers (Jackson et al., 1973; White, 1974).

LABORATORY DIAGNOSIS OF CHBA

General Parameters of Hemolysis

Patients with CHBA, like those with other types of chronic hemolysis, will have reticulocytosis accompanied by increased

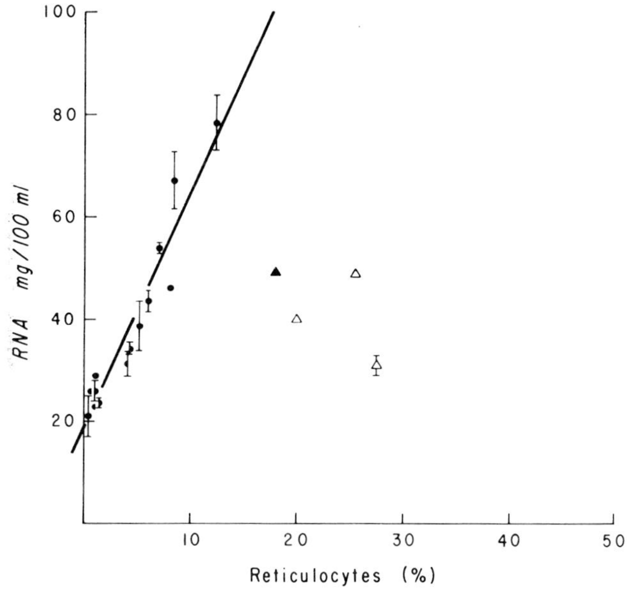

Figure 5–6. The relationship between reticulocytes estimated by supravital stain (abscissa) and by measurement of RNA (ordinate). Normal reticulocytes (●) have a linear relationship between these two measurements. Patients with an unstable hemoglobin variant (Hb Casper) have a falsely high reticulocyte count both prior to (△) and following (▲) splenectomy. (From Koler, R. T., et al.: Amer. J. Med. 55:549, 1973.)

serum bilirubin and decreased haptoglobin. However, the extent of hemolysis is often difficult to evaluate in patients having an unstable hemoglobin. Because the precipitated variant takes up supravital stains, Heinz body–containing cells may be mistaken for reticulocytes. Thus, the estimate of reticulocytes by ordinary methods may be falsely high. As Figure 5–6 shows, measurement of red cell RNA will give a truer indication of reticulocyte number (Koler et al., 1973). In like manner, measurements of red cell life span by tagging red cells with ^{51}Cr are very difficult to interpret. There is no correlation between ^{51}Cr red cell survival and degree of hemolysis in CHBA (Bentley and Lewis, 1974). As mentioned above, ^{51}Cr will bind preferentially to the variant hemoglobin, compared to Hb A (White and Dacie, 1972). Secondly, the isotope appears to elute more readily from the abnormal hemoglobin (Pederson et al., 1973). Finally, as we have discussed, precipitates containing the unstable variant are selectively pitted from red cells during in vivo circulation. These factors make the rate of disappearance of ^{51}Cr radioactivity greatly exceed the rate of red cell destruction. The use of radioactive amino acid precursor (Honig et al., 1973) (Fig. 5–7) or DF^{32}P labeling (Bentley and Lewis, 1974; Hutchinson et al., 1974) will give a more reliable indication of red cell survival.

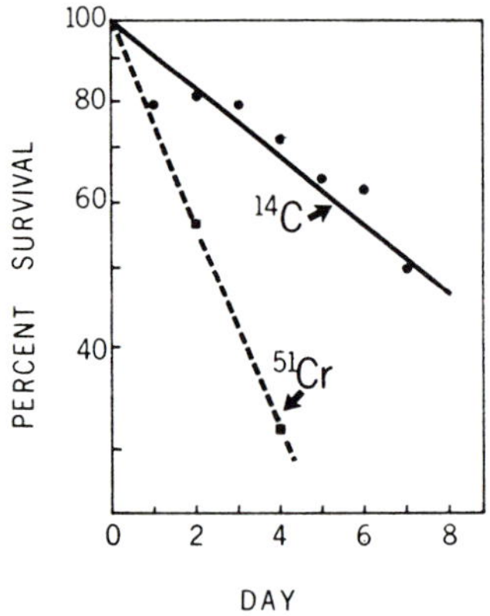

Figure 5–7. Red cell survival of a patient with an unstable hemoglobin variant (Hb Abraham Lincoln) measured by ^{14}C-amino acid labeling of reticulocytes and ^{51}Cr labeling of whole blood. (From Honig, G., et al.: J. Clin. Invest. 52:1748, 1974.)

Red Cell Morphology

Congenital Heinz body anemia red cells may appear entirely normal on a Wright's stained blood film. Often, however, the cells are hypochromic (low MCHC) despite having a normal mean corpuscular volume. This may be a reflection of the pitting function of the spleen. The red cells often show more variation in size and shape than normal, and prominent basophilic stippling may be seen (Fig. 5–8). In some patients the red cells appear as if a bite had been taken from the margin. Again, this may be a morphological sequela of splenic pitting.

The demonstration of Heinz bodies requires the use of a supravital stain such as crystal violet or new methylene blue. Their presence is highly variable. In the most mild forms of CHBA, it may be necessary to incubate red cells for long time periods, either in the presence of an oxidant such as acetylphenylhydrazine or in the absence of substrate (glucose), before Heinz bodies can be demonstrated. It is important to have normal controls for comparison, since numbers of Heinz bodies may be elicited in normal red cells by these maneuvers. Heinz bodies are more readily demonstrable in patients with severe CHBA. In all cases they are much more abundant following splenectomy. They appear as irregular blue-purple inclusions, 0.5 to 2.0μ, often solitary and adjacent to the inner surface of the red cell membrane (Fig. 5–8). In contrast, inclusions generated by the oxidant dye tend to be smaller and multiple. Recent evidence indicates that in CHBA, these bodies are not irreversibly bound to the membrane (Winterbourn and Carrell, 1973). Heinz bodies are not specific for CHBA. They can also be seen in the red cells of patients with some forms of α or β thalassemia and in the red cells of patients exposed to an oxidant stress, particularly those deficient in an enzyme involved in the pentose-phosphate pathway (HMP shunt) or in the synthesis of glutathione.

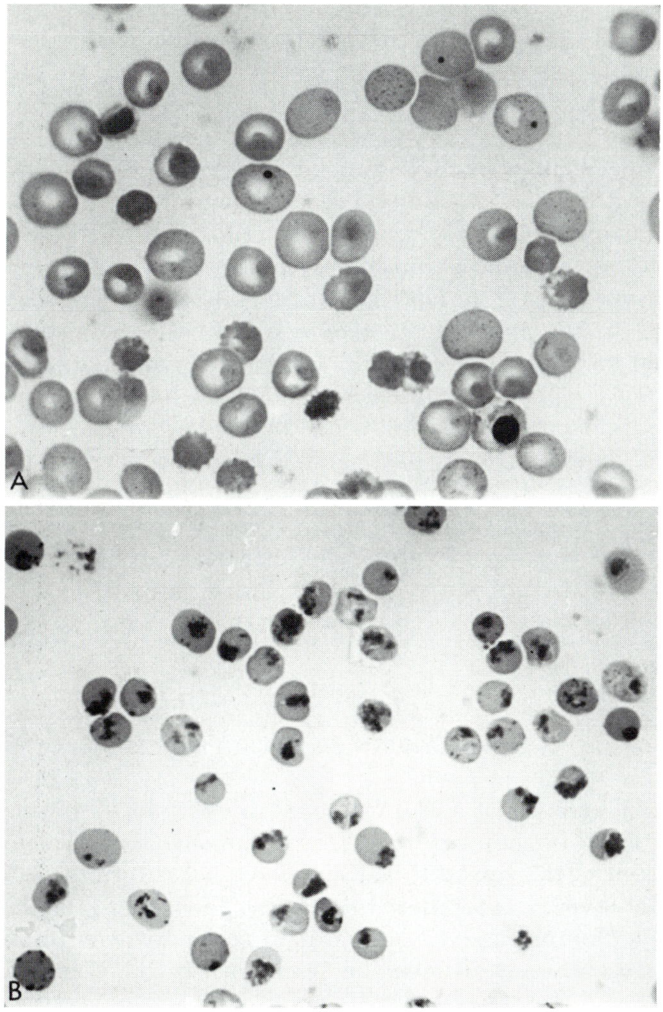

Figure 5–8. *A*, Photomicrograph of peripheral blood from a patient with an unstable hemoglobin variant (Hb Abraham Lincoln). Note basophilic stippling, Howell-Jolly bodies, and normoblast. *B*, Following incubation of blood for 30 minutes with new methylene blue. Most red cells contain large Heinz bodies. (From Honig, G., et al.: J. Clin. Invest. 52:1748, 1974.)

Hemoglobin Denaturation

The diagnosis of CHBA can often be established by the demonstration of denatured hemoglobin in the hemolysate. In most cases the hemoglobin variant will form a flocculent precipitate when a 1 per cent solution of the hemolysate is incubated in a neutral phosphate buffer at 50° C for 1 to 2 hours (Grimes and Meisler, 1962; Grimes et al., 1964). In the preparation of the hemolysate, the stroma should not be removed with organic solvents (White, 1974). The sensitivity of the test may be enhanced by the use of TRIS buffer (Schneiderman et al., 1970), although we have been unable to notice any advantage in this method for the unstable variants which we have tested. Carrell and Kay (1972) showed that incubation of hemolysates in 17 per cent isopropanol at 37° C provides enhanced sensitivity. This test is easy to perform and should be available in clinical laboratories for routine screening. The addition of the sulfhydryl reagent *p*-mercuribenzoate to the hemolysate can result in the precipitation of the abnormal subunit (Rieder et al., 1969; Huisman et al., 1971a; Honig et al., 1973). Those unstable variants which have an increased tendency to dissociate into subunits can be readily attacked by sulfhydryl reagents. This approach has been used to prepare unstable hemoglobin subunits that cannot be separated by conventional means (Huisman et al., 1971a; Honig et al., 1973). In view of the tendency of unstable hemoglobins to denature under a variety of experimental conditions, it is not surprising that the Sickledex Test may give a false-positive result in CHBA (Fairbanks and Pettit, 1972).

Hemoglobin Electrophoresis

The diagnosis of CHBA is confirmed if an abnormal band is demonstrated on hemoglobin electrophoresis. However, only about 45 per cent of the unstable variants have substitutions (or deletions) which involve an alteration in charge. Thus, many of these abnormal hemoglobins are very difficult to separate by ordinary electrophoretic techniques. It may be necessary to try electrophoresis in different media and several pH's before an optimal separation can be achieved. If hemes are lost or displaced from the abnormal subunit, one or more bands (or a smear) migrating less rapidly toward the anode than the intact hemoglobin (i.e., a more positive net charge) may appear. The anomalous electrophoretic behavior of a number of the unstable variants may be related to heme depletion of the abnormal subunits. Another type of electrophoretic heterogeneity was demonstrated in studies on Hb Rush (Adams et al., 1974). Analysis of the hemolysate on cellulose acetate at pH 8.6 revealed two bands migrating cathodally to Hb A. Re-electrophoresis of the middle band produced a pattern similar to that of the whole hemolysate, suggesting that this component was the hybrid tetramer $\alpha_2\beta^A\beta^{Rush}$, and upon re-electrophoresis it dissociated and recombined to form the two parent tetramers.

Hb A_2 may be increased somewhat in patients with CHBA

(White and Dacie, 1972; Honig et al., 1973). This is probably a reflection of the fact that the variant hemoglobin is selectively removed from the red cell as discussed previously, leaving a higher ratio of Hb A_2 to total hemoglobin (Rieder et al., 1965). Similar to other types of chronic hemolysis, Hb F levels may be modestly elevated in CHBA. In some unstable variants, free α chains can be demonstrated on electrophoresis, since the unstable β chains may be selectively precipitated (see previous section on biosynthesis).

If an unstable variant is difficult to separate electrophoretically, it will also be difficult to purify by standard preparative procedures such as column chromatography. For this reason, it may be necessary to take advantage of the relative insolubility or enhanced denaturation of the variant in order to purify it and study its properties. This has been done by *p*-mercuribenzoate precipitation (see above) or isopropanol precipitation (deWeinstein et al., 1973).

OXYGEN EQUILIBRIA

The unstable hemoglobins tend to have abnormal oxygen affinity. Whole blood oxygen saturation curves have been determined for about half the various unstable variants (Table 5–1). Of these, the oxygen affinity is normal in 20 per cent, decreased in 30 per cent, and increased in 50 per cent. The lattermost finding is not surprising, since the tertiary structure of the variant subunit may be so altered that it cannot form a stable t structure. If the oxygen affinity of the variant hemoglobin differs significantly from that of Hb A, the whole blood oxygen saturation curve will be biphasic (Fig. 5–9).

As Bellingham and Huehns (1968) have pointed out, oxygen affinity may be an important determinant of red cell mass in patients with CHBA. The hemoglobin of individuals with Hb Köln exhibits significantly increased oxygen affinity and, as a consequence, impaired release of oxygen during capillary circulation. The resultant tissue hypoxia stimulates erythropoiesis, presumably via regulation by erythropoietin. As a result, individuals with Hb Köln have minimal anemia, despite a significant amount of hemolysis. One patient actually developed an increase in oxygen affinity and erythrocytosis following splenectomy (Egan and Fairbanks, 1973). Thus, oxygen delivery may not have been improved by the operation (Desforges, 1973). Woodson et al. (1974) have studied oxygen transport in two individuals with Hb Köln. These patients had normal oxygen consumption, hemoglobin concentration, and cardiac output. From the Fick equation discussed in Chapter 1, it follows that A-V oxygen extraction must also be normal. However, because of the increase in red cell oxygen affinity, oxygen delivery could only be achieved at the expense of a significant reduction in mixed venous PO_2. This was

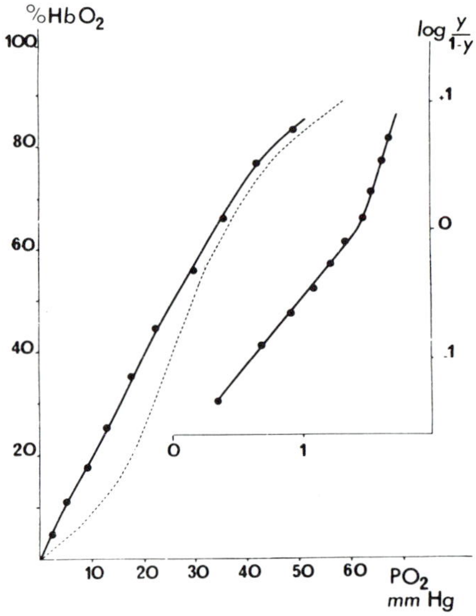

Figure 5–9. Oxygen dissociation curve of blood of a patient with Hb Tours. (Dotted line indicates normal curve.) The Hill plot shown in an inset on the right shows a biphasic curve. The left-hand portion of the curve shows increased oxygen affinity due to the presence of the hemoglobin variant. The right-hand portion of the curve reflects oxygenation of Hb A in the patient's red cells. (From Wajcman, H., et al.: Biochim. Biophys. Acta 295:495, 1973a.)

documented by direct measurement. The marked increase in urinary erythropoietin in one patient and evidence for redistribution of blood flow to vital organs indicated that these individuals were on the verge of hypoxia.

In contrast, patients with Hb Hammersmith have decreased O_2 affinity (Wajcman et al., 1973b) and severe anemia. Those with Hb Seattle also have a "shift to the right" (Stamatoyannopoulos et al., 1969b), although much less hemolysis than the Hammersmith patients. Because oxygen unloading is enhanced, there is less stimulation to erythropoiesis. The red cell mass of these individuals is thus set at a subnormal level appropriate for their hemoglobin function (Stamatoyannopoulos et al., 1969). This relationship appears to be a general phenomenon among patients with CHBA. As Figure 5–10 shows, those individuals who have unstable variants with increased oxygen affinity tend to have normal or near normal hemoglobin values while those with decreased oxygen affinity may have significant anemia.

It is often difficult to study the functional properties of unstable hemoglobins in detail. During the process of separation from normal Hb A the variant may become irreversibly denatured. Some unstable variants such as Hb Köln (Wajcman et al., 1971; Pederson et al., 1973; Sharma et al., 1974), Hb Savannah (Huisman et al., 1971a), Hb Bibba (Smith et al., 1970), and Hb Istanbul (Aksoy et al., 1972) have an increased tendency to dissociate into dimers. This process appears to be related to the displacement or loss of heme from the β chains. The initial measurements of the oxygen equilibria of purified

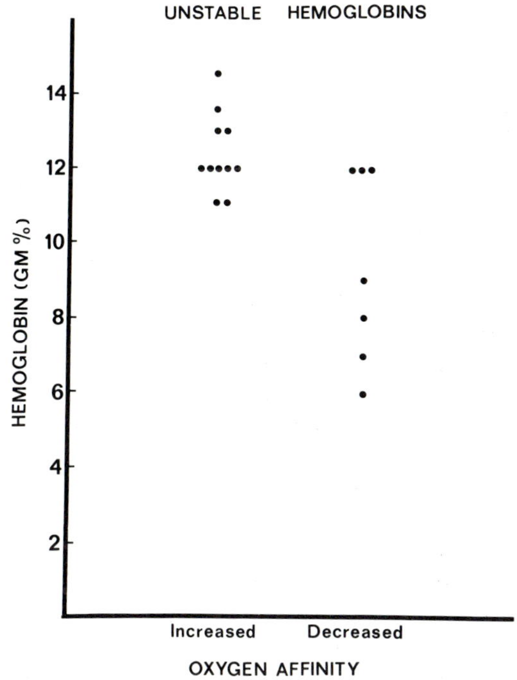

Figure 5–10. Comparison of hemoglobin levels in CHBA patients having increased and decreased oxygen affinity.

Hb Köln by Wajcman et al. (1971) showed it to have high oxygen affinity, low heme-heme interaction, and decreased reactivity with 2,3-DPG. In contrast, DeFuria and Miller (1972) showed that in the presence of added hemin, hemoglobin Köln had a higher degree of heme-heme interaction and normal 2,3-DPG reactivity. Sharma et al. (1974) measured the kinetics of binding of carbon monoxide to Hb Köln and found that in the absence of added hemin, the reaction was fast and monophasic, indicating that deoxy Köln was largely in the R structure. Following the addition of hemin, a biphasic curve was obtained, with the slow component resembling Hb A. These results indicate that the addition of hemin permits Hb Köln to assume the T ("deoxy") conformation and help to explain the conflicting observations on oxygen equilibria noted above.

Besides Hb Köln, two other unstable hemoglobins have been shown to have impaired interaction with 2,3-DPG (May and Huehns, 1972a; Nagel et al., 1973). Hb Leiden ($\alpha_2\beta_2^{6 \text{ or } 7\ \text{Glu}\rightarrow 0}$) (Nagel et al., 1973) probably has weak binding to 2,3-DPG because the deletion increases the distance between the two N termini of the β chains (see Chapter 1). The mechanism for the diminished response of Hb Shepherds Bush ($\alpha_2\beta^{74\ \text{Gly}\rightarrow\text{Asp}}$) to 2,3-DPG is less clear (May and Huehns, 1972a).

TREATMENT

Most individuals with CHBA do not require treatment. Those with severe hemolysis derive benefit from general supportive measures such as folic acid and prompt attention to infections. Oxidant drugs should be avoided. Transfusions are indicated only rarely such as during an aplastic crisis in which erythropoiesis has been suppressed.

As discussed in the section on pathogenesis, the spleen has been shown to sequester CHBA red cells. During the circulation through the spleen Heinz bodies may be "pitted" from the cell, leaving the remainder of the red cell intact. Other cells do not escape from the splenic cords and are destroyed in situ. From these considerations, splenectomy seems to be a reasonable approach in selected cases. In a recent review of the literature, Koler et al. (1973) concluded that splenectomy may be beneficial in severely affected patients. As Figure 5–11 shows, some patients have achieved a significant increase in hemoglobin following splenectomy. Others with equally severe hemolysis have not benefited. It is difficult to predict preoperatively which patients will respond. Measurements of ^{51}Cr red cell survival and splenic uptake are very difficult to interpret (see above). The decision on whether a patient with CHBA should undergo splenectomy may sometimes be resolved by ascertaining whether other patients with the same variant were benefited (see Koler et al., 1973,

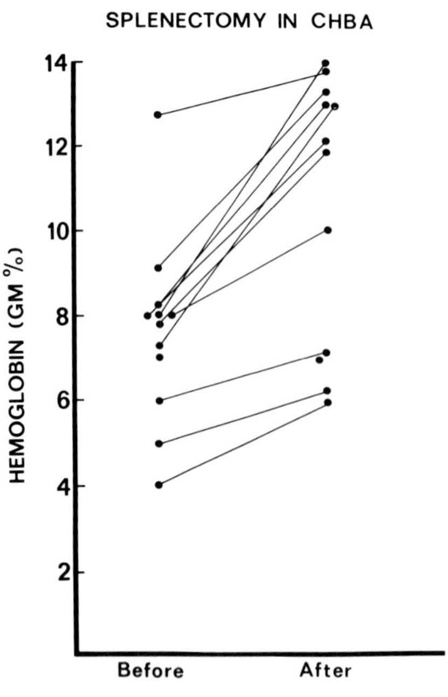

Figure 5–11. Effect of splenectomy on hemoglobin levels in patients with CHBA.

and Figure 5–11). As mentioned earlier, one patient with Hb Köln actually developed polycythemia following splenectomy (Egan and Fairbanks, 1973), probably as a result of the increased oxygen affinity of this variant (see above). It is difficult to appraise the significance of CHBA in the reported deaths of two patients, presumed to have Hb Duarte, following splenectomy, since many relevant details of the hematological status of the individuals either pre- or postoperatively are not known (Beutler et al., 1974b). Splenectomy should not be performed on young children (<6 years of age), since they are at increased risk of developing septicemia following surgery. One 6-year-old child with Hb Hammersmith died of pneumococcal septicemia four years after undergoing a splenectomy (White, 1974).

Chapter 6

HEMOGLOBINOPATHY DUE TO ABNORMAL OXYGEN BINDING*

In 1966, Charache, Weatherall, and Clegg described an individual with unexplained erythrocytosis in association with a hemoglobin variant. Their patient was an 81-year-old man who presented with mild angina pectoris that developed late in life. He had no other significant clinical problems. By chance, he was initially seen in the hematology clinic at Johns Hopkins Hospital (Charache, 1974b). In this setting, Dr. Charache discovered that he had a hemoglobin of 19.9 g/100 ml and an abnormal hemoglobin band on electrophoresis. In an attempt to relate these two findings, Dr. Charache and Dr. Andre Helleghers determined an oxygen dissociation curve on the patient's blood and found that it was significantly displaced to the left. This observation suggested the intriguing possibility that the patient's erythrocytosis might be a secondary compensation to a primary defect in oxygen unloading. A thorough family study revealed 15 other members with both erythrocytosis and the electrophoretically abnormal hemoglobin. Charache then purified the hemoglobin variant and confirmed that it had a marked increase in oxygen affinity. Clegg and Weatherall established that hemoglobin Chesapeake is an α-chain variant with a substitution of leucine for arginine at position 93 (Clegg et al., 1966). This series of observations opened up a new chapter in the developing story of hemoglobin.

Nineteen other variants with increased oxygen affinity have been encountered thus far in individuals with secondary erythrocy-

*This subject has recently been discussed in two excellent reviews (Charache, 1974a; Nagel and Bookchin, 1974b).

TABLE 6–1. *Hemoglobin Variants Associated With Familial Erythrocytosis*

Variant	Structure	Area Affected	Severity	Bohr Effect	Max. Hb. Conc. (g/100 ml)	Reference
Chesapeake	α92 (FG4) Arg→Leu	$\alpha_1\beta_2$	3+	Normal	19.9	Charache et al., 1966
J-Cape Town	α92 (FG4) Arg→Gln	$\alpha_1\beta_2$	+	Normal	16.6	Lines and McIntosh, 1967
Olympia	β20 (B2) Val→Met	$\alpha_1\beta_2$	3+		20.7	Stamatoyannopoulos et al., 1973
Rahere	β82 (EF6) Lys→Thr		2+	Normal	20.0	Lorkin et al., 1975
Creteil	β89 (F5) Ser→Asn					Gavel et al., 1974
Malmö	β97 (FG4) His→Gln	$\alpha_1\beta_2$	3+	Normal	21.3	Fairbanks et al., 1971
Wood	β97 (FG4) His→Leu	$\alpha_1\beta_2$				Taketa et al., 1976
Yakima	β99 (G1) Asp→His	$\alpha_1\beta_2$	3+	Normal	22.9	Jones et al., 1967
Kempsey	β99 (G1) Asp→Asn	$\alpha_1\beta_2$	3+	↓	21.3	Reed et al., 1968
Ypsilanti	β99 (G1) Asp→Tyr	$\alpha_1\beta_2$	2+		22.0	Glynn et al., 1968
Brigham	β100 (G2) Pro→Leu	$\alpha_1\beta_2$	2+	Normal	20.0	Lokich et al., 1973
Heathrow	β103 (G5) Phe→Leu	Heme	3+	Normal	21.0	White et al., 1973
San Diego	β109 (G11) Val→Met	$\alpha_1\beta_2$	2+		18.1	Nute et al., 1974b
Little Rock	β143 (H21) His→Gln	$\beta\beta$	3+	Normal	23.0	Perutz, 1973
Syracuse	β143 (H21) His→Pro	$\beta\beta$	3+	↓	23.8	Jensen et al., 1975
Andrew-Minneapolis	β144 (HC1) Lys→Asn	$\beta\beta$			19.8	Zak et al., 1974
Rainier	β145 (HC2) Tyr→Cys	$\beta\beta$	3+	↓	21.0	Adamson et al., 1969
Bethesda	β145 (HC2) Tyr→His	$\beta\beta$	3+	↓	20.5	Hayashi et al., 1971
Osler (Fort Gordon)	β145 (HC2) Tyr→Asp	$\beta\beta$	3+	↓	22.0	Charache et al., 1975a; Kleckner et al., 1975; Jacon et al., 1975
Hiroshima	β146 (HC3) His→Asp	$\beta\beta$	2+	↓	17.4	Hamilton et al., 1969

tosis (Table 6–1). These variants generally have amino acid substitutions at sites crucial to hemoglobin function. Indeed, the understanding of structural-functional relationships of human hemoglobin is sufficiently advanced that, in most cases, the abnormal oxygen binding of the variant can be readily explained by its specific structural alteration (see below). In addition, a number of other variants are known to have increased oxygen affinity, though they are not associated with secondary erythrocytosis. These variants, shown in Table 6–2, generally do not have such marked increases in oxygen affinity as those listed in Table 6–1. Among the 120-odd variants unassociated with any relevant clinical manifestations, there are probably additional hemoglobins with abnormal functional properties. Until recently, oxygen affinity measurements were not generally included in studies on new hemoglobin variants.

About 30 per cent of the 50-odd unstable hemoglobin variants have significantly increased oxygen affinity (see Table 5–1). In fact, some of these mutant hemoglobins have higher oxygen affinity than those listed in Table 6–1. However, the predominant clinical manifestations are due to accelerated red cell destruction. The oxygen affinity of unstable hemoglobins appears to be an important determinant of the degree to which the patient's hemolysis is compensated: those patients with CHBA due to a variant with high affinity tend to have higher hemoglobin levels than those with normal or decreased oxygen affinity (see Bellingham and Huehns, 1968, and Chapter 5).

MOLECULAR PATHOGENESIS

The functional behavior of normal hemoglobin depends on a transition in its three-dimensional conformation which accompanies the addition and removal of oxygen. This process is discussed in detail in Chapter 1. As formulated in the allosteric model of Monod,

TABLE 6–2. *Hemoglobin Variants Having Increased Oxygen Affinity Without Erythrocytosis*

Variant	Structure	Area Affected	Bohr Effect	References
G-Norfolk	α85 (F6) Asp→Asn		Normal	Cohen-Solal et al., 1975
Denmark Hill	α95 (G2) Pro→Ala	$\alpha_1\beta_2$	↓	Wiltshire et al., 1972
Rampa	α95 (G2) Pro→Ser	$\alpha_1\beta_2$		DeJong et al., 1971
G-Georgia	α95 (G2) Pro→Leu	$\alpha_1\beta_2$	↓	
Hirose	β37 (C3) Trp→Ser	$\alpha_1\beta_2$		
Abruzzo	β143 (H21) His→Arg	$\beta\beta$		

Wyman, and Changeux (MWC) (1965), the hemoglobin tetramer exists in equilibrium between two quaternary conformations: R and T. When normal hemoglobin is fully deoxygenated, it is about 99.99 per cent in the T or "tense" structure. In this state, hemoglobin has a relatively low affinity for oxygen and other heme ligands and a relatively high affinity for allosteric effectors such as Bohr protons and 2,3-DPG. Conversely, normal oxyhemoglobin exists almost exclusively in the R or "relaxed" conformation. In this state it has a relatively high affinity for heme ligands such as oxygen and a low affinity for Bohr protons and 2,3-DPG. The transition between these two conformers involves a considerable free energy change, reflected as cooperativity between subunits or "heme-heme interaction" (Chapter 1). The change from the T to the R conformation involves a rather well-defined series of structural changes including the rupture of the salt bonds that stabilize the T conformation and the rotation of the β chains relative to the α chains. A considerable amount of intramolecular "movement" during this conformational isomerization occurs at the $\alpha_1\beta_2$ interface.

A structural alteration which affects the equilibrium between the R and T states would be expected to have a marked effect on hemoglobin function. Thus, if a specific amino acid substitution decreases the stability of the T structure, the transition to the R state will occur at an earlier stage in ligation, and the hemoglobin will have increased oxygen affinity and decreased heme-heme interaction. This has been demonstrated for a number of chemically modified hemoglobins as well as many of the high-affinity mutants. Hemoglobin Kempsey is a particularly well studied example (Reed et al., 1968; Ogata et al., 1972; Lindstrom et al., 1973; Bunn et al., 1974; Perutz et al., 1974). It is a β-chain variant in which β99-aspartic acid has been substituted by asparagine. In deoxyhemoglobin A this aspartic acid residue normally forms an important hydrogen bond with α42-tyrosine at the $\alpha_1\beta_2$ interface (Fig. 6–1). Upon oxygenation, the two subunits shift in a dovetail fashion, so that the β99-α42 hydrogen bond is broken and another one forms between α94-aspartic acid and β102-asparagine (Perutz, 1972). In hemoglobin Kempsey, the substitution at β99 prevents the formation of the former hydrogen bond, and lessens the stability of the "deoxy" or T structure. Thus, when hemoglobin Kempsey is fully deoxygenated it remains partly in the R state. (The equilibrium constant L in the MWC model is drastically reduced.) This has been verified experimentally in a number of ways. There are a number of physical and chemical properties which distinguish normal oxy- and deoxyhemoglobin. In fact, these can be considered to be properties which distinguish the R and T conformations. In many respects, deoxygenated hemoglobin Kempsey bears more resemblance to oxyhemoglobin A than to deoxyhemoglobin A. These include kinetics of ligand binding, sulf-

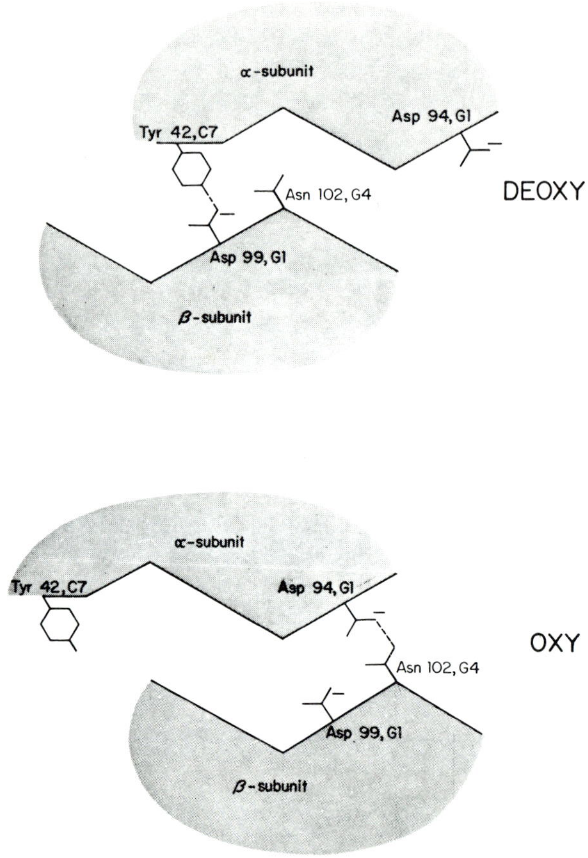

Figure 6–1. Changes at a portion of the $\alpha_2\beta_2$ interface upon oxygenation. The area of contact shifts in a dovetail fashion. Deoxyhemoglobin is stabilized by a hydrogen bond between α42 Tyr and β99 Asp. This bond cannot form in Hb Kempsey (β99 Asp→Asn). Likewise, oxyhemoglobin is stabilized by a bond between α94 Asp and β102 Asn. This bond cannot form in Hb Kansas (β102 Asn→Thr), Hb Beth Israel (β102 Asn→Thr), and Hb Titusville (α94 Asp→Asn). (From Perutz, M. F.: New Scient. Sci. J., June, 1971.)

hydryl reactivity, extent of dissociation into αβ dimers, and binding to haptoglobin (Bunn et al., 1974). In addition, physical probes such as nuclear magnetic resonance spectroscopy (Lindstrom et al., 1973) and circular dichroism (Perutz et al., 1974a, b) support the conclusion that deoxygenated Hb Kempsey is partially in the R conformation.

Most of the high-affinity variants thus far encountered have substitutions at either of two regions that are crucial to hemoglobin function (see Tables 6–1 and 6–2):

1. The $\alpha_1\beta_2$ interface.
2. The C-terminal end of the β chain.

As discussed in Chapter 1, the C-terminal portions of the α and β chains contribute greatly to the overall stability of the "deoxy" or T conformation (Perutz, 1970). The penultimate tyrosine of both chains

(α140, β145) is anchored in a cleft between the F and H helices. In the α chain, the C-terminal arginine is involved in two salt bonds: the guanido group is linked to an aspartate (residue 126) of the α chain and the carboxyl group may be linked to the N-terminal amino group of the other α chain. The C-terminal end of the β chain plays an equally important role. The C-terminal histidine (β146) forms two salt bonds: its carboxyl group is linked to the ϵ amino group of α40-lysine, while its imidazole group forms an intrasubunit bond with the carboxyl of β94-aspartate. In addition, β143-histidine is an important binding site for 2,3-DPG. All these interactions are oxygen-linked. The bonds break upon oxygenation and the molecule then assumes the relaxed (R) conformation. It is not surprising that variants having substitutions at the C-terminal portion of the β chain can have abnormal functional properties, including high oxygen affinity, decreased heme-heme interaction, decreased Bohr effect, and impaired interaction with 2,3-DPG. These will be discussed in more detail in the next section.

PROPERTIES OF THE HIGH-AFFINITY VARIANTS

Oxygen Equilibrium

By definition, this group of hemoglobin variants is associated with a shift to the left of the whole blood oxygen dissociation curve. Under physiologic conditions of pH (7.4) and temperature (37° C), normal red cells in plasma have a P_{50} of 26 mm Hg. That is, at an oxygen tension of 26 mm Hg, hemoglobin in these cells will be half saturated. Increased oxygen affinity is associated with low P_{50}.

In patients with erythrocytosis due to abnormal hemoglobins, whole blood P_{50} values have ranged from 12 mm Hg (hemoglobin Yakima, Novy et al., 1967) to 18 mm Hg (hemoglobin Brigham, Lokich et al., 1973). Figure 6–2 shows a whole blood oxygen dissociation curve from a girl with hemoglobin Bethesda. The red cell organic phosphates were within normal limits. Therefore, the marked shift to the left in the oxygen binding curves indicates the presence of functionally abnormal hemoglobin. From a Hill plot of the data shown in Figure 6–2, it is apparent that the patient has a biphasic curve (Fig. 6–3). The lower portion of the curve is due to the presence of hemoglobin Bethesda. An inflection point is seen at about 50 per cent saturation. The slope of the Hill plot at this point is low, as is the case for a mixture of any two hemoglobins of widely different oxygen affinities. This particular "n" value is *not* a reflection of heme-heme interaction, contrary to some statements in the literature. The upper portion of the patient's curve in Figure 6–3 approaches the normal curve asymptotically and reflects the oxygen-

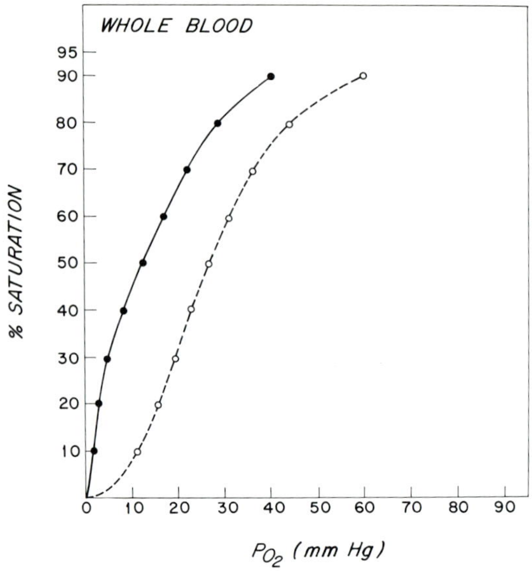

Figure 6–2. Oxygen binding curves of a normal individual ○----○ ($P_{50} = 26.5$ mm Hg) and of a patient with Hb Bethesda ●——● ($P_{50} = 12.8$ mm Hg). (Courtesy of Dr. M. B. Laver.)

ation of normal hemoglobin A which coexists in the red cells with an equal amount of hemoglobin Bethesda.

Although the whole blood oxygen dissociation curve provides information which is physiologically relevant, it does not give precise information on the functional properties of the variant hemoglobin. The whole blood curve is determined by the relative oxygen affinities and proportions of the normal and abnormal hemoglobins, as well as by intracellular factors such as organic phosphates, pH, and

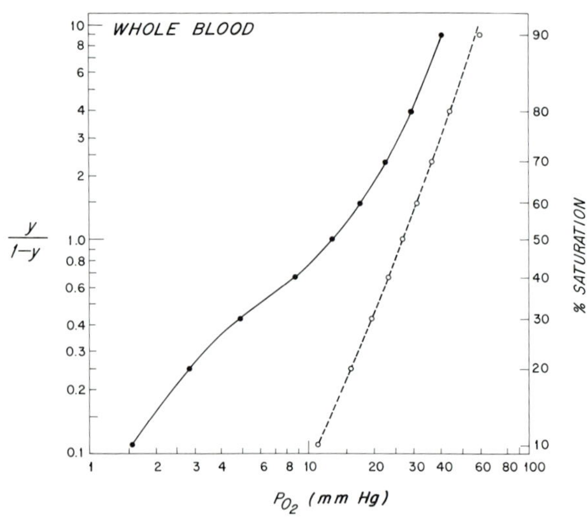

Figure 6–3. Hill plots of data shown in Figure 6–2. Normal (○----○); patient (●——●). Note biphasic curve. (Courtesy of Dr. M. B. Laver.)

TABLE 6–3. *Comparison of Functional Properties of High-Affinity Variants Studied under Identical Conditions*

Hemoglobin Variant	Phosphate-free Hemolysate		Purified Hemoglobin			
	% Abnormal	P_{50}* *(mm Hg)*	P_{50}* *(mm Hg)*	*n**	*Bohr Effect***	$P_{50}DPG/P_{50}$†
Chesapeake	30		0.55	1.4		
Kempsey	45	1.2	0.23	1.1	−0.22	1.6
Bethesda	50	1.3	0.18	1.1	−0.21	1.6
Brigham	50	2.7	#			
Hiroshima	50		0.90	2.2		
Syracuse	45	1.5	0.33	1.1	−0.24	1.4
A (Normal)	0	4.0	3.4	2.8	−0.55	2.4
α^A Chains			0.45	1.0		
β^A Chains			0.24	1.0		

*0.05 M bis-TRIS buffer (0.1 M Cl^-), pH 7.2, 20° C; hemoglobin concentration = 0.1 mM tetramer.

**$\Delta \log P_{50}/\Delta pH$.

† P_{50} (1 mM 2,3-DPG)/P_{50} (no. 2,3-DPG).

Hemoglobin Brigham cannot be separated from Hb A by conventional techniques.

carbon dioxide tension. These latter variables are eliminated if measurements are made on a phosphate-free hemolysate. A fuller investigation of the variant requires its isolation by some preparative technique such as column chromatography prior to the measurement of its functional properties. It is difficult to compare the 20-odd high-affinity variants because they have been studied in a number of laboratories by a variety of techniques and under different experimental conditions. In Table 6–3 we show a comparison of the oxygen equilibria of the variants which have been studied in our laboratory. Some of these mutant hemoglobins have oxygen binding properties approaching those of isolated subunits of hemoglobin A. Generally those variants having the highest oxygen affinity have the lowest heme-heme interaction. This abnormality reflects a perturbation in the equilibrium between conformational isomers. These hemoglobins flip from T to R at a relatively early stage in ligation. The reduction in the overall energy of interaction between subunits results in a low *n* value (see Chapter 1). If the $R \rightleftharpoons T$ equilibrium can be shifted back toward T, then the energy of subunit interaction will be enhanced and Hill's *n* will increase. For example, the subunit cooperativity of several of the high-affinity variants can be significantly increased by the addition of organic phosphates such as 2,3-DPG and inositol hexaphosphate (Olson and Gibson, 1972; Bunn et al., 1974b) (Fig. 6–4).

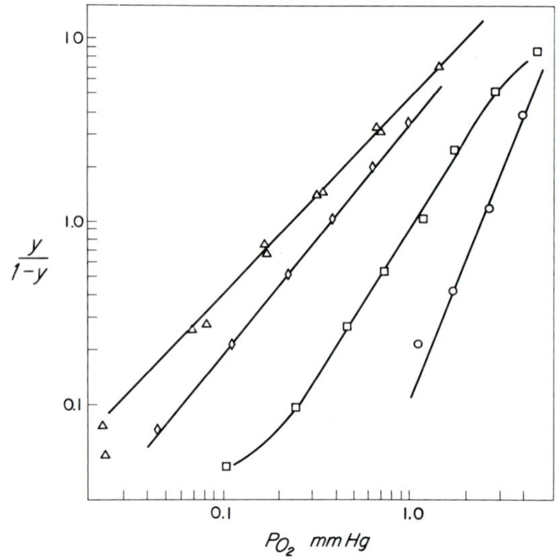

Figure 6–4. Oxygen equilibria of hemoglobin Kempsey and hemoglobin A (isolated from the same column). Hemoglobin (0.4 mM heme) in 0.05 M bis-TRIS buffer, pH 7.2, 0.1 M Cl^-, 20° C.

	P_{50} mm Hg	n
△ Kempsey	0.23	1.1
◇ Kempsey + 1 mM 2,3-DPG	0.37	1.3
□ Kempsey + 1 mM inositol hexaphosphate	1.1	1.7
○ A	2.4	2.6

(From Bunn, H. F., et al.: J. Biol. Chem. *249*:7402, 1974.)

Bohr Effect

Many of the high-affinity hemoglobins have a decreased alkaline Bohr effect (Tables 6–1 and 6–3). In the first place, those variants having substitutions at the C-terminal end of the β chain may have a decreased value because of failure to form the important salt bond (in deoxyhemoglobin) between the imidazole of β146-histidine and the carboxyl group of β94-aspartic acid. This interaction contributes about 50 per cent to the normal alkaline Bohr effect. In hemoglobin Hiroshima, the substitution of aspartic acid for histidine at β146 prevents the formation of this salt bond. The Bohr effect of Hb Hiroshima is half normal. On the other hand, certain variants have a reduced Bohr effect, even though their structural alterations are not at or near one of the residues which are known to contribute Bohr protons. For example, hemoglobin Kempsey (in the absence of organic phosphates) cannot assume a fully T structure upon deoxygenation and thus does not liberate a full complement of Bohr protons upon oxygenation.

INTERACTION WITH 2,3-DPG

Red cell 2,3-DPG has been measured in about half of these variants and has been consistently normal. However, several of these variants have been shown to have a diminished interaction with 2,3-DPG. Two variants, hemoglobins Little Rock and Syracuse, have amino acid substitutions at β143-histidine, one of the residues responsible for the binding of 2,3-DPG to deoxyhemoglobin. Hemoglobin Little Rock ($a_2\beta_2{}^{143\ His\rightarrow Gln}$) is of particular interest, since it has near normal heme-heme interaction and Bohr effect (Bromberg et al., 1973). Its high oxygen affinity may be due to *enhanced* stability of the R structure (Perutz, 1973). Bare et al. (1974) have done careful and extensive oxygen binding studies on hemoglobin Little Rock in the absence and presence of varying concentrations of 2,3-DPG. They have found that deoxyhemoglobin Little Rock binds 2,3-DPG somewhat more weakly than deoxyhemoglobin A. However, the binding of oxyhemoglobin Little Rock with 2,3-DPG is even weaker than that of oxyhemoglobin A with 2,3-DPG, so the overall effect of 2,3-DPG on the oxygenation of hemoglobin Little Rock is normal or even increased. In contrast, hemoglobin Syracuse ($\alpha_2\beta_2{}^{143\ His\rightarrow Pro}$) has decreased 2,3-DPG reactivity, as measured by oxygen affinities (Jensen et al., 1975). The oxygen binding experiments on hemoglobin Syracuse are difficult to interpret in terms of 2,3-DPG interaction with a hemoglobin lacking β143-histidine, because the proline substitution probably disrupts the H helix at position 143 and greatly weakens the overall stability of the T structure.

Beta 82-lysine is another residue involved in the binding of hemoglobin 2,3-DPG (see Figure 1–6). Two variants have recently been encountered which have amino acid substitutions at this site: Hb Rahere ($\alpha_2\beta_2{}^{82\ Lys\rightarrow Thr}$) Lorkin et al., 1975) and Hb Providence ($\alpha_2\beta_2{}^{82\ Lys\rightarrow Asn,\ Asp}$)* (Charache et al., 1975d). Both hemoglobins have nearly normal oxygen affinity in the absence of organic phosphates, but have very little change in P_{50} upon the addition of 2,3-DPG. As a result, heterozygotes have increased whole blood oxygen affinity. The individual with Hb Rahere had a marked increase in hemoglobin (20 g/100 ml) yet his red cell mass was not significantly elevated.

KINETICS OF LIGAND BINDING

Measurement of the rate of binding of oxygen or other ligands to hemoglobin provides information beyond that obtained from equilibrium determinations. In particular, kinetic data have provided insights into the conformational transition that occurs on ligand bind-

*Asparagine is partially deamidated to aspartic acid as a post-translational modification.

ing and into the differential reactivity of the α and β subunits. Gibson and his colleagues have developed very sophisticated methods for studying these fast reactions and have applied them not only to normal human hemoglobin A but to chemically modified hemoglobin and some of the functionally abnormal variants. Those studied in detail at this time include hemoglobins Chesapeake (Nagel et al., 1967; Gibson and Nagel, 1974), Rainier (Amiconi et al., 1972; Salhany, 1972), Hiroshima (Olson et al., 1972), Bethesda (Olson and Gibson, 1972), Kempsey (Bunn et al., 1974), and Syracuse (McDonald and Gibson, unpublished observations). In general, these variants when fully liganded behave like hemoglobin A. The reaction

$$Hb(O_2)_4 \xrightarrow{k_4} Hb(O_2)_3 + O_2$$

is very similar among these hemoglobins. (The value of k_4 is somewhat low for hemoglobin Hiroshima [Olson et al., 1972] and Syracuse [McDonald and Gibson, unpublished observations] but normal for the others.) Thus, these variants when fully liganded appear to assume a normal R conformation. When deoxygenated, these variants tend to have a rapid and monophasic reaction with heme ligands (such as carbon monoxide), indicating that the deoxygenated hemoglobin exists at least partially in the R state. In contrast, deoxyhemoglobin A has a slow and biphasic reaction with heme ligands, indicating the transition from T to R during heme ligation. In some variants such as Hiroshima (Olson et al., 1972), the abnormal subunit shows particularly fast ligand binding, suggesting that the amino acid substitution has drastically altered the tertiary conformation of the subunit and has exaggerated the asymmetry between α and β chain reactivity for heme ligands. Other variants such as hemoglobin Kempsey do not show such asymmetry between subunits (Bunn et al., 1974).

X-Ray Crystallography

The precise delineation of the high-affinity variants in three-dimensional space should provide the most direct information on structural-functional relationships. The structure of normal and variant hemoglobins can be compared by difference Fourier analysis. From such information, electron-density maps can be constructed which indicate specific sites where the two molecules differ. Since the three-dimensional structure of deoxyhuman hemoglobin A has been solved at high resolution (2.4 Å), difference Fourier analyses can be obtained by examining crystals prepared from deoxygenated variants. At this time no comparable structural information on the oxygenated forms of these variants is available. X-ray studies have been done on the following high-affinity variants: J-Capetown and Chesapeake (Greer, 1971c), Yakima (Pulsinelli, 1973), Rainier (Greer and Perutz, 1971), Hiroshima (Perutz et al., 1971), Kempsey (Perutz et al., 1974), and San Diego (Anderson, 1974). In general, difference Fourier analyses of these variants in the deoxy state show marked differences from hemoglobin A that extend beyond the site of amino acid substitution and indicate alterations in both the tertiary structure of the subunit and, in some cases, the quaternary structure of the tetramer. Hemoglobin Chesapeake appears to be an exception. Its deoxy structure appears to differ very little from that of hemoglobin A. In contrast, electron-density maps of the oxy structure at low resolution show marked differences. On occasion, the x-ray studies have provided very specific information. The difference Fourier analysis of deoxyhemoglobin Rainier showed a disulfide bridge between cysteine introduced by mutation at β145 and the cysteine at β93 (Greer and Perutz, 1971). These results indicated that the original structural analysis of hemoglobin Rainier was incorrect. Likewise, x-ray crystallography identified the amino acid substitution of hemoglobin Hiroshima as β146 (Perutz et al., 1971) rather than β143, as was first reported.

Physical Studies

Nuclear magnetic resonance (NMR) and electron paramagnetic resonance (EPR) have proved to be useful conformational probes not only of functionally normal hemoglobin but especially of the high-affinity variants (Davis et al., 1971; Ho and Lindstrom, 1972; Lindstrom et al., 1972b). Since the primary structural alteration in each of these variants is known, a comparison of its NMR spectrum with that of normal hemoglobin under identical conditions permits an assignment of certain peaks to specific structural loci. For example, NMR spectra of hyperfine shifted proton resonance have demonstrated that the environments around the α- and β-chain heme groups are structurally different. From the change in spectra upon partial saturation with ligand, the differential binding to α and β hemes can be demonstrated. This approach was used to show that the β chains of hemoglobin Kempsey have a higher affinity for carbon monoxide than the α chains (Lindstrom et al., 1973). From ring current shift resonances of the carboxy derivatives, assignments can be made to certain residues adjacent to the hemes. Recently, specific NMR signals have also been attributed to certain protons involved in hydrogen bonds at the subunit interfaces. These assignments have been largely based on comparisons with certain high-affinity variants which have amino acid substitutions at these sites (Fung and Ho, 1975).

Synthetic molecules that have paramagnetic resonance (spin labels) have been used to probe the conformation of normal and variant hemoglobins. Spin labels have been employed in several ways: (a) 2,3-DPG analogues (Ogata et al., 1972; Ogata and McConnell, 1972); (b) sulfhydryl reagents (Baldassare et al., 1970); and (c) the heme ligand, nitric oxide (Salhany et al., 1975). Both the binding of organic phosphates to hemoglobin and the environment around the reactive $\beta 93$ sulfhydryl group appear to be strongly dependent upon quaternary structure. Therefore, these measurements can provide a means of monitoring the transition from the T to R structure during ligation of the hemes. Such information on both normal and high-affinity hemoglobins has been useful in testing models of allosteric behavior.

SUBUNIT DISSOCIATION

As discussed in Chapter 1, fully liganded hemoglobin* in solution dissociates readily into dimers:

$$\alpha_2\beta_2 \rightleftharpoons 2\alpha\beta$$

There is ample evidence that the molecule splits at the $\alpha_1\beta_2$ interface. Extremes of pH or denaturing solvent conditions are required to cleave the molecule at the $\alpha_1\beta_1$ interface. In contrast to liganded hemoglobins, deoxyhemoglobin dissociates much less readily into dimers. This difference is due primarily to the inter-subunit salt bonds which stabilize the T structure (Perutz, 1970). As mentioned above and in Table 6–1, many of the high-affinity variants have substitutions at the $\alpha_1\beta_2$ interface. Such structural alterations might be expected to affect the dissociation of the tetramer into dimers. There is convincing evidence that hemoglobins Bethesda (Olson and Gibson, 1972), Kempsey (Bunn et al., 1974), and Chesapeake (Nagel and Gibson, 1972), when fully deoxygenated, dissociate more readily into dimers than does deoxyhemoglobin A. These observations are in accord with other evidence that neither deoxy Bethesda nor deoxy Kempsey can form a stable T quaternary structure. Furthermore, hemoglobin Chesapeake in the liganded state has *decreased* subunit dissociation (Bunn, 1970), indicating that its R structure is relatively more stable than that of hemoglobin A.

The energy of interaction between hemoglobin subunits in the oxy and deoxy states can be linked thermodynamically to the cooperative binding of ligand to hemes (Briehl, 1964; Noble, 1969; Ackers and Halvorson, 1974). As Figure 6–5 indicates, the oxygen affinity of a mutant or chemically modified hemoglobin will be affected if the

*Oxyhemoglobin, carboxyhemoglobin, cyanmethemoglobin.

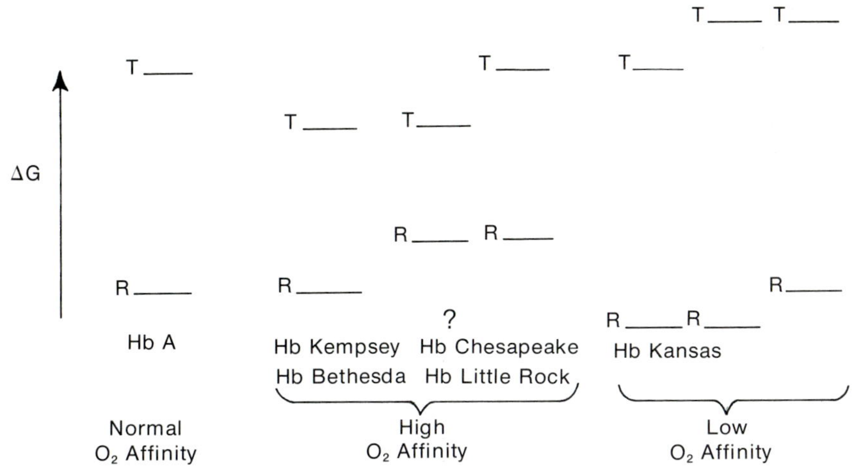

Figure 6–5. Comparison of subunit bonding energies (ΔG) of normal and variant hemoglobins in the oxy (R) and deoxy (T) conformations.

relative stabilities of the R and T structure differ significantly from those of native hemoglobin A. Variants having a relatively unstable T structure like Bethesda and Kempsey will have high oxygen affinity. Similarly, enhanced stability of the R state should also result in high oxygen affinity. Perutz has suggested that the presence of an additional hydrogen bond in oxyhemoglobin Little Rock may be the basis for its high oxygen affinity (Perutz, 1973). If so, this variant in its liganded state should have decreased dissociation into dimers. As mentioned above, this appears to be true for hemoglobin Chesapeake. Greer (1971c) has presented crystallographic evidence that the conformation of oxyhemoglobin Chesapeake differs markedly from that of oxyhemoglobin A, whereas the deoxygenated hemoglobins have very similar three-dimensional structures. However, there are both kinetic (Nagel et al., 1967; Gibson and Nagel, 1974) and NMR data (Ho and Lindstrom, 1972) indicating that deoxy Chesapeake differs significantly from deoxy A. It is likely that both the T and the R forms of this variant have abnormal conformation and subunit interaction. Such a situation is depicted in Figure 6–5.

PHYSIOLOGICAL ASPECTS

In normal man, the oxygen dissociation curve is appropriately poised to permit efficient loading and unloading of oxygen during rest and exercise. Chapter 1 discusses the pathophysiological consequences of significant displacements of the oxygen binding curve. Most commonly, a "shift to the left" or "shift to the right" can be explained by intracellular factors such as alterations in pH and red cell 2,3-DPG or modification of the heme groups, as in carbon monoxide poisoning or methemoglobinemia. In many instances the change in oxygen affinity constitutes an adaptation to some form of environmental stress such as hypoxia. In contrast, individuals with hemoglobin variants of high oxygen affinity exhibit a *primary* displacement of the whole blood oxygen dissociation curve and respond to this molecular lesion with appropriate physiological adjustments. According to the Fick equation cited in Chapter 1, oxygen delivery to tissues (VO_2) is a function of three independent variables:

$$VO_2 = 0.139 \cdot Q \cdot Hb \cdot (S_aO_2 - S_{\bar{v}}O_2)$$

The primary shift to the left in the oxygen dissociation curve results in a marked decrease in oxygen extraction per gram of hemoglobin ($S_aO_2 - S_{\bar{v}}O_2$). Consequently, tissue oxygenation can be maintained by two adjustments: increase in circulating hemoglobin concentration (Hb) or increase in blood flow (Q).

The primary form of compensation appears to be erythrocytosis. An individual with a stable high-affinity variant (normal red cell life span) will have an increase in red cell mass roughly proportional to the "shift to the left" of the whole blood oxygen dissociation curve. This response appears to be mediated through erythropoietin. Adamson et al. (1968, 1969, 1972) have studied individuals with hemoglobins Rainier, Yakima, and Bethesda. The urinary erythropoietin

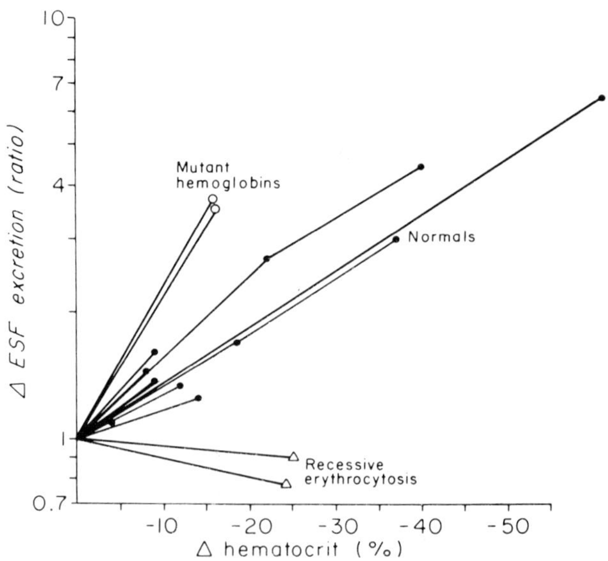

Figure 6–6. Effect of phlebotomy on erythropoietin (ESF) excretion in normal volunteers (●), individuals with high-affinity hemoglobin variants (○), and individuals with autosomal recessive erythrocytosis (△) (see Table 6–4). (From Adamson, J. W., et al.: Blood *41*:641, 1973.)

(ESF) of these polycythemic subjects was normal. However, when these individuals were bled down to a "normal" red cell mass, urinary ESF increased markedly (Fig. 6–6). Similar results have been reported in a patient with hemoglobin Little Rock (Bromberg et al., 1971). These observations attest to the significant hypoxia that these individuals will develop if they are robbed of an important mode of compensation.

Individuals with high-affinity variants have normal arterial oxygen tension. The fact that they develop enhanced erythropoietin production indicates that the sensor for this hormonal regulation must be located in the postarterial region of the renal vasculature (Adamson, 1975).

It is more difficult to assess alterations in blood flow of individuals with high-affinity variants. Total cardiac output and oxygen consumption were found to be normal in a patient with hemoglobin Yakima, whereas the calculated mixed venous oxygen tension was somewhat decreased (Novy et al., 1967). A patient with hemoglobin Little Rock also had a normal resting cardiac output and oxygen consumption but slightly decreased mixed venous oxygen tension (Bromberg et al., 1971). The $P_{\bar{v}}O_2$ dropped more than anticipated when the patient underwent graded exercise. Individuals with hemoglobins Heathrow (White et al., 1973) and Syracuse (Oski, unpublished observations) have been found to have somewhat elevated resting cardiac outputs. The latter patient showed a marked increase in cardiac output during graded exercise. After this patient had been bled down to a normal red cell mass, these measurements became even more abnormal. Changes in total cardiac output do not reflect adjustments in blood flow to specific organs. Individuals with high-affinity variants may have appropriate alterations in regional circulation in order to preserve adequate oxygenation of vital tissues. Recently, a patient with hemoglobin Malmö was shown to have myocardial blood flow that was greater than normal (Kan et al., 1974).

In Chapter 1, a case is made for the importance of red cell 2,3-DPG in the adaptation to hypoxia. However, the high-affinity variants represent one type of hypoxia in which this adaptation does not occur. Red cell 2,3-DPG has been measured in about half the different high-affinity variants and has been consistently normal. It is possible that erythrocytosis provides adequate compensation; however, individuals with this disorder should theoretically derive some benefit from increased red cell 2,3-DPG. An extreme example is depicted in Figure 6–7: these red cells contain half normal hemoglobin A. The remainder of the hemoglobin has extremely high oxygen affinity which fails to form stable mixed hybrid tetramers with normal hemoglobin (e.g., $\alpha_2\beta^A\beta^X$). Such a lack of interaction has been demonstrated for hemoglobins Bethesda (Bunn et al., 1972a) and Kempsey (Bunn et al., 1974b), two variants which are unable to form a

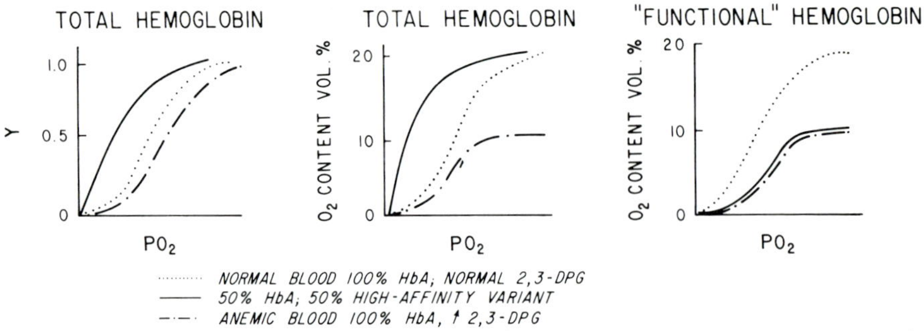

Figure 6–7. Oxygen binding curves of a normal individual (·····), a patient with anemia and increased red cell 2,3-DPG (—·—·—), and a patient with a high affinity variant (———).

stable T structure. In red cells containing such a mixture, the two hemoglobins are oxygenated independently. Furthermore, the high O_2 affinity hemoglobin remains almost fully saturated in all parts of the circulation. Therefore, the abnormal hemoglobin lacks any physiological function and might as well be albumin or some other space-occupying colloid. If so, the individual has a functioning hemoglobin level that is half the total. Such an "anemic" patient should benefit from the interaction of 2,3-DPG on the normal functioning hemoglobin. Actually, in such individuals, red cell 2,3-DPG should be expressed as moles per mole of hemoglobin A, since under physiologic conditions the abnormal hemoglobin remains in the R conformation and fails to interact strongly with 2,3-DPG. Furthermore, several of these variants have impaired interaction with 2,3-DPG (Bunn et al., 1972a, 1974b; Jensen et al., 1975). Viewed in this way, the individual with a high-affinity variant has elevated red cell 2,3-DPG, similar to other patients with anemia!

CLINICAL MANIFESTATIONS

Genetics

Like other structurally abnormal hemoglobins, the high-affinity variants follow an autosomal dominant pattern of inheritance. All affected individuals are heterozygotes; their red cells contain at least as much normal hemoglobin A as the abnormal variant. In most instances the homozygous state would be incompatible with life. A positive family history is very helpful in evaluating a patient for the presence of a high-affinity hemoglobin. However, spontaneous mutations undoubtedly exist. We have seen a girl with hemoglobin Bethesda whose parents were both normal (Bunn et al., 1972a).

Clinical Presentation

The great majority of affected individuals are entirely asymptomatic. Physical examination is unremarkable except for the occasional presence of ruddy complexion. Most commonly, erythrocytosis is detected on a routine blood count. The increase in packed cell volume and red cell mass is generally not severe. Accordingly, affected individuals do not usually have symptoms due to hyperviscosity of the blood. Some individuals with hemoglobin Malmö may be an exception. One patient reliably reported subjective improvement following phlebotomy (Kan et al., 1974). This patient had severe cardiac dysfunction with a history of myocardial infarction, angina, dyspnea, and decreased exercise tolerance. Interestingly, coronary angiography revealed patent vessels except an isolated narrow segment in a branch of the right posterior descending artery. As mentioned in the beginning of this chapter, the first patient in whom this disorder was established had mild angina. However, a survey of the 100-odd individuals that have been reported to date does not indicate a high incidence of myocardial ischemia or any other form of tissue hypoxia.

Some have speculated that in a pregnant woman with a high-affinity variant, the transplacental transport of oxygen may be impaired. In both humans and nearly all other mammals which have been tested, the oxygen affinity of fetal blood is significantly higher than that of maternal blood. The physiological importance of this phenomenon is not well established. There are several instances in which the oxygen binding curve of the mother was shifted to the left of that of the fetus because of an abnormal hemoglobin; these pregnancies were perfectly uneventful and the babies were healthy. An increased incidence of fetal mortality has been reported in a family with hemoglobin Yakima (Jones et al., 1967), but the significance of this is not clear.

Diagnosis

Affected individuals come to the attention of physicians because of unexplained erythrocytosis. Hemoglobin values vary considerably with a mean of about 20 g/100 ml. The increase in red cell mass is less marked than that seen in patients with polycythemia vera. The white count and platelet count are normal and the peripheral blood smear is unremarkable. During the initial evaluation a number of diagnostic possibilities must be ruled out. Table 6–4 is one approach to classifying various types of erythrocytosis. If appropriate clinical and laboratory information does not suggest one of the more common etiologies, the possibility remains that the patient's erythrocytosis is

TABLE 6–4. Differential Diagnosis of Erythrocytosis

I. Autonomous erythroid proliferation (↓ ESF); polycythemia vera
II. Secondary erythroid proliferation
  A. Autonomous or inappropriate increase in ESF
    1. Neoplasm
    2. Renal lesions
    3. Familial erythrocytosis (autosomal recessive inheritance)
  B. Secondary increase in ESF
    1. Hypoxemia (↓ arterial PO_2)
      a. High altitude
      b. Alveolar hypoventilation
      c. Pulmonary disease
      d. Cardiac R→L shunt
    2. Abnormal hemoglobin function (normal arterial PO_2)
      a. High-affinity variants (autosomal dominant inheritance)
      b. Congenital methemoglobinemia
      c. Carboxyhemoglobin (smokers)

due to the presence of a functionally abnormal hemoglobin. The likelihood is considerably strengthened if other blood relatives also have unexplained erythrocytosis. However, not all familial erythrocytosis is due to the presence of a functionally abnormal hemoglobin variant. Adamson (1975) has recently reviewed this subject. There is a very rare entity in which familial erythrocytosis is due to a defect in the humoral regulation of red cell mass (Adamson et al., 1973). Unlike the high-affinity variants, this disorder has an autosomal recessive pattern of inheritance.

If hemoglobin electrophoresis reveals the presence of an abnormal band, the diagnosis is virtually established. However, the failure to demonstrate any electrophoretic abnormality by no means rules out the diagnosis. As Table 6–5 shows, only about half the high-affinity variants that have been reported to date can be separated from hemoglobin A by routine electrophoresis on cellulose acetate or starch gel at pH 8.6. Some variants can be detected if other types of electrophoresis are employed, such as agar gel (pH 6.0) or gel electrofocusing. There remains a group that appear to be electrophoretically silent. These include hemoglobins Olympia, Heathrow, Brigham, and Creteil. Certain tricks can be employed to "separate the unseparable." Garel and his colleagues (1974) have taken advantage of the fact that high-affinity mutants may have an altered reactivity to sulfhydryl reagents. This selective chemical modification permits the hemoglobin variant to be separated on the basis of the surface charge.[1] Variants with reduced Bohr effect will have less of a change in isoelectric point upon deoxygenation than has hemoglobin A. Figure 6–8 shows how this approach was used to enhance the

[1]Rieder et al. (1969) have utilized differential sulfhydryl reactivity to isolate hemoglobin Philly, an unstable variant with a neutral substitution.

TABLE 6–5. *Electrophoretic Properties of High-Affinity Hemoglobin Variants**

Hemoglobin Variant	Electrophoretic Separation from Hb A: *Starch Gel (pH 8.6)*	*Agar Gel (pH 6.0)*	*Gel Electrofocusing*	Reference
Chesapeake (α92 Arg→Leu)	Yes	Yes	Yes	
J-Cape Town (α92 Arg→Gln)	Yes			
Yakima (β99 Asp→His)	Yes			
Kempsey (β99 Asp→Asn)	Yes		Yes	
Ypsilanti (β99 Asp→Tyr)	Yes			
Hiroshima (β146 His→Asp)	Yes	Yes	Yes	
Andrew-Minneapolis (β144 Lys→Asn)	Yes		Yes	
Abruzzo (β143 His→Arg)	Yes			
Rainier (β145 Tyr→Cys)	No	Yes		
Bethesda (β145 Tyr→His)	No	Yes	No	
Little Rock (β143 His→Gln)	No	Yes	Yes	
Malmö (β97 His→Gln)	No	No	Yes	Jeppson and Berglund, 1972
Wood (β97 His→Leu)	No		Yes	Taketa et al., 1975
Syracuse (β143 His→Pro)	No	No	Yes	Jensen et al., 1975
San Diego (B109 Val→Met)	No	No	Yes	Monte et al., 1976
Creteil (β89 Ser→Asn)	No	No	Yes	Monte et al., 1976
Olympia (β20 Val→Met)	No	No	No	
Brigham (β100 Pro→Leu)	No	No	No	
Heathrow (β103 Phe→Leu)	No	No	No	

*Taken from Jensen et al., 1975.

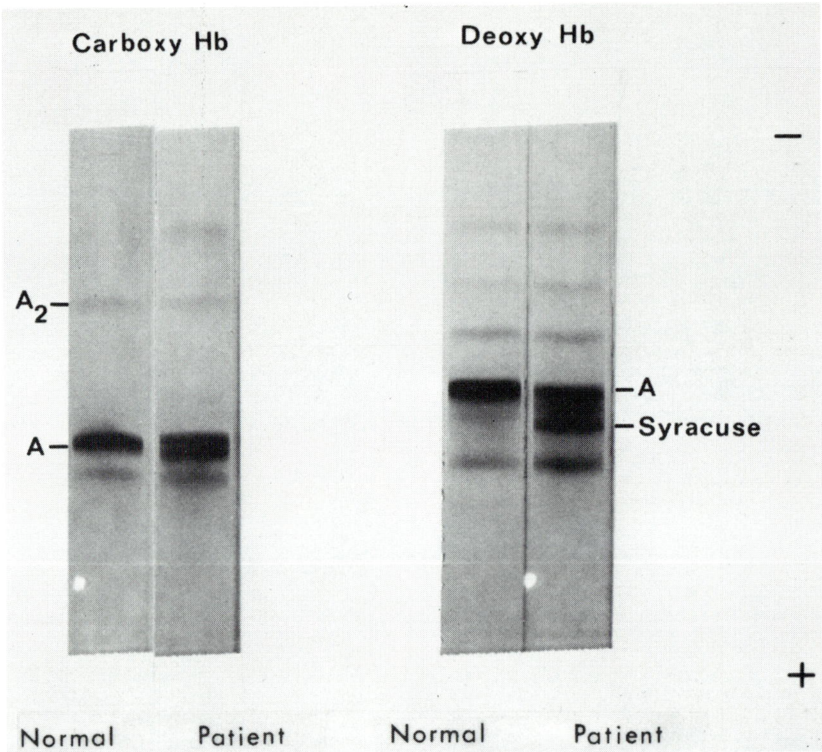

Figure 6–8. Comparison of gel electrofocusing patterns of normal hemolysate and hemolysate of a patient with hemoglobin Syracuse. *Left*, Hemoglobin with CO. *Right*, Deoxygenated hemoglobin. The improved separation of Hb Syracuse from Hb A following deoxygenation is a reflection of the fact that Hb Syracuse has a decreased Bohr effect (see text). (From Jensen, M., et al.: J. Clin. Invest. 55:469, 1975.)

electrophoretic separation of hemoglobin Syracuse from hemoglobin A (Jensen et al., 1975).

Since high-affinity hemoglobins may not be detectable by electrophoresis, measurement of oxygen affinity is required to establish the diagnosis. The relative merits of measurements on whole blood versus phosphate-free hemolysate are discussed in a previous section. If the patient's erythrocytosis is due to a hemoglobin variant, there will be a marked and reproducible "shift to the left" of the oxygen dissociation curve. It is advisable to measure red cell 2,3-DPG to rule out the possibility that the increase in whole blood oxygen affinity is due to an abnormality in red cell metabolism, leading to deficiency of 2,3-DPG. Such a finding would be quite unexpected, since most red cell enzymopathies are associated with nonspherocytic hemolytic anemia. This uncertainty is obviated if oxygen affinity is measured on hemolysate stripped of organic phosphates.

TREATMENT

Once the diagnosis is established, all affected family members should be reassured that they have a benign condition. The great majority of individuals require no treatment at all. However, it is prudent to perform follow-up blood counts at regular intervals. A minority of patients may develop a hematocrit high enough that the viscosity of the blood poses a potential threat. As mentioned earlier, occasional patients have derived subjective benefit from phlebotomy. However, this treatment should be used sparingly, since the increased cell mass is an important mode of compensation. Some affected individuals have been "treated" with radiomimetic drugs such as phosphorus-32 or phenylalanine mustard because they were thought to have polycythemia vera. As Charache (1974a) has pointed out, the avoidance of such inappropriate therapy is one of the important reasons to establish a diagnosis in these patients.

VARIANTS HAVING LOW OXYGEN AFFINITY

The six stable hemoglobin variants that have been found to have abnormally low oxygen affinity are listed in Table 6–6. In addition, a number of the unstable variants and some of the M hemoglobins have been found to have decreased oxygen affinity (see Chapters 5 and 7).

Hemoglobin Kansas is of particular interest, since it has the most abnormal functional properties. In 1961, Reissman, Ruth, and Nomura studied a mother and son with unexplained cyanosis. The subjects were otherwise asymptomatic and had normal hemoglobin levels without any evidence of hemolysis. The cyanosis was explained by an oxygen saturation of only 60 per cent in samples of arterial blood, despite a P_aO_2 of 100 mm Hg. Upon breathing 100 per cent O_2, the oxygen saturation increased by about 35 per cent. These results indicated a marked decrease in whole blood oxygen affinity. At first glance, it is surprising that the red cell mass is "set" at a normal level, in view of such abnormal oxygenation of hemoglobin. However, the amount of oxygen unloaded during the circulation through capillaries is probably within normal limits. Despite the reduced oxygen content of the arterial blood, the shape of the curve permits adequate oxygen release. However, it seems likely that individuals with hemoglobin Kansas would have a limited tolerance to strenuous muscular exercise, which depends upon a marked increase in oxygen unloading.

The structure-function relationships of hemoglobin Kansas have been studied in considerable detail. Bonaventura and Riggs (1968) showed that the structural abnormality was a substitution of threo-

TABLE 6–6. *Stable Hemoglobin Variants Having Decreased Oxygen Affinity*

Variant	Structure	Area Affected	Bohr Effect	Comment	Reference
Titusville	α94 (G1) Asp→Asn	$\alpha_1\beta_2$	Low		Schneider et al., 1975
Providence	β82 (EF6) Leu→Asn,Asp		Low		Charache et al., 1975
Agenogi	β90 (F6) Glu→Lys				Imai et al., 1970
Kansas	β102 (G4) Asn→Thr	$\alpha_1\beta_2$	Normal	Familial cyanosis	Reissman et al., 1961 Bonaventura and Riggs, 1968
Beth Israel	β102 (G4) Asn→Ser	$\alpha_1\beta_2$	Normal	Cyanosis	Nagel et al., 1976
Yoshizuka	β108 (G10) Asn→Asp	$\alpha_1\beta_2$			Imamura et al., 1969

nine for asparagine at β102. Like many of the high-affinity variants, this site is at the $\alpha_1\beta_2$ interface. Indeed, as shown in Figure 6–1, when normal hemoglobin A is oxygenated, β102 Asn forms a hydrogen bond with α94 Asp. Such a bond is not possible in oxyhemoglobin Kansas. Therefore, it is interesting to note that oxyhemoglobin Kansas dissociates more readily into $\alpha\beta$ dimers than does oxyhemoglobin A (Bonaventura and Riggs, 1968). Its low oxygen affinity appears to be due in part to a relatively unstable R structure. In hemoglobin Kansas, the transition from the T to the R structure occurs relatively late in heme ligation. Indeed, in the presence of organic phosphates such as 2,3-DPG and inositol hexaphosphate, fully liganded hemoglobin Kansas has the NMR characteristics of the T structure (Ogawa et al., 1972). Difference Fourier analyses of crystals of deoxyhemoglobin Kansas indicate widespread abnormalities in the T structure (Greer, 1971a). Furthermore, isolated β chains of Kansas subunits also have relatively low oxygen affinity (Riggs and Gibson, 1973). The interpretation of these results is complicated by the fact that these preparations of β subunits showed a considerable amount of kinetic heterogeneity that is unexplained.

Recently, Nagel et al. (1976) have reported a patient with cyanosis due to Hb Beth Israel (β102 Asn $\rightarrow$ Ser). This variant has an amino acid substitution at the same site as Hb Kansas. The functional properties of the two variants are very similar. Hb Beth Israel probably arose as a spontaneous mutation, since neither parent is cyanotic.

Hb Titusville (α94 Asp $\rightarrow$ Asn) (Schneider et al., 1975) appears to have an oxygen affinity nearly as low as that of Hb Kansas and Hb Beth Israel. The amino acid substitution prevents the formation of the bond between α94 and β102 which normally stabilizes oxyhemoglobin (Figure 6–1). As a result, Hb Titusville resembles Hb Kansas in having enhanced dissociation of tetramer into dimers. The proposita had no apparent clinical or hematological abnormalities.

Hemoglobins Yoshizuka (Imamura et al., 1969) and Agenogi (Imai et al., 1970) also have decreased O_2 affinity, although less marked than Hbs Kansas, Beth Israel, or Titusville. Some affected family members have slightly decreased hemoglobin levels. It may be that this "anemia" is the opposite of the polycythemia found in association with high-affinity variants; the enhanced oxygen release provided by the right-shifted curve would reduce the erythropoietin-mediated stimulus to erythropoiesis. Such a mechanism has been offered to explain the anemia in patients with hemoglobin Seattle (Stamatoyannopoulos et al., 1969b), an unstable variant. However, this situation is more complex, since the shortened red cell survival in these individuals also contributes to the reduction in their red cell mass.

Chapter 7

M HEMOGLOBINS

In 1948, a young physician, H. Hörlein, and a medical student, G. Weber, described a family in which certain members had congenital cyanosis. The abnormality was transmitted as an autosomal dominant trait through four generations. The affected individuals had a "lavender-blue" appearance while their blood appeared brown. Hemolysates had absorption spectra which were similar but not identical to that of methemoglobin. Hörlein and Weber proved that the abnormality lay with the globin and not with the heme by forming hybrids of patient's globin with normal heme and patient's heme with normal globin. Only the former produced the spectral changes present in the native hemolysate. These results provided the first convincing evidence of a familial hemoglobinopathy, antedating by one year Itano and Pauling's discovery of the abnormal electrophoretic behavior of Hb S.

In 1955, Singer designated this type of hemoglobin variant as Hb M. Subsequently other examples of Hb M were discovered (Kiese et al., 1956; Gerald et al., 1957; Pisciotta et al., 1959) and were found to have abnormal electrophoretic (Gerald, 1958) as well as spectral properties.

The existence of familial cyanosis having an autosomal dominant inheritance pattern has been recognized in Japan since 1800 (Shibata et al., 1967a). This disorder, called "Kochikuro" (black mouth), was restricted to the prefecture of Iwate in the northeast corner of Honshu. In the 1950's there were about 70 affected individuals residing in this region who had blood "as black as Japanese soy sauce."

The structural analysis of the M hemoglobins was first completed by Gerald and Efron (1961). They identified three variants: M-Boston ($\alpha^{58\ His \rightarrow Tyr}\beta_2$), M-Saskatoon ($\alpha_2\beta_2^{63\ His \rightarrow Tyr}$), and M-Milwaukee-1 ($\alpha_2\beta_2{}^{67\ \mathrm{Val}\rightarrow\mathrm{Glu}}$). Subsequently, the family described by Hörlein and Weber (1948) was shown to have Hb M-Saskatoon. The Japanese with "Kochikuro" were found to have a fourth variant, Hb M-Iwate ($\alpha_2{}^{87\ \mathrm{His}\rightarrow\mathrm{Tyr}}\beta_2$) (Shibata et al., 1964). In 1966, Heller et al. described a fifth M hemoglobin: Hyde Park ($\alpha_2\beta_2{}^{92\ \mathrm{His}\rightarrow\mathrm{Tyr}}$). No other new M hemoglobins have been discovered in subsequent years. The unstable variant Hb St. Louis almost qualifies as an M hemoglobin. The substitution of glutamine for leucine at β28 causes the heme iron in the abnormal subunits to become completely oxidized to methemoglobin (Cohen-Solal et al., 1975). In addition, another unstable variant, Hb Freiburg ($\alpha_2\beta_2{}^{23\ \mathrm{Val}\rightarrow 0}$), has an enhanced tendency toward auto-oxidation (Jones et al., 1966). However, these two hemoglobins lack the clinical, electrophoretic, and spectral properties shared by the five M hemoglobins.

Because individuals affected with one of the M hemoglobins have a distinctive physical appearance they have been discovered

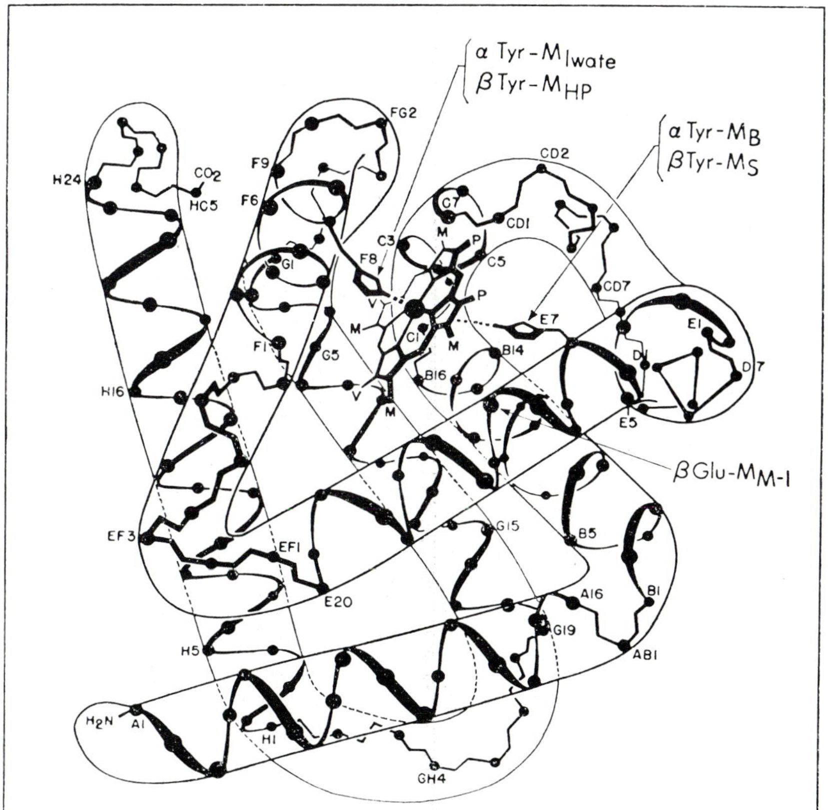

Figure 7–1. Three-dimensional model of hemoglobin subunit modified from Dickerson (1963) showing substituted sites in the M hemoglobins. (From Ranney, H. M., et al.: Proc. First Inter-Am. Symp. on Hemoglobins, 1971.) $M_{HP} = M_{Hyde\ Park}$; $M_{M\text{-}1} = M_{Milwaukee\text{-}1}$; $M_B = M_{Boston}$; $M_S = M_{Saskatoon}$.

quite readily in far-flung parts of the globe. For example, Hb M-Saskatoon has been found in Germany, Canada, Britain, the United States, France, Denmark, Norway, Poland, Italy, South Africa, and Japan (Vella et al., 1974). The various exotic names that have been applied to the M hemoglobins (Table 3–2) provide further testimony to the worldwide distribution of these variants. Understandably, Hb M has only rarely been recognized in blacks (Heller et al., 1966).

As discussed in detail in Chapter 1, the iron atom of the heme group is normally linked to the imidazole group of the proximal (F8) histidine of the α and β chains. Another histidine residue at position E7 is situated on the opposite side, near the sixth coordination position of the heme iron, where oxygen normally binds. Its imidazole group does not form a bond with heme iron unless hemichrome is engendered during hemoglobin denaturation (see Chapter 5). As shown in Figure 7–1, four of the five M hemoglobins involve a substitution of a tyrosine for either the proximal (F8) or distal (E7) histidine in the α or β chain. Gerald and Efron (1961) postulated that the phenolic group of the tyrosine residues are able to form a covalent link with the heme iron, thus stabilizing the atom in the oxidized (Fe^{+++}) form.

STRUCTURE-FUNCTION RELATIONSHIPS

Studies on chemically modified hemoglobins have provided important insights into how the protein functions. Among the most thoroughly investigated are the valence hybrids in which the heme iron of either the α or the β chain has been selectively oxidized and then stabilized by the addition of a heme ligand such as cyanide. For example, in $\alpha_2^{CNMet}\beta_2$, the α-chain hemes are frozen in the oxidized state and only the β chains are able to bind oxygen. These valence hybrids may be suitable analogues of partially oxygenated intermediates such as $Hb(O_2)_2$ which have been so difficult to study. Comparable attention has been devoted to the functional properties of the M hemoglobins which are naturally occurring valence hybrids.

Oxygen Equilibria

Because of the close homology between the structure of the α and β chains, one might expect that mutants having a substitution (His→Tyr) at the proximal heme binding site (F8) would have functional properties similar to each other, yet different from those having the substitution at the distal heme binding site (E7). In fact, the experimental results are totally contrary to this expectation. The oxygen equilibria of the M hemoglobins depend primarily upon which subunit is affected, rather than whether the substitution is at the

TABLE 7–1. *Properties of M Hemoglobins*

	M-Boston	M-Iwate	M-Saskatoon	M-Hyde Park	M-Milwaukee-1
Structure	$\alpha_2^{58\ \mathrm{His \to Tyr}}\beta_2$	$\alpha_2^{87\ \mathrm{His \to Tyr}}\beta_2$	$\alpha_2\beta_2^{63\ \mathrm{His \to Tyr}}$	$\alpha_2\beta_2^{92\ \mathrm{His \to Tyr}}$	$\alpha_2\beta_2^{67\ \mathrm{Val \to Glu}}$
Helical residue	E7	F8	E7	F8	E11
O_2 affinity at P_{50}	Low	Low	Normal	Normal	Low
Bohr effect	Low	Low	Present	Present	Present
Hill's *n*	1.2	1.1	1.2	1.3	1.1–1.3
Quaternary Structure					
Deoxygenated	T*	T*		T*	T*
Oxygenated	T**	T**		R**	R**
Rate of reduction of Fe^{+++} in abn chains†	↓↓	↓↓	↓		↓
Rate of binding of Fe^{+++} in abn chains with cyanide	↓↓	↓↓	↓	↓	
Rate of heat denaturation	↓		↑	↑	Normal

*Determined from x-ray data.

**Assumed but unproved (see text).

†Rate of reduction of Fe^{+++} in abnormal chains with dithionite in presence of CO.

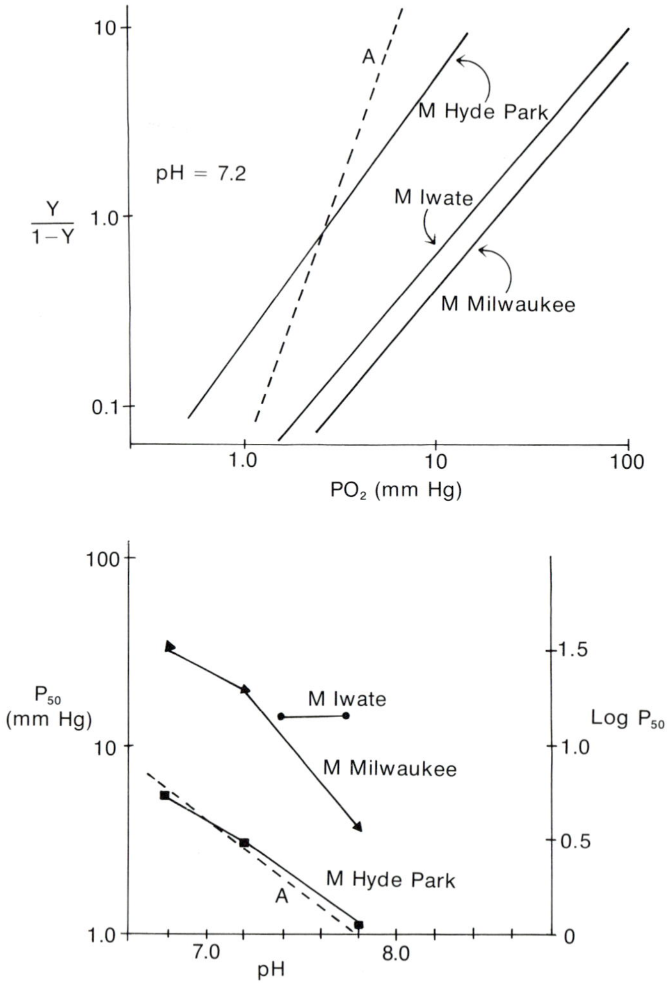

Figure 7–2. Oxygen equilibria of M hemoglobins.

Top Panel, Hill plots of Hbs M Hyde Park (β92 Tyr), M Iwate (α87 Tyr), and M Milwaukee (β67 Glu). Note that all the M hemoglobins have decreased subunit cooperativity as shown by slopes of Hill plots ($n = 1.1–1.3$). In contrast Hb A (– – –) has n of 2.9 (0.1 M PO_4, pH 7.2, 10° C).

Bottom Panel, Relationship of P_{50} to pH. Note that Hb M Hyde Park (■) and Hb M Milwaukee (▲) appear to have a normal Bohr effect ($\Delta \log P_{50}/\Delta$ pH). However, since the M hemoglobins bind only two oxygen molecules, the total number of protons re-upon oxygenation of Hb A is 4 ($\Delta \log P_{50}/\Delta$ pH). Thus, the alkaline Bohr effect of Hbs M Hyde Park and M Milwaukee is about half normal. It is nearly absent in Hb M Iwate (●).

(This figure was constructed from the data of Ranney, H. M., et al.: Biochem. Biophys. Acta *160*:112, 1968b, and Udem, L., et al.: J. Mol. Biol. *48*:489, 1970.)

proximal or distal histidine. The α-chain M hemoglobins (Boston and Iwate), in which only the β chains react with oxygen, have low oxygen affinity and nearly absent Bohr effect (Kikuchi et al., 1964; Suzuki et al., 1965). In contrast, the β-chain variants (Saskatoon and Hyde Park), which carry O_2 only on the α chains, have nearly normal P_{50} and a substantial Bohr effect. (Suzuki et al., 1966; Ranney et al., 1968b.) Representative oxygen binding curves are shown in Figure 7–2. Hemoglobin M-Milwaukee-1 differs from the other two β variants in having low oxygen affinity (Udem et al., 1970) (Table 7–1).

Hill plots of oxygen binding curves of the M hemoglobins reveal n values ranging from 1.1 to 1.3. Since only two of the subunits can bind oxygen, the maximal value of n is 2.0, rather than 4.0 as for Hb A. Even so, the M hemoglobins have markedly reduced subunit cooperativity compared to Hb A.

Whole blood oxygen binding curves of individuals with M hemoglobin tend to be markedly right-shifted, particularly if the variant has low oxygen affinity or if red cell 2,3-DPG is markedly elevated (Byckova et al., 1971). Because of low subunit cooperativity, the M hemoglobin is less saturated at high oxygen tensions compared to Hb A. These factors increase the amount of deoxyhemoglobin in arterial blood and may contribute to the individual's cyanosis.

X-RAY CRYSTALLOGRAPHY

Analysis of the three-dimensional structure of the M hemoglobins by x-ray crystallography has proved useful in explaining their puzzling functional properties. Thus far four of the variants have been examined: M-Hyde Park (Greer, 1971b), M-Iwate (Greer, 1971b), M-Milwaukee-1 (Perutz et al., 1972), and M-Boston (Pulsinelli et al., 1973).

When deoxygenated, both Hb M-Hyde Park (βF8 Tyr) and Hb M-Iwate (αF8 Tyr) are isomorphous with deoxy Hb A. This means that the abnormal oxidized subunit assumes the t tertiary conformation. Hb M-Iwate remains in the T quaternary conformation, even after it is fully oxidized. It is likely that the oxygenated form of Hb M-Iwate ($\alpha_2^M\beta_2^{O_2}$) would also remain in the T structure. The stable T structure of Hb M-Iwate and the failure to switch to the R structure upon oxygen binding explains the low oxygen affinity and absent Bohr effect of this hemoglobin variant. There is some uncertainty about the interaction of the heme group with the tyrosine at F8 or with histidine at E7, since the analysis of Hb M-Iwate was done at relatively low resolution (5.5 Å).

Hb M-Hyde Park differs from Hb M-Iwate in its ability to assume an R conformation when fully oxidized. In view of its full Bohr effect, Hb M-Hyde Park probably switches from the T to the R conformation upon full oxygenation. The x-ray data indicated a loss of about 20 to 30 per cent of the β-chain heme groups. This observation helps to explain the relative instability of Hb M-Hyde Park (Hayashi et al., 1968b). Because of heme loss, the resolution in the vicinity of the β hemes of Hb M-Hyde Park was reduced and therefore the position of the tyrosine at βF8 remains uncertain. However, from the position of the heme group relative to E7-histidine, F8-tyrosine probably does not act as an internal ligand stabilizing the Fe^{+++} atom. On the other hand, the x-ray data on Hb M-Iwate do indicate that such a linkage occurs as predicted by Gerald and Efron (1961). There are kinetic data which support the structural evidence for a difference between Hb M-Hyde Park and Hb M-Iwate in the stability of the internal ligand at F8. For example, both Hb M-Iwate and the other α variant, Hb M-Boston, have a much slower rate of reduction of the abnormal subunit's heme Fe^{+++} than have M-Hyde Park and the other two β-chain M hemoglobins (Shibata et al., 1967; Hayashi et al., 1968a). Secondly, the α-chain M hemoglobins have a very slow rate of reaction with cyanide in keeping with the presence of a strong internal ligand (Hayashi et al., 1967) (see Table 7–1).

The x-ray analysis of Hb M-Boston (αE7 Tyr) produced quite surprising results (Pulsinelli et al., 1973). Deoxygenated Hb M-Boston was isomorphous with deoxyhemoglobin A. The α heme Fe^{+++} was bonded to the phenolate group of E7-tyrosine! The iron atom is displaced to the distal side of the porphyrin ring and is no longer bonded to the proximal (F8) histidine. Thus the Fe^{+++} heme of the abnormal subunit is five-coordinated. These relationships are shown diagrammatically in Figure 7–3. It is likely that Hb M-Boston remains in the T conformation even after it is oxygenated. Pulsinelli et al. (1973) found that the x-ray diffraction pattern of the deoxy crystals

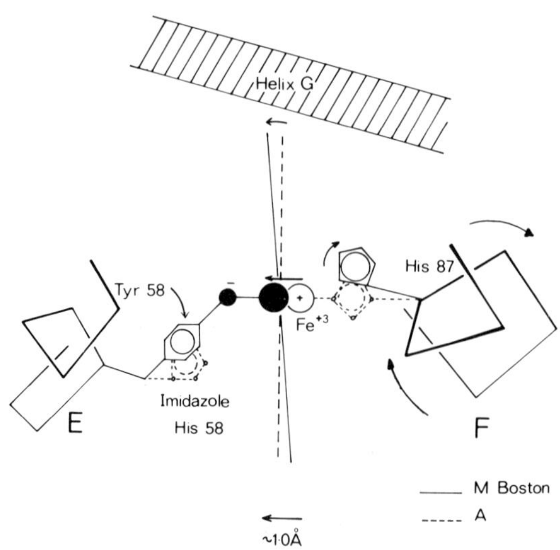

Figure 7–3. Schematic diagram of the abnormal β chain of Hb M Boston showing the relationship of the iron atom to the plane of the porphyrin ring (shown as straight and dotted lines) and the substituted tyrosine at α58 (E7) forming a bond with the iron atom. (From Pulsinelli, P. D., et al.: Proc. Natl. Acad. Sci. USA *70*:3870, 1973.)

was preserved even after exposure to air. Failure to undergo a switch to the R conformation would explain the low oxygen affinity and absent Bohr effect of Hb M-Boston. When Hb M-Boston is chemically reduced to $\alpha_2^{++}\beta_2^{++}$, it has normal heme-heme interaction and near normal Bohr effect (Nishikura et al., 1975). It is likely that the reduced iron (Fe^{++}) binds to the proximal (F8) histidine, since the phenolate group has a relatively weak affinity for Fe^{++}. If so, the iron atom would have to go through the porphyrin ring and come out the other side!

When deoxygenated, Hb M-Milwaukee-1 (βE11 Glu) had a quaternary (T) structure like that of deoxyhemoglobin A (Perutz et al., 1972). The carboxyl group of the substituted glutamic acid at β67 was shown to be coordinated with the heme iron at the sixth position. In contrast, when fully oxidized, Hb M-Milwaukee-1 assumed an R quaternary structure isomorphous with that of oxyhemoglobin A. Thus, the abnormal β chains of Hb M-Milwaukee-1 can form either the t or the r tertiary structure, dependent upon the state of the normal α chain. This conclusion gained strong independent support from optical data (Perutz et al., 1972) showing a shift in the red absorption spectrum contributed by the abnormal β chains when the normal α chains reacted with carbon monoxide. In addition, NMR data of Lindstrom et al. (1972a) indicate that such a change in quaternary conformation occurs when deoxyhemoglobin M-Milwaukee is treated with carbon monoxide. The fact that Hb M-Milwaukee-1 has a substantial Bohr effect is also consistent with this conclusion.

CLINICAL MANIFESTATIONS

Patients have obvious cyanosis but are otherwise totally asymptomatic. A family history will often elicit a dominant inheritance pattern. However, in a number of affected individuals, the M hemoglobin has apparently arisen as a spontaneous mutation (Josephson et al., 1962; Farmer et al., 1964; Becroft et al., 1968; Stavem et al., 1972; Kohne et al., 1975). If the individual's cyanosis was apparent at birth, an α-chain M hemoglobin is likely. The β-chain M hemoglobins do not present clinically until the γ chain has been replaced by β chains at about six months of age.

The blood has a chocolate brown appearance and does not "pink up" when equilibrated with room air. Routine hematological parameters are usually within normal limits. Some but not all individuals with the β-chain M hemoglobins (Hyde Park and Saskatoon) have a mild compensated hemolytic state (Josephson et al., 1962; Hobolth, 1965a, b; Shibata et al., 1967b; Heller, 1969; Stavem et al., 1972), reflecting the fact that these two hemoglobin variants are slightly unstable (Hayashi et al., 1968a). The fact that x-ray crystallography of Hb

M-Hyde Park revealed a partial loss of hemes from the β chains supports this contention. One individual with Hb M-Saskatoon had a significant decrease in hemoglobin following the ingestion of an oxidant drug (Stavem et al., 1972).

Diagnosis

The presumptive diagnosis of M hemoglobin is made from absorption spectra of hemolysate and hemoglobin electrophoresis.

Spectral abnormalities of the M hemoglobins are best seen if all the hemoglobin is oxidized to the Fe^{+++} state with ferricyanide. As Figure 7–4 shows, the absorption spectrum of each of the M hemoglobins differs slightly from the others and can be readily distin-

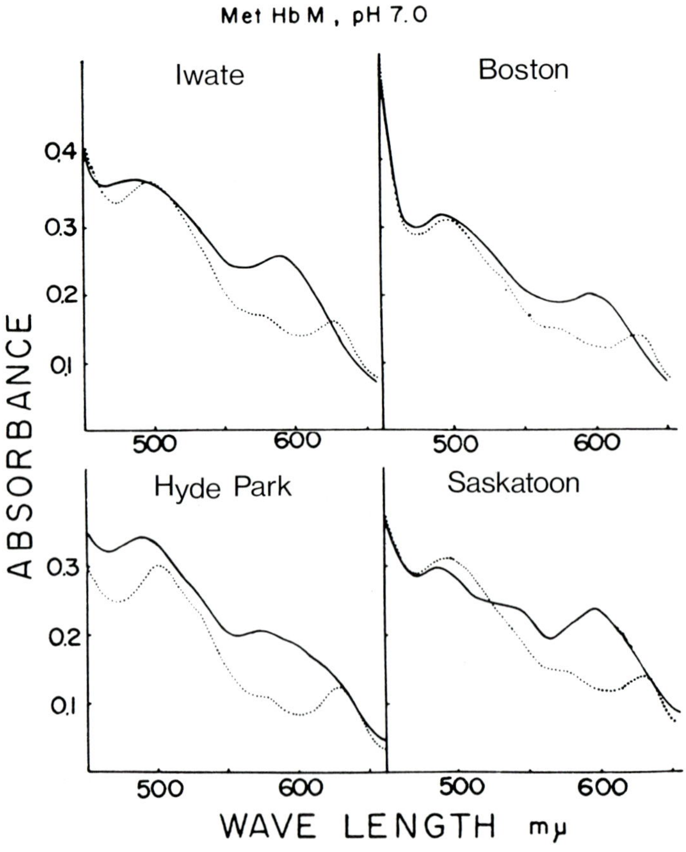

Figure 7–4. Absorption spectra of purified M hemoglobins after they had been fully oxidized with ferricyanide. The absorption spectrum of normal methemoglobin A is shown by the dotted line. (From Shibata, S., et al.: Bull. Yamaguchi Med. Sch. *14*:141, 1967a.)

guished from that of normal methemoglobin. However, it is not possible to identify any of the M hemoglobins on the basis of absorption spectra, since the results are affected by differences in the composition of the buffer and the purity of the sample. Shibata et al. (1967a) have published a very thorough treatment of the spectroscopy of the M hemoglobins. Hayashi et al. (1966) have shown that EPR spectroscopy provides a more specific identification of several of the M hemoglobins.

ELECTROPHORESIS. The M hemoglobins can also be demonstrated by electrophoresis under appropriate conditions. Routine electrophoresis of the oxygenated hemolysate at pH 8.6 usually fails to separate the normal and abnormal hemoglobins. However, electrophoresis on agar gel at pH 7.1 will generally reveal a brown band (Hb M) running slightly on the anodal side of a red band (Hb A). A much sharper pattern can be obtained with gel electrofocusing (Fig. 7–5). A wider separation of M and A hemoglobins is achieved if the hemolysate is oxidized with ferricyanide (Gerald, 1958). Methemoglobin A has a much higher isoelectric point (more positive surface charge) than methemoglobin M, since the Fe^{+++} atoms of the abnormal subunits are neutralized by an internal ligand.

The *differential diagnosis* rests between hemoglobin M and congenital methemoglobinemia (diaphorase I deficiency). The former has a dominant inheritance pattern while the latter has a recessive pattern. The two disorders can be readily distinguished by a spectral analysis of the hemolysate and hemoglobin electrophoresis. Diaphorase I deficiency is discussed in Chapter 1.

Once the presumptive diagnosis of Hb M is made, it is necessary to identify the structural abnormality. The M hemoglobins can be purified by chromatography on Biorex-70. In Dr. Ranney's laboratory the hemolysate is applied to a column equilibrated with sodium phosphate buffer (0.130 M Na^+, pH 6.42) at room temperature. The red Hb A elutes faster than the brown Hbs M, which remain at the top of the column. It is convenient to split the column, once the separation has been achieved, and then elute the purified components. Usually the α-chain M hemoglobins make up 15 to 30 per cent of the total while the β-chain variants make up 40 to 50 per cent (see Figure 3–4). The structural abnormality can be identified from peptide maps of tryptic digests of the abnormal subunit. Specific stains for histidine and tyrosine are very useful in interpreting the fingerprints.

TREATMENT

No specific treatment of these individuals is either indicated or possible. It is important that the patient be thoroughly informed of the benign nature of the disorder. The primary reason for establish-

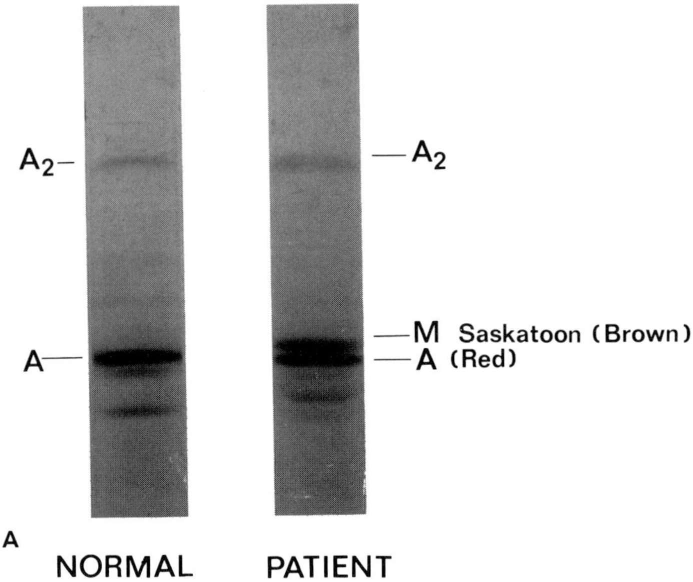

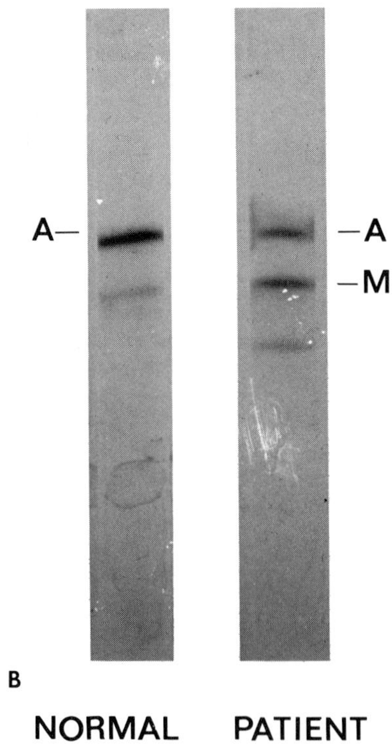

Figure 7–5. Gel electrofocusing patterns obtained on hemolysate of patient with Hb M Saskatoon. *A*, Pattern obtained on oxygenated specimens showing separation of red Hb A band and brown Hb M Saskatoon band. *B*, Pattern obtained after ferricyanide, showing wider separation of Hbs A and M Saskatoon. (The structural analysis of Hb M Saskatoon was done by Dr. Thomas Bradley.)

ing the diagnosis is to provide adequate reassurance and prevent iatrogenic misadventures that might arise under the mistaken impression that the patient has a cardiac or pulmonary disorder. One member of the original family described by Hörlein and Weber was barred from military service during the Franco-Prussian war. Individuals with M hemoglobins have undergone cardiac catheterization (Overly et al., 1967) and even exploratory surgery (Nagel and Bookchin, 1974) because of presumed heart disease. One woman in labor was refused anesthesia because "she was already cyanotic" (Vella et al., 1974). A patient believing she had heart disease declined to have abdominal surgery (Baltzan and Sugarman, 1950). Another unfortunate subject was confined to a bed and chair existence because his solicitous family felt he had a life-threatening illness (Huntsman and Lehmann, 1974).

REFERENCES

Abramson, R. K., Rucknagel, D. L., Shreffler, D. C., et al.: Homozygous Hb J Tongariki: evidence for only one alpha chain structural locus in Melanesians. Science *169*:194, 1970.

Ackers, G. K., and Halvorson, H. R.: Linkage between oxygenation and subunit dissociation in human hemoglobin. Proc. Natl. Acad. Sci. USA *71*:4312, 1974.

Adams, J. G., III: Hemoglobin Ann Arbor: Disturbance in the coordinated biosynthesis of globin chains? Ann. NY Acad. Sci. *241*:232, 1974.

Adams, J. G., III, Winter, W. P., Rucknagel, D. L., et al.: Biosynthesis of hemoglobin Ann Arbor: Evidence for catabolic and feedback regulation. Science *176*:1427, 1972.

Adams, J. G., III, Winter, W. P., Tausk, K., et al.: Hemoglobin Rush (β101[G3] Glutamine): A new unstable hemoglobin causing mild hemolytic anemia. Blood *43*:261, 1974.

Adamson, J. W.: Familial polycythemia. Semin. Hematol. *12*:383, 1975.

Adamson, J. W., and Finch, C. A.: Erythropoietin and the polycythemias. Ann. NY Acad. Sci. *149*:560, 1968.

Adamson, J. W., and Finch, C. A.: Hemoglobin function, oxygen affinity and erythropoietin. Ann. Rev. Physiol. *37*:351, 1975.

Adamson, J. W., and Stamatoyannopoulos, G.: Activation of hemoglobin C synthesis in sheep marrow culture. Science *180*:130, 1973.

Adamson, J. W., Parer, J. T., and Stamatoyannopoulos, G.: Erythrocytosis associated with hemoglobin Rainier: oxygen equilibria and marrow regulation. J. Clin. Invest. *48*:1376, 1969.

Adamson, J. W., Stamatoyannopoulos, G., Kontras, S., et al.: Recessive familial erythrocytosis: aspects of marrow regulation in two families. Blood *41*:641, 1973.

Adamson, S. D., Howard, G. A., and Herbert, E.: The ribosome cycle in a reconstituted cell-free system from reticulocytes. Cold Spring Harbor Symp. Quant. Biol. *37*:547, 1969.

Adamson, S. D., Yau, P. M., Herbert, E., et al.: Involvement of hemin, a stimulatory fraction from ribosomes and a protein synthesis inhibitor in the regulation of hemoglobin synthesis. J. Mol. Biol. *63*:247, 1972.

Akerblöm, O., De Verdier, C. H., Garby, L., et al.: Restoration of defective oxygen-transport function of stored red blood cells by addition of inosine. Scand. J. Clin. Lab. Invest. *21*:245, 1968.

Aksoy, M.: The hemoglobin E syndromes. II. Sickle-cell–hemoglobin E disease. Blood *15*:610, 1960.

Aksoy, M.: The first observation of homozygous hemoglobin S–alpha thalassemia disease and two types of sickle cell thalassemia disease: (a) Sickle cell–alpha thalassemia disease; (b) sickle cell–beta thalassemia disease. Blood *22*:757, 1963.

Aksoy, M.: Thalassemia intermedia: a genetic study in 11 patients. J. Med. Genet. 7:47, 1970.

Aksoy, M., and Erdem, S.: Some problems of hemoglobin patterns in different thalassemic syndromes showing the heterogeneity of beta-thalassemia genes. Ann. NY Acad. Sci. *165*:13, 1969.

Aksoy, M., Erdem, S., Efremov, G. D., et al.: Hemoglobin Istanbul: Substitution of glutamine for histidine in a proximal histidine (F8[92]β). J. Clin. Invest. *51*:2380, 1972.

Alavi, A., Bond, J. P., Kuhl, D. E., et al.: Scan detection of bone marrow infarcts in sickle cell disorders. J. Nucl. Med. *15*:1003, 1974.

Alexanian, R., and Nadell, J.: Oxymetholone treatment for sickle cell anemia. Blood *45*:769, 1975.

Alkjaersig, N., Fletcher, A., Joist, H., and Chaplin, H.: Hemostatic alterations accompanying sickle cell pain crises. J. Lab. Clin. Med. *88*:440, 1976.

Allen, D. W., and Wyman, J.: Equilibre de l'hémoglobine de drepanocytose avec l'oxygène. Rev. Hématol. *9*:155, 1954.

Allison, A. C.: Protection afforded by sickle cell trait against subtertian malarial infection. Br. Med. J. *1*:290, 1954.

Allison, A. C.: Observations on the sickling phenomenon and on the distribution of different haemoglobin types in erythrocyte populations. Clin. Sci. *15*:497, 1956.

Allison, A. C.: Malaria in carriers of the sickle-cell trait and in newborn children. Exp. Parasitol. *6*:418, 1957a.

Allison, A. C.: Properties of sickle-cell haemoglobin. Biochem. J. *65*:212, 1957b.

Alter, B. P., Rappeport, J. M., Huisman, T. H. J., et al.: Fetal erythropoiesis following bone marrow transplantation. Blood *46*:1054, 1975, and Blood *48*:843, 1976.

Alter, B. P., Friedman, S., Hobbins, J. C., et al.: Prenatal diagnosis of sickle-cell anemia and alpha G-Philadelphia. N. Engl. J. Med. *294*:1040, 1976a.

Alter, B. P., Sherman, A. S., Hobbins, J. C., et al.: Prenatal diagnosis of hemoglobinopathies: experience in 17 cases. Clin. Res. *24*:293A, 1976b, and N. Engl. J. Med. *295*: 1437, 1976.

Amiconi, G., Winterhalter, K. H., Antonini, E., et al.: Functional properties of hemoglobin Rainier. FEBS Lett., *21*:341, 1972.

Anderson, N. L.: Hemoglobin San Diego (β109[G11] Val→Met): crystal structure of the deoxy form. J. Clin. Invest. *53*:329, 1974.

Anderson, W. F., Steggles, A., Wilson, G., et al.: Cell-free transcription of human bone marrow chromatin. Ann. NY Acad. Sci. *241*:262, 1974.

Andre, R., Naiman, A., Duhamel, G., et al.: Erythro-leucemie avec hémoglobine H acquise et anomalies des antigènes erythrocytaires. Nouv. Rev. Fr. Hematol. *12*:29, 1972.

Antonovych, T. T.: Ultrastructural changes in glomeruli of patients with sickle cell disease and nephrotic syndrome. In Abstracts, Fifth Annual Meeting, Washington, D.C. The American Society of Nephrology, 1971, p. 3.

Armaly, M. F.: Ocular manifestations in sickle cell disease. Arch. Intern. Med. *133*:670, 1974.

Arnone, A.: X-ray diffraction study of binding of 2,3-diphosphoglycerate to human deoxyhaemoglobin. Nature *237*:146, 1972.

Arnone, A., and Perutz, M. F.: Structure of inositol hexaphosphate—human deoxyhaemoglobin complex. Nature *249*:34, 1974.

Asakura, T., Agarwal, P. L., Relman, D. A., et al.: Mechanical instability of the oxyform of sickle haemoglobin. Nature *244*:437, 1973.

Asakura, T., Ohnishi, T., Friedman, S., et al.: Abnormal precipitation of oxyhemoglobin S by mechanical shaking. Proc. Natl. Acad. Sci. USA *71*:1594, 1974.

Attah, E. B., and Ekere, M. C.: Death patterns in sickle cell anemia. JAMA *233*:889, 1975.

Atwater, J., Schwartz, I. R., Erslev, A. J., et al.: Sickling of erythrocytes in a patient with thalassemia-hemoglobin I disease. N. Engl. J. Med. *263*:1215, 1960.

Azevêdo, E.: Historical note on inheritance of sickle cell anemia. Am. J. Hum. Genet. *25*:457, 1973.

Badr, F. M., Lorkin, P. A., and Lehmann, H.: Haemoglobin P-Nilotic containing a β-δ chain. Nature [New Biol.] *242*:107, 1973.

Baglioni, C.: Chemical studies on haemoglobin D. Biochim. Biophys. Acta *59*:437, 1962a.

Baglioni, C.: The fusion of two peptide chains in hemoglobin Lepore and its interpretation as a genetic deletion. Proc. Natl. Acad. Sci. USA *48*:1880, 1962b.

Baglioni, C.: Correlations between genetics and chemistry of human hemoglobins. In Taylor, H. J. (ed.): Molecular Genetics, Part I. New York, Academic Press, 1963, pp. 405–475.
Baglioni, C., Colombo, B., and Jacobs-Lorena, M.: Chain termination: a test for a possible explanation of thalassemia. Ann. NY Acad. Sci. *165*:212, 1969.
Baine, R. M., Rucknagel, D. L., Dublin, P. A., et al.: Trimodality in the proportion of hemoglobin G Philadelphia in heterozygotes: evidence for heterogeneity in the number of human alpha chain loci. Proc. Natl. Acad. Sci. USA *73*:3633, 1976.
Baker, R., Powers, D., and Haywood, L. J.: Restoration of the deformability of "irreversibly" sickled cells by procaine hydrochloride. Biochem. Biophys. Res. Commun. *59*:548, 1974.
Baldassare, J. J., Charache, S., Jones, R. T., and Ho, C.: Electron paramagnetic resonance studies of spin-labeled hemoglobins. II. Roles of subunit interactions and of intermediate structures in the cooperative oxygenation of hemoglobin and the results on hemoglobin Yakima, hemoglobin J Cape Town and carboxypeptidases A– and B–treated hemoglobin A. Biochemistry *9*:4707, 1970.
Ball, G. V., and Sorenson, L. B.: The pathogenesis of hyperuricemia and gout in sickle cell anemia. Arthritis Rheum. *13*:846, 1970.
Baltzman, D. M., and Sugarman, H.: Hereditary cyanosis. Can. Med. Assoc. J. *62*:348, 1950.
Bank, A., and Marks, P. A.: Excess alpha chain synthesis relative to beta chain synthesis in thalassemia major and minor. Nature *212*:1158, 1966a.
Bank, A., and Marks, P. A.: Protein synthesis in a cell-free human reticulocyte system: ribosome function in thalassemia, J. Clin. Invest. *45*:330, 1966b.
Bank, A., Braverman, S., O'Donnell, J. V., and Marks, P. A.: Absolute rates of globin chain synthesis in thalassemia. Blood *31*:226, 1968.
Bank, A., O'Donnell, J. V., and Braverman, A. D.: Globin chain synthesis in heterozygotes for beta chain mutations. J. Lab. Clin. Med. *76*:616, 1970.
Bank, A., Mears, G., Weiss, R., et al.: Preferential binding of β^S globin chains associated with stroma in sickle cell disorder. J. Clin. Invest. *54*:805, 1974.
Bannerman, R. M.: Abnormalities of heme and pyrrole metabolism in thalassemia. Ann. NY Acad. Sci. *119*:503, 1964.
Bannerman, R. M., Grinstein, M., and Moore, C. V.: Haemoglobin synthesis in thalassemia; *in vitro* studies. Br. J. Haematol. *5*:102, 1959.
Bannerman, R. M., Callender, S. T., Hardisty, R. M., et al.: Iron absorption in thalassemia. Br. J. Haematol. *10*:490, 1964.
Bard, H.: Études préliminaire de la synthèse des hémoglobines foetales et adultes chez le prémature. Union Medicale du Canada *100*:1097, 1971.
Bard, H.: Postnatal fetal and adult hemoglobin synthesis in D1 trisomy syndrome. Blood *40*:523, 1972.
Bard, H.: Postnatal, fetal and adult hemoglobin synthesis in early preterm newborn infants. J. Clin. Invest. *52*:1789, 1973.
Bard, H.: The postnatal decline of hemoglobin F synthesis in normal full-term infants. J. Clin. Invest. *55*:395, 1975.
Bard, H., Makowski, E. L., Meschia, G., et al.: The relative rates of synthesis of hemoglobin A and F in immature red cells of newborn infants. Pediatrics *45*:766, 1970.
Bare, G. H., Alben, J., Bromberg, P. A., et al.: Hemoglobin Little Rock (β143 [H21] His→Gln). Effects of an amino acid substitution at the 2,3-diphosphoglycerate binding site. J. Biol. Chem. *249*:773, 1974.
Bargellesi, A., Pontremoli, S., and Conconi, F.: Absence of beta-globin synthesis and excess of alpha-globin synthesis in homozygous beta-thalassemia. Eur. J. Biochem. *1*:73, 1967.
Bargellesi, A., Pontremoli, S., Menini, C., et al.: Excess of alpha globin synthesis in homozygous beta-thalassemia and its removal from the red blood cell cytoplasm. Eur. J. Biochem. *3*:364, 1968.
Barnes, P. M., Hendrickse, R. G., and Watson-Williams, E. J.: Low-molecular-weight dextran in treatment of bone-pain crises in sickle cell disease: a double-blind trial. Lancet *2*:1271, 1965.
Barnicot, N. A., Wade, P. T., and Cohen, P.: Evidence for a second haemoglobin α-locus duplication in Macaca irus. Nature (London) *228*:379, 1970.

Barreras, L., Diggs, L. W., and Bell, A.: Erythrocyte morphology in patients with sickle cell anemia and pulmonary emboli. JAMA *203*:569, 1968.

Barrett-Connor, E.: Cholelithiasis in sickle cell anemia. Am. J. Med. *45*:889, 1968.

Barrett-Connor, E.: Bacterial infection and sickle cell anemia. Medicine (Baltimore) *50*:97, 1971.

Barrett-Connor, E.: Anemia and infection. Am. J. Med. *52*:242, 1972.

Barrett-Connor, E.: Pneumonia and pulmonary infarction in sickle cell anemia. JAMA *224*:997, 1973.

Barry, M., Flynn, D. M., Letsky, E. A., et al.: Long-term chelation therapy in thalassemia major: effect on liver iron concentration, liver histology and clinical progress. Br. Med. J. *2*:16, 1974.

Basch, R. A.: Hemoglobin synthesis in short term cultures of human fetal hematopoietic tissues. Blood *39*:530, 1972.

Basu, A. K., and Woodruff, A. W.: Effect of pyrexia on sicklaemic states. Lancet *ii*:1088, 1963.

Bauer, C.: Antagonistic influence of CO_2 and 2,3-diphosphoglycerate on the Bohr effect of human haemoglobin. Life Sci. *8*:1041, 1969.

Bauer, C., Ludwig, I., and Ludwig, M.: Different effects of 2,3-diphosphoglycerate and adenosine triphosphate on the oxygen affinity of adult and foetal human haemoglobin. Life Sci. *7*:1339, 1968.

Baur, E. W., and Motulsky, A. G.: Hemoglobin Tacoma—a β chain variant associated with increased Hb A_2. Humangenetik *1*:621, 1965.

Beard, M. E. J., Necheles, T. F., and Allen, D. M.: Clinical experience with intensive transfusion therapy in Cooley's anemia. Ann. NY Acad. Sci. *165*:415, 1969.

Beaven, G. H., Stevens, B. L., Dance, H., and White, J. C.: Occurrence of haemoglobin H in leukaemia. Nature *199*:1297, 1963.

Beaven, G. H., Hornabrook, R. W., Fox, R. H., et al.: Occurrence of heterozygotes and homozygotes for the alpha chain haemoglobin variant Hb J (Tongariki) in New Guinea. Nature (London) *235*:46, 1972.

Beck, W. S. (ed.): Hematology. 2nd ed. Boston, MIT Press, 1976.

Becroft, D. M. O., Douglas, R., Carrell, R. W., and Lehmann, H.: Haemoglobin M Hyde Park: A hereditary methaemoglobinaemia in a Caucasian child. NZ Med. J. *68*:72, 1968.

Beet, E. A.: The genetics of the sickle cell trait in a Bantu tribe. Ann. Eugen. *14*:279, 1949.

Bellingham, A. J., and Huehns, E. R.: Compensation in haemolytic anaemias caused by abnormal haemoglobins. Nature *218*:924, 1968.

Bellingham, A. J., Detter, J. C., and Lenfant, C.: The role of hemoglobin affinity for oxygen and red-cell 2,3-diphosphoglycerate in the management of diabetic ketoacidosis. Trans. Assoc. Am. Physicians *83*:113, 1970.

Bellingham, A. J., Detter, J. C., and Lenfant, C.: Regulatory mechanisms of hemoglobin oxygen affinity in acidosis and alkalosis. J. Clin. Invest. *50*:700, 1971.

Beltrami, C. A., Bearzi, I., and Fabris, G.: Storage cells of spleen and bone marrow in thalassemia: an ultrastructural study. Blood *41*:901, 1973.

Benesch, R., and Benesch, R. E.: The effect of organic phosphates from the human erythrocyte on the allosteric properties of hemoglobin. Biochem. Biophys. Res. Commun. *26*:162, 1967.

Benesch, R., and Benesch, R. E.: Intracellular organic phosphates as regulators of oxygen release by haemoglobin. Nature (London) *221*:618, 1969.

Benesch, R., Benesch, R. E., and Yung, S.: Chemical modifications that inhibit gelation of sickle hemoglobin. Proc. Natl. Acad. Sci. USA *71*:1504, 1974.

Benesch, R. E., Yung, S., Benesch, R., et al.: α-Chain contacts in the polymerisation of sickle haemoglobin. Nature *260*:219, 1976.

Bennett, M. A., Heslop, R. W., and Meynell, M. J.. Massive haematuria associated with sickle-cell trait. Br. Med. J. *1*:677, 1967.

Bentley, S. A., Lewis, S. M., and White, J. M.: Red cell survival studies in patients with unstable hemoglobin disorders. Br. J. Haematol. *26*:85, 1974.

Benz, E. J., Jr., and Forget, B. G.: Defect in messenger RNA for human hemoglobin synthesis in beta thalassemia. J. Clin. Invest. *50*:2755, 1971.

Benz, E. J., Jr., and Forget, B. G.: The biosynthesis of hemoglobin. Semin. Hematol. *11*:463, 1974.

Benz, E. J., Jr., and Forget, B. G.: The molecular genetics of the thalassemia syndromes. *In* Brown, E. B. (ed.): Progress in Hematology. New York, Grune & Stratton, Vol IX, p. 107, 1975.

Benz, E. J., Jr., Swerdlow, P. S., and Forget, B. G.: Globin messenger RNA in Hb H disease. Blood *42*:825, 1973.

Benz, E. J., Jr., Housman, D., Pritchard, J., and Forget, B. G.: Non-functioning globin messenger RNA for Lepore globin chains in Hb Lepore-β°-thalassemia. Clin. Res. *23*:269A, 1975a.

Benz, E. J., Jr., Swerdlow, P. S., and Forget, B. G.: Absence of functional messenger RNA activity for beta globin chain synthesis in β^{0}-thalassemia. Blood *45*:1, 1975b.

Beresford, C. H., Clegg, J. B., and Weatherall, D. J.: Haemoglobin Ocho Rios (β52 (D3) aspartic acid→alanine): A new β chain variant of haemoglobin A found in combination with haemoglobin S. J. Med. Genet. *9*:151, 1972.

Beretta, A., Prato, V., Gallo, E., and Lehmann, H.: Haemoglobin Torino – α43 (CD1) phenylalanine→valine. Nature *217*:1016, 1968.

Bernini, L., Colucci, C. F., deMichele, D., et al.: A possible case of alpha-beta thalassemia. Acta Genet. Stat. Med. *12*:202, 1962.

Berns, A., Salden, M., Bogdanovsky, D., et al.: Non-specific stimulation of cell-free protein synthesis by a dialyzable factor isolated from reticulocyte initiation factors (iRNA). Proc. Natl. Acad. Sci. USA *72*:714, 1975.

Bernstein, J., and Whitten, C. F.: A histologic appraisal of the kidney in sickle cell anemia. Arch. Pathol. *70*:407, 1960.

Bertles, J. F., and Döbler, J.: Reversible and irreversible sickling: A distinction by electron microscopy. Blood *33*:884, 1969.

Bertles, J. F., and Milner, P. F. A.: Irreversibly sickled erythrocytes: a consequence of the heterogeneous distribution of hemoglobin types in sickle cell anemia. J. Clin. Invest. *47*:1731, 1968.

Bertles, J. F., Rabinowitz, R., and Döbler, J.: Hemoglobin interaction: modification of solid phase composition in the sickling phenomenon. Science *169*:375, 1970.

Beutler, E.: The effect of methemoglobin formation in sickle cell disease. J. Clin. Invest. *40*:1856, 1961.

Beutler, E., and Wood, L. A.: The in vivo regeneration of red cell 2,3-diphosphoglyceric acid after transfusion of stored blood. J. Lab. Clin. Med. *74*:300, 1969.

Beutler, E., Johnson, C., Powars, D., and West, C.: Prevalence of glucose-6-phosphate dehydrogenase deficiency in sickle cell disease. N. Engl. J. Med. *290*:826, 1974a.

Beutler, E., Lang, A., and Lehmann, H.: Hemoglobin Duarte ($\alpha_2\beta_2{}^{62}$ [E6] Ala→Pro): A new unstable hemoglobin with increased oxygen affinity. Blood *43*:527, 1974b.

Beuzard, Y., Courvalin, J. C., Cohen-Solal, M., et al.: Structural studies on hemoglobin St. Etienne (β92 [F8] His→Gln): a new abnormal hemoglobin with loss of β proximal histidine and absence of heme on the β chain. FEBS Lett. *27*:76, 1972.

Bhoyroo, S. I., and Storrs, C. N.: Adult and fetal haemoglobin haemolytic disease of the newborn. Arch. Dis. Child. *46*:570, 1971.

Bilinski, R. T., Kandel, G. L., and Rabiner, S. F.: Epsilon aminocaproic acid therapy of hematuria due to heterozygous sickle cell diseases. J. Urol. *102*:93, 1969.

Bird, G. W. G., and Lehmann, H.: Haemoglobin D in India. Br. Med. J. *1*:514, 1956.

Bishop, J. O., and Jones, K. W.: Chromosomal localization of human haemoglobin structural genes. Nature *240*:149, 1972.

Bishop, J. O., and Rosbash, M.: Reiteration frequency of duck haemoglobin genes. Nature [New Biol.] *241*:204, 1973.

Blendis, L. M., Modell, C. B., Bowdler, A. J., and Williams, R.: Some effects of splenectomy in thalassaemia major. Br. J. Haematol. *28*:77, 1974.

Blum, N., Maleknia, M., Schapira, G., et al.: α- et β-globines libres et biosynthèse de l'hémoglobine. Biochim. Biophys. Acta *199*:236, 1970.

Blum, M., Kneip, B., and Schapira, G.: Influence d'origine specifique des chaines α d'hémoglobine sur la biosynthèse de l'hémoglobine de lapin. Biochimie *54*:1121, 1972.

Blunt, M. H., and Evans, J. V.: Changes in the concentration of potassium in the erythrocyte and in haemoglobin type in Merino sheep under a severe anaemic stress. Nature *200*:1215, 1963.

Boggs, D. R., Hyde, F., and Srodes C.: An unusual pattern of neutrophil kinetics in sickle cell anemia. Blood *41*:59, 1973.

Bohr, C., Hasselbalch, K., and Krogh, A.: Ueber einen in biologischer Beziehung wichtigen Einfluss, den die Kohlensäurespannung des Blutes auf dessen Sauerstoffbindung übt. Skand. Arch. Physiol. *16*:402, 1904.

Bonaventura, J., and Riggs, A.: Hemoglobin Kansas, a human hemoglobin with a neutral amino acid substitution and an abnormal oxygen equilibrium. J. Biol. Chem. *243*: 980, 1968.

Bookchin, R. M., and Nagel, R. L.: Ligand-induced conformational dependence of hemoglobin in sickling interactions. J. Mol. Biol. *60*:263, 1971.

Bookchin, R. M., and Nagel, R. L.: Conformational requirements for the polymerization of hemoglobin S: Studies of mixed liganded hybrids. J. Mol. Biol. *76*:233, 1973a.

Bookchin, R., and Nagel, R. L.: Molecular interactions of sickling hemoglobins. In Abramson, H., Bertles, J. F., and Wethers, D. L. (eds.): Sickle Cell Disease. St. Louis, The C. V. Mosby Co., 1973b, p. 140.

Bookchin, R. M., Nagel, R. L., and Ranney, H. M.: Structure and properties of hemoglobin C-Harlem, a human hemoglobin variant with amino acid substitutions in 2 residues of the β-polypeptide chain. J. Biol. Chem. *242*:248, 1967.

Bookchin, R. M., Nagel, R. L., and Ranney, H. M.: The effect of $\beta^{73\ \mathrm{Asn}}$ on the interactions of sickling hemoglobins. Biochim. Biophys. Acta *221*:373, 1970.

Bookchin, R. M., Nagel, R. L., and Balazs, T.: Role of hybrid tetramers in gelation of deoxy Hb mixtures containing hemoglobin S. Blood *44*:942 (Abst.), 1974.

Bookchin, R. M., Nagel, R. L., and Balazs, T.: Role of hybrid tetramer formation in gelation of haemoglobin S. Nature *256*:667, 1975.

Boyer, S. H., Rucknagel, D. L., Weatherall, D. J., et al.: Further evidence for linkage between the β and δ loci governing human hemoglobin and the population dynamics of linked genes. Am. J. Hum. Genet. *15*:438, 1963.

Boyer, S. H., Hathaway, P., Pascasio, F., et al.: Differences in the amino acid sequences of tryptic peptides from three sheep hemoglobin β chains. J. Biol. Chem. *242*:2211, 1967.

Boyer, S. H., Belding, T. K., Margolet, L., and Noyes, A. N.: Fetal hemoglobin restriction to a few erythrocytes (F cells) in normal human adults. Science *188*:361, 1975.

Bradley, T. B., and Rieder, R. F.: Hemoglobin Gun Hill: a β chain abnormality associated with a hemolytic state. Blood *28*:975, 1966.

Bradley, T. B., Brawner, J. N., and Conley, C. L.: Further observations on an inherited anomaly characterized by persistence of fetal hemoglobin. Bull. Johns Hopkins Hosp. *108*:242, 1961.

Bradley, T. B., Wohl, R. C., and Rieder, R. F.: Hemoglobin Gun Hill: Deletion of five amino acid residues and impaired heme-globin binding. Science *157*:1581, 1967.

Bradley, T. B., Wohl, R. C., Murphy, S. B., et al.: Properties of hemoglobin Bryn Mawr, $\beta^{85\ \mathrm{Phe} \rightarrow \mathrm{Ser}}$, a new spontaneous mutation producing an unstable hemoglobin with high oxygen affinity. Blood *40*:947, 1972.

Bradley, T. B., Wohl, R. C., and Smith, G. J.: Elongation of the α-globin chain in a Black family: interaction with Hb G-Philadelphia. Clin. Res. *23*:131A, 1975.

Bratu, V., Lorkin, P. A., Lehmann, H., and Predescu, C.: Haemoglobin Buchuresti, β42 (CD1) Phe→Leu, a cause of unstable haemoglobin haemolytic anaemia. Biochim. Biophys. Acta *251*:1, 1971.

Braverman, A. S., and Bank, A.: Changing rates of globin chain synthesis during erythroid cell maturation in thalassemia. J. Mol. Biol. *42*:57, 1969.

Braverman, A. S., McCurdy, P. R., Manos, O., et al.: Homozygous beta-thalassemia in American blacks: the problem of mild thalassemia. J. Lab. Clin. Med. *81*:857, 1973.

Brewer, G. J., and Oelshlegel, F. J., Jr.: Antisickling effects of zinc. Biochem. Biophys. Res. Commun. *58*:854, 1974.

Briehl, R. W., and Ewert, S.: Effects of pH, 2,3-diphosphoglycerate and salts on gelation of sickle cell deoxyhemoglobin. J. Mol. Biol. *80*:445, 1973.

Briehl, R. W., and Ewert, S. M.: Gelation of sickle cell hemoglobin. II. Methemoglobin. J. Mol. Biol. *89*:759, 1974.

Briehl, R. W., and Salhany, J. M.: R-T conformational switch in nitrosyl hemoglobin S as judged by gelation. Fed. Proc. *34*:654, (Abst. 2471) 1975.

Brimhall, B., Jones, R. T., Baur, E. W., and Motulsky, A. G.: Structural characterization of hemoglobin Tacoma. Biochemistry *8*:2125, 1969.

Brittain, H. P., de la Torre, A., and Willey, E. N.: A case of sickle cell disease with an abscess arising in an infarct of the liver. Ann. Intern. Med. *65*:560, 1966.

Brittenham, G., Lozoff, B., and Narasimhan, S.: Sickle cell disease among the Veddoid groups of South India. In Hechter, J. I., Schechter, A. N., Eaton, W. A., et al. (eds.): Proceedings of First National Symposium on Sickle Cell Disease. Washington, D.C. DHEW Pub. No. 75–723 (NIH), Bethesda, Md., 1974, p. 257.
Brody, J. I., Goldsmith, M. H., Park, S. K., et al.: Symptomatic crises of sickle cell anemia treated by limited exchange transfusion. Ann. Intern. Med: *72*:327, 1970.
Bromberg, P. A.: Pulmonary aspects of sickle cell disease. Arch. Intern. Med. *133*:652, 1974.
Bromberg, P. A., and Jensen, W. N.: Arterial oxygen unsaturation in sickle cell disease. Am. Rev. Respir. Dis. *96*:400, 1967a.
Bromberg, P. A., and Jensen, W. N.: Blood oxygen dissociation curves in sickle cell disease. J. Lab. Clin. Med. *70*:480, 1967b.
Bromberg, P. A., Padilla, F., Guy, J. T., and Balcerzak, S. P.: Effect of a new hemoglobin (Hb Little Rock) on the physiology of oxygen delivery. J. Lab. Clin. Med. *78*:837, 1971.
Bromberg, P. A., Alben, T. O., Bare, G. H., et al.: High oxygen affinity variant of haemoglobin Little Rock with unique properties. Nature [New Biol.] *243*:177, 1973.
Bromberg, Y. M., Abrahamov, A., and Salzberger, M.: The effect of maternal anoxaemia on the foetal haemoglobin of the newborn. J. Obstet. Gynaecol. Br. Commonw. *63*: 875, 1956.
Brook, C. G. D., Thompson, E. N., Marshall, W. C., et al.: Growth in children with thalassemia major and effect of two different transfusion regimens. Arch. Dis. Child. *44*:612, 1969.
Brown, M. J., Weatherall, D. J., Clegg, J. B., et al.: Benign sickle cell anaemia. Br. J. Haematol. *22*:635, 1972.
Bruns, G. P., and London, I. M.: The effect of hemin on the synthesis of globin. Biochem. Biophys. Res. Commun. *18*:236, 1965.
Buckalew, V. M., and Someren, A.: Renal manifestations of sickle cell disease. Arch. Intern. Med. *133*:660, 1974.
Bunn, H. F.: Effect of sulfhydryl reagents on binding of human hemoglobin to haptoglobin. J. Lab. Clin. Med. *70*:606, 1967.
Bunn, H. F.: Dissociation of haemoglobin Chesapeake into subunits. Nature *227*:839, 1970.
Bunn, H. F.: The interaction of sickle hemoglobin with DPG, CO_2 and with other hemoglobins: formation of asymmetrical hybrids. In Brewer, G. J. (ed.): Hemoglobin and Red Cell Structure and Function. New York, Plenum Press, 1972, p. 41. (Adv. Exp. Med. Biol., Vol. 28.)
Bunn, H. F., and Briehl, R. W.: The interaction of 2,3-diphosphoglycerate with various human hemoglobins. J. Clin. Invest. *49*:1088, 1970.
Bunn, H. F., and Jandl, J. H.: Exchange of heme among hemoglobins and between hemoglobin and albumin. J. Biol. Chem. *243*:465, 1968.
Bunn, H. F., and Kitchen, H.: Hemoglobin function in the horse: the role of 2,3-diphosphoglycerate in modifying the oxygen affinity of maternal and fetal blood. Blood *42*:471, 1973.
Bunn, H. F., and McDonough, M.: Asymmetrical hemoglobin hybrids. An approach to the study of subunit interactions. Biochemistry *13*:988, 1974.
Bunn, H. F., Esham, W. T., and Bull, R. W.: The renal handling of hemoglobin. I. Glomerular filtration. J. Exp. Med. *129*:909, 1969a.
Bunn, H. F., May, M. H., Kocholaty, W., and Shields, C. E.: Hemoglobin function in stored blood. J. Clin. Invest. *48*:311, 1969b.
Bunn, H. F., Ransil, B. J., and Chao, A.: The interaction between erythrocyte organic phosphates, magnesium ion and hemoglobin. J. Biol. Chem. *246*:5273, 1971.
Bunn, H. F., Bradley, T. B., Davis, W. E., et al.: Structural and functional studies on hemoglobin Bethesda ($\alpha_2\beta_2{}^{145\ His}$), a variant associated with compensatory erythrocytosis. J. Clin. Invest. *51*:2299, 1972a.
Bunn, H. F., Meriwether, W. D., Balcerzak, S. P., and Rucknagel, D. L.: Oxygen equilibrium of hemoglobin E. J. Clin. Invest. *51*:2984, 1972b.
Bunn, H. F., Wohl, R. C., Bradley, T. B., et al.: Functional properties of hemoglobin Kempsey. J. Biol. Chem. *249*:7402, 1974b.
Bunn, H. F., Haney, D. N., Gabbay, K. H., and Gallop, P.: Further identification of the nature and linkage of the carbohydrate in hemoglobin A_{Ic}. Biochem. Biophys. Res. Commun. *67*:103, 1975a.

Bunn, H. F., Schmidt, G. J., Haney, D. N., et al.: Hemoglobin Cranston, an unstable variant having an elongated β chain due to nonhomologous crossover between two normal β chain genes. Proc. Natl. Acad. Sci. USA *72*:3609, 1975b.

Burka, E. R., and Marks, P. A.: Ribosomes active in protein synthesis in human reticulocytes: a defect in thalassemia major. Nature *199*:706, 1963.

Burkert, L. B., Sharma, V. S., Pisciotta, A. V., et al.: Hemoglobin Mequon β41 (C7) Phenylalanine→Tyrosine. Clin. Res. *22*:176 (Abst.), 1974.

Byckova, V., Wajcman, H., Labie, D., et al.: Hemoglobin M Saskatoon: further data on biophysics and oxygen equilibrium. Biochim. Biophys. Acta *243*:117, 1971.

Campbell, J. H., and Cummins, S. D.: Priapism in sickle cell anemia. J. Urol. *66*:697, 1951.

Capp, G. L., Rigas, D. A., and Jones, R. T.: Hemoglobin Portland 1: a new human hemoglobin unique in structure. Science *157*:65, 1967.

Capp, G. L., Rigas, D. A., and Jones, R. T.: Evidence for a new haemoglobin chain (ζ-chain). Nature *228*:278, 1970.

Card, R., and Brain, M.: The "anemia" of childhood. N. Engl. J. Med. *288*:388, 1973.

Carrell, R. W., and Kay, R.: A simple method for the detection of unstable hemoglobins. Br. J. Haematol. *23*:615, 1972.

Carrell, R. W., and Owen, M. C.: A new approach to haemoglobin variant identification. Haemoglobin Christchurch β71 (E15) Phenylalanine→Serine. Biochim. Biophys. Acta *236*:507, 1971.

Carrell, R. W., Lehmann, H., and Hutchison, H. E.: Haemoglobin Köln (β98 Valine→ Methionine): an unstable protein causing inclusion-body anaemia. Nature *210*:915, 1966.

Carrell, R. W., Lehmann, H., Lorkin, P. A., et al.: Haemoglobin Sydney: β67 (E11) Valine→Alanine: An emerging pattern of unstable haemoglobins. Nature *215*:626, 1967.

Cathie, I. A. B.: Apparent idiopathic Heinz body anemia. Great Ormond St. J. *3*:43, 1952.

Cerami, A., and Manning, J. M.: Potassium cyanate as an inhibitor of the sickling of erythrocytes *in vitro*. Proc. Natl. Acad. Sci. USA *68*:1180, 1971.

Chalevelakis, G., Clegg, J. B., and Weatherall, D. J.: Imbalanced globin chain synthesis in heterozygous β-thalassemic bone marrow. Proc. Natl. Acad. Sci. USA *72*:3853, 1975.

Chan, E., and Desforges, J.: Role of disulfide bonds in Heinz body attachment to membranes. Blood *44*:921, 1974.

Chang, H., Hobbins, J. C., Cividalli, G., et al.: In utero diagnosis of hemoglobinopathies. Hemoglobin synthesis in fetal red cells. N. Engl. J. Med. *290*:1067, 1974.

Chang, H., Modell, C. B., Alter, B. P., et al.: Expression of the β-thalassemia gene in the first trimester fetus. Proc. Natl. Acad. Sci. USA *72*:3633, 1975.

Chanutin, A., and Curnish, R. R.: Effect of organic and inorganic phosphates on the oxygen equilibrium of human erythrocytes. Arch. Biochem. Biophys. *121*:96, 1967.

Charache, S.: Haemoglobins with altered oxygen affinity. Clin. Haematol. *3*:357, 1974a.

Charache, S.: A manifestation of abnormal hemoglobins of man: altered oxygen affinity. Hemoglobin Chesapeake: from the clinic to the laboratory and back again. Ann. NY Acad. Sci. *241*:449, 1974b.

Charache, S.: The treatment of sickle cell anemia. Arch. Intern. Med. *133*:698, 1974c.

Charache, S., and Conley, C. L.: Rate of sickling of red cells during deoxygenation of blood from persons with various sickling disorders. Blood *24*:25, 1964.

Charache, S., and Conley, C. L.: Factors leading to vascular occlusion in sickle cell anemia. In Brewer, G. J. (ed.): Erythrocyte Structure and Function. (Third International Conference on Red Cell Metabolism and Function, University of Michigan, 1974–1975.) A. R. Liss, 1975, p. 243.

Charache, S., and Page, D. L.: Infarction of bone marrow in the sickle cell disorders. Ann. Intern. Med. *67*:1195, 1967.

Charache, S., and Weatherall, D. J.: Fast hemoglobin in lead poisoning. Blood *28*:377, 1966.

Charache, S., Weatherall, D. J., and Clegg, J. B.: Polycythemia associated with a hemoglobinopathy. J. Clin. Invest. *45*:813, 1966.

Charache, S., Conley, C. L., Waugh, D. F., et al.: Pathogenesis of hemolytic anemia in homozygous hemoglobin C disease. J. Clin. Invest. *46*:1795, 1967.

Charache, S., Mondzac, A. M., and Gessner, U.: Hemoglobin Hasharon ($\alpha_2^{47\ \mathrm{His}}$ [CD5] β_2): a hemoglobin found in low concentration. J. Clin. Invest. *48*:834, 1969.

Charache, S., Grisolia, S., Fiedler, A. J., and Hellegers, A.: Effect of 2,3-diphosphoglycerate on oxygen affinity of blood in sickle cell anemia. J. Clin. Invest. *49*:806, 1970.
Charache, S., Brimhall, B., and Milner, P.: Hemoglobin Okaloosa (β48(CD7) Leucine→Arginine): An unstable variant with low oxygen affinity. J. Clin. Invest. *52*:2858, 1973.
Charache, S., Brimhall, B., and Jones, R. T.: Polycythemia produced by hemoglobin Osler (β145 [HC2] Tyr→Asp). Johns Hopkins Med. J. *136*:132, 1975a.
Charache, S., Clegg, J. B., Weatherall, D. J., and Conley, C. L.: Unbalanced globin synthesis in hereditary persistence of fetal hemoglobin. Clin. Res. *23*:587A, 1975b.
Charache, S., Duffy, T. R., Jander, N., et al.: Toxic-therapeutic ratio of sodium cyanate. Arch. Intern. Med. *135*:1043, 1975c.
Charache, S., McCurdy, P., and Fox, J.: Hemoglobin Providence (Hb Prov), a fetal-like hemoglobin. Blood *46*:1030, 1975d.
Chernoff, A. I.: The human hemoglobins in health and disease. N. Engl. J. Med. *253*: 365, 1955.
Chernoff, A. I.: Studies of hemoglobin E. I. The clinical, hematologic and genetic characteristics of the hemoglobin E syndromes. J. Lab. Clin. Med. *47*:455, 1956.
Chernoff, A. I.: The hemoglobin D syndromes. Blood *13*:116, 1958.
Chernoff, A. I.: A method for the quantitative determination of HgB A_2. Ann. NY Acad. Sci. *119*:557, 1964.
Chernoff, A. I., and Singer, K.: Studies on abnormal hemoglobins. IV. Persistence of fetal hemoglobin in the erythrocytes of normal children. Pediatrics *9*:469, 1952.
Chien, S., Usami, S., and Bertles, J. F.: Abnormal rheology of oxygenated blood in sickle cell anemia. J. Clin. Invest. *49*:623, 1970.
Chillar, R. K., Slawsky, P., and Desforges, J. F.: Red cell 2,3-diphosphoglycerate and adenosine triphosphate in patients with shock. Br. J. Haematol. *21*:183, 1971.
Chou, P. Y., and Fasman, G. D.: Prediction of protein conformation. Biochemistry *13*: 222, 1974.
Chuang, A. H., Waterman, M. R., Yamaoka, K., et al.: Effect of pH, carbamylation and other hemoglobins on deoxyhemoglobin S aggregation inside intact erythrocytes as detected by proton relaxation rate measurements. Arch. Biochem. Biophys. *167*:145, 1975.
Cividalli, G., Nathan, D. G., Kan, Y. W., et al.: Relation of beta to gamma synthesis during the first trimester: An approach to prenatal diagnosis of thalassemia. Pediatr. Res. *8*:553, 1974a.
Cividalli, G., Nathan, D. G., and Lodish, H. F.: Translational control of hemoglobin synthesis in thalassemic bone marrow. J. Clin. Invest. *53*:955, 1974b.
Clark, M. R., and Shohet, S. B.: Hybrid erythrocytes for membrane studies in sickle cell disease. Blood *47*:121, 1976.
Clegg, J. B., and Weatherall, D. J.: Hemoglobin synthesis in α-thalassemia (haemoglobin H disease). Nature *215*:1241, 1967.
Clegg, J. B., and Weatherall, D. J.: Hemoglobin synthesis during erythroid maturation in β-thalassemia. Nature [New Biol.] *240*:190, 1972.
Clegg, J. B., Weatherall, D. J., Na-Nakorn, S., et al.: Haemoglobin synthesis in beta thalassemia. Nature *220*:664, 1968.
Clegg, J. B., Weatherall, D. J., and Eunson, C. E.: The distribution of nascent globin chains on human reticulocyte polysomes. Biochim. Biophys. Acta *247*:109, 1971a.
Clegg, J. B., Weatherall, D. J., and Milner, P. F.: Haemoglobin Constant Spring—a chain-termination mutant? Nature *234*:337, 1971b.
Clegg, J. B., Weatherall, D. J., Contopolou-Griva, I., et al.: Haemoglobin Icaria, a new chain-termination mutant which causes α-thalassaemia. Nature *251*:245, 1974a.
Clegg, J. B., Weatherall, D. J., Smith, D. H., et al.: Hb Kenya: a clue to the genetic control of human foetal haemoglobin synthesis. Br. J. Haematol. *28*:141, 1974b.
Coburn, R. F. (ed.): Biological effects of carbon monoxide. Ann. NY Acad. Sci. *174*:all, 1970.
Cohen, R. J., Sachs, J. R., Wicker, D. J., et al.: Methemoglobinemia provoked by malarial chemoprophylaxis in Vietnam. N. Engl. J. Med. *279*:1127, 1968.
Cohen-Solal, M., Thillet, J., Gaillardon, J., et al.: Functional properties of hemoglobin Saint Etienne, a variant carrying heme only on α chains. Rev. Eur. Etud. Clin. Biol. *17*:988, 1972.

Cohen-Solal, M., Seligmann, M., Thillet, J., and Rosa, J.: Haemoglobin Saint Louis β28 (B10) leucine→glutamine. A new unstable haemoglobin only present in a ferri form. FEBS Lett. *33*:37, 1973.

Cohen-Solal, M., Manesse, B., Thillet, J., and Rosa, J.: Haemoglobin G-Norfolk α85(F6) Asp→Asn. Structural characterization by sequenator analysis and functional properties of a new variant with high oxygen affinity. FEBS Lett. *50*:163, 1975.

Cohen-Solal, M., Blouquit, Y., Garel, M. C., et al.: Haemoglobin Lyon (β17–18 [A14–15] Lys→Val→0). Determination by sequenator analysis. Biochim. Biophys. Acta *351*:306, 1974.

Colombo, B., Kim, B., Perez Atencio, R., et al.: The pattern of fetal haeomoglobin disappearance after birth. Br. J. Haematol. *32*:79, 1976.

Conconi, F., and Del Senno, L.: The molecular defect of Ferrara β-thalassemia. Ann. NY Acad. Sci. *232*:54, 1974.

Conconi, F., Bargellesi, A., Del Senno, L., et al.: Globin chain synthesis in Sicilian thalassaemic subjects. Br. J. Haematol. *19*:469, 1970.

Conconi, F., Rowley, P. T., Del Senno, L., et al.: Induction of β-globin synthesis in the β-thalassaemia of Ferrara. Nature [New Biol.] *238*:83, 1972.

Conconi, F., Del Senno, L., Ferrarese, P., et al.: Appearance of β globin synthesis in erythroid cells of Ferrara β^0-thalassaemic patients following blood transfusion. Nature *254*:256, 1975.

Condon, P. I., and Serjeant, G. R.: Ocular findings in homozygous sickle cell anemia in Jamaica. Am. J. Ophthalmol. *73*:533, 1972a.

Condon, P. I., and Serjeant, G. R.: Ocular findings in hemoglobin sickle cell disease in Jamaica. Am. J. Ophthalmol. *74*:921, 1972b.

Conley, C. L., Weatherall, D. J., Richardson, S. N., et al.: Hereditary persistence of fetal hemoglobin: A study of 79 affected persons in 15 Negro families in Baltimore. Blood *21*:261, 1963.

Constantoulakis, M., Economidou, J., Karagiorga, M., et al.: Combined long term treatment of hemosiderosis with desferrioxamine and DTPA in homozygous β-thalassemia. Ann. NY Acad. Sci. *232*:193, 1974.

Cooper, H. A., and Hoagland, H. C.: Fetal hemoglobin. Mayo Clin. Proc. *47*:402, 1972.

Cooper, M. R., Kraus, A. P., Felts, J. H., et al.: A third case of hemoglobin Memphis/sickle cell disease: whole blood viscosity used as a screening test. Am. J. Med. *55*:535, 1973.

Cooperative Urea Trials Group: Clinical trials of therapy for sickle cell vaso-occlusive crises. JAMA *228*:1120, 1974.

Cottam, G. L., Valentine, K. M., Yamaoka, K., and Waterman, M. R.: The gelatin of deoxyhemoglobin S in erythrocytes as detected by transverse water proton relaxation measurements. Arch. Biochem. Biophys. *162*:487, 1974.

Craddock, P. R. Hunt, F. A., and Rozenberg, M. C.: The effective use of oxymetholone in the therapy of thalassaemia with anaemia. Med. J. Aust. *2*:199, 1972.

Crookston, J. H., Farquharson, H. A., Beale, D., et al.: Hemoglobin Etobicoke: α84 (F5) serine replaced by arginine. Can. J. Biochem. *47*:143, 1969.

Crystal, R. G., Elson, N. A., Nienhuis, A. W., et al.: Initiation of globin synthesis in β-thalassemia. N. Engl. J. Med. *288*:1091, 1973.

Dacie, J. V., Shinton, N. K., Gaffney, P. J., et al.: Haemoglobin Hammersmith (β42 [CD1] Phe→Ser). Nature (London) *216*:663, 1967.

Davis, D. G., Lindstrom, T. R., Mock, N. H., et al.: Nuclear magnetic resonance studies of hemoglobins. VI. Heme proton spectra of human deoxyhemoglobins and their relevance to the nature of cooperative oxygenation of hemoglobin. J. Mol. Biol. *60*:101, 1971.

Dayhoff, M. O.: Computer analysis of protein evolution. Sci. Am. *221*:86, 1969.

Dayhoff, M. O.: Atlas of Protein Sequence and Structure. Vol. 5. Washington, D.C., National Biomedical Research Foundation, 1972.

DeFuria, F. G., and Miller, D. R.: Oxygen affinity in hemoglobin Köln disease. Blood *39*:398, 1972.

DeFuria, F. G., Miller, D. R., and Canale, V. C.: Red blood cell metabolism and function in transfused β-thalassemia. Ann. NY Acad. Sci. *232*:323, 1974.

Deisseroth, A., Velez, R., and Nienhuis, A. W.: Hemoglobin synthesis in somatic cell hybrids: independent segregation of the human alpha- and beta-globin genes. Science *191*:1262, 1976.

DeJong, W. W. W.: Structure of the δ-chain of chimpanzee haemoglobin A_2. Nature [New Biol.] *234*:176, 1971.

DeJong, W. W. W., Went, L. N., and Bernini, L. F.: Haemoglobin Leiden: Deletion of β6 or 7 glutamic acid. Nature *220*:788, 1968.

DeJong, W. W. W., Bernini, L. F., and Khan, P. M.: Haemoglobin Rampa: α95 Pro→Ser. Biochim. Biophys. Acta *236*:197, 1971.

DeJong, W. W. W., Khan, P. M., and Bernini, L. F.: Hemoglobin Koya Dora: High frequency of a chain termination mutant. Am. J. Hum. Genet. *27*:81, 1975.

Desforges, J. F.: Unstable oxygen delivery. N. Engl. J. Med. *288*:965, 1973.

DeSimone, J., Kleve, L., Longley, M. A., and Shaeffer, J.: Rapid turnover of newly-synthesized β^S chains in reticulocytes from individuals with sickle cell trait. Biochem. Biophys. Res. Commun. *57*:248, 1974a.

DeSimone, J., Kleve, L., Longley, M. A., et al.: Unbalanced globin chain synthesis in reticulocytes of sickle cell trait individuals. Biochem. Biophys. Res. Commun. *59*:564, 1974b.

deVerdier, C. H., and Garby, L.: Glucose metabolism in normal erythrocytes: II. Factors influencing the hexokinase step. Scand. J. Haematol. *2*:305, 1965.

deVerdier, C. H., and Garby, L.: Low binding of 2,3-diphosphoglycerate to haemoglobin F: a contribution to the knowledge of the binding site and an explanation for the high oxygen affinity of foetal blood. Scand. J. Clin. Lab. Invest. *23*:149, 1969.

deVerdier, C. H., Garby, L., and Hjelm, M.: The role of 2,3-diphosphoglycerate in the erythrocyte as a regulator of tissue oxygen tension. Försvarsmedicin *5*:258, 1969.

de Weinstein, B. I., White, J. M., Wiltshire, B. G., and Lehmann, H.: A new unstable haemoglobin: Hb Buenos Aires, β85 (F1) Phe→Ser. Acta Haematol. *50*:357, 1973.

Diamond, H. S., Meisel, A., Sharon, E., et al.: Hyperuricosuria and increased tubular secretion of urate in sickle cell anemia. Am. J. Med. *59*:796, 1976.

Diamond, M. P., Cotgrove, I., and Parker, A.: Case of intrauterine death due to α-thalassemia. Br. Med. J. *2*:278, 1965.

Dickerman, J. D., Holtzman, N. A., and Zinkham, W. H.: Hemoglobin Zürich. A third family presenting with hemolytic reactions to sulfonamides. Am. J. Med. *55*:638, 1973a.

Dickerson, R. E.: X-ray analysis and protein structure. In Neurath, H. (ed.): The Proteins: Composition, Structure and Function. Vol. II. 2nd ed. New York, Academic Press, 1963, p. 603.

Diederich, D., Gill, P., and Larsen, W.: The irreversibly sickled erythrocyte: response to *in vitro* carbamylation. In Hercules, J. I., Schechter, A. N., Eaton, W. A., et al. (eds.): Proceedings of First National Symposium on Sickle Cell Disease, Washington, D.C. DHEW Pub. No. 75–723 (NIH), Bethesda, Md., 1974, p. 53.

Diggs, L. W.: Pulmonary lesions in sickle cell anemia. Blood *34*:734, 1969.

Diggs, L. W.: Anatomic lesions in sickle cell disease. *In* Abramson, H., Bertles, J. F., and Wethers, D. L. (eds.): Sickle Cell Disease: Diagnosis, Management, Education and Research. St. Louis, The C. V. Mosby Co., 1973, p. 189.

Diggs, L. W., and Bell, A.: Intraerythrocytic hemoglobin crystals in sickle cell-hemoglobin C disease. Blood *25*:218, 1965.

Donahue, R. P., Bias, W. B., Renwick, J. H., and McKusick, V. A.: Probable assignment of the Duffy blood group locus to chromosome 1 in man. Proc. Natl. Acad. Sci. USA *61*:949, 1968.

Dos-Santos, W. D., and Lehmann, H.: Acetazolamide in sickle-cell anaemia. Br. Med. J. *2*:139, 1959.

Douglas, R. H., and Hultquist, D. E.: Evidence that two forms of bovine erythrocyte cytochrome b_5 are identical to segments of microsomal cytochrome b_5. Proc. Natl. Acad. Sci. USA, in press, 1976.

Dow, L., Terada, M., Natta, C., et al.: Globin synthesis of intact cells and activity of isolated mRNA in β-thalassemia. Nature [New Biol.] *243*:114, 1973.

Dreyfus, J. C., Labie, D., Vibert, M., et al.: An attempt at demonstrating the existence of a nonsense mutation in β-thalassemia. Eur. J. Biochem. *27*:291, 1972.

Eaton, J. W., Skelton, T. D., Swofford, H. S., et al.: Elevated erythrocyte calcium in sickle cell disease. Nature *246*:105, 1973.

Eaton, J. W., White, J. G., Jacob, H. S., et al.: Ca^{2+}-induced maintenance of sickling in Hb SS erythrocytes. Blood *46*:1051, 1975.

Economidou, J., Constantoulakis, M., Augoustaki, O., et al.: Frequency of antibodies to various antigenic determinants in polytransfused patients with homozygous thalassemia in Greece. Vox Sang. *20*:252, 1971.

Edelstein, S. J., Telford, J. N., and Crepeaw, R. H.: Structure of fibers of sickle cell hemoglobin. Proc. Natl. Acad. Sci. USA *70*:1104, 1973.

Efremov, G. D., Huisman, T. H. J., Smith, L. L., et al.: Haemoglobin Richmond, a human hemoglobin which forms asymmetric hybrids with other hemoglobins. J. Biol. Chem. *244*:6105, 1969.
Egan, E. L., and Fairbanks, V. F.: Postsplenectomy erythrocytosis in hemoglobin Köln disease. N. Engl. J. Med. *288*:929, 1973.
Elbaum, D., Nagel, R. L., Bookchin, R. M., et al.: Effect of alkylureas on the polymerization of hemoglobin S. Proc. Natl. Acad. Sci. USA *71*:4718, 1974.
Engelhard, D., Cividalli, G., and Rachmilewitz, E. A.: Splenectomy in homozygous beta thalassaemia: a retrospective study of 30 pateints. Br. J. Haematol. *31*:391, 1975.
England, J. M., and Fraser, P. M.: Differentiation of iron deficiency from thalassaemia trait by routine blood-count. Lancet *1*:449, 1973.
Engle, M. A.: Cardiac involvement in Cooley's anemia. Ann. NY Acad. Sci. *119*:694, 1964.
Eraklis, A. J., Kevy, S. V., Diamond, L. K., et al.: Hazard of overwhelming infection after splenectomy in childhood. N. Engl. J. Med. *276*:1225, 1967.
Erlandson, M. E., Walden, B., Stern, G., et al.: Studies on congenital hemolytic syndrome: IV. Gastrointestinal absorption of iron. Blood *19*:359, 1962.
Ernst, V., and Arnstein, H. R. V.: Synthesis of α and β globin directed by messenger ribonucleoprotein from rabbit reticulocytes. Biochim. Biophys. Acta *378*:251, 1975.
Esan, G. J. F., Morgan, F. J., O'Donnell, J. V. et al.: Diminished synthesis of an alpha chain mutant, hemoglobin I (α16 Lys→Glu). J. Clin. Invest. *49*:2218, 1970.
Fairbanks, V. F., and Pettit, R. M.: Sickledex test in unstable hemoglobin disorders. JAMA *220*:128, 1972.
Fairbanks, V. F., Opfell, R. W., and Burgert, E. O.: Three families with unstable hemoglobinopathies (Köln, Olmsted and Santa Ana) causing hemolytic anemia with inclusion bodies and pigmenturia. Am. J. Med. *46*:344, 1969.
Fairbanks, V. F., Maldanado, J. E., Charache, S., et al.: Familial erythrocytosis due to electrophoretically undetectable hemoglobin with impaired oxygen dissociation (Hemoglobin Malmö, $\alpha_2\beta_2^{97Gln}$). Mayo Clin. Proc. *46*:721, 1971.
Farmer, M. B., Lehmann, H., and Raine, D. N.: Two unrelated patients with congenital cyanosis due to haemoglobinopathy M. Lancet *II*:786, 1964.
Feig, S. A., Nathan, D. G., Gerald, P. S., et al.: Congenital methemoglobinemia: the result of age dependent decay of methemoglobin reductase. Blood *39*:407, 1972.
Fernandez, L. A., and Erslev, A. J.: Oxygen affinity and compensated hemolysis in hereditary spherocytosis. J. Lab. Clin. Med. *80*:780, 1972.
Fessas, P.: Inclusions of hemoglobin in erythroblasts and erythrocytes of thalassemia. Blood *21*:21, 1963.
Fessas, P.: Forms of thalassemia. In Jonxis, J. H. P. (ed.): Abnormal Hemoglobins in Africa. Oxford, Blackwell Scientific Publications, 1965, p. 71.
Fessas, P., and Loukopoulos, D.: Alpha-chain of human hemoglobin: occurrence *in vivo*. Science *143*:590, 1964.
Fessas, P., and Stamatoyannopoulos, G.: Absence of hemoglobin A_2 in an adult. Nature *195*:1215, 1962.
Fessas, P., and Stamatoyannopoulos, G.: Hereditary persistence of fetal hemoglobin in Greece. A study and a comparison. Blood *24*:223, 1964.
Fessas, P., and Yataganas, X.: Intraerythroblastic instability of hemoglobin β_4 (Hgb H). Blood *31*:323, 1968.
Fessas, P., Loukopoulos, D., and Kaltsoya, A.: Peptide analysis of the inclusions of erythroid cells in β-thalassemia. Biochim. Biophys. Acta *124*:430, 1966.
Finch, C. A., and Lenfant, C.: Oxygen transport in man. N. Engl. J. Med. *286*:407, 1972.
Finch, C. A., Deubelbeiss, K., Cook, J. D., et al.: Ferrokinetics in man. Medicine (Baltimore) *49*:17, 1970.
Finch, J. T., Perutz, M. F., Bertles, J. F., and Döbler, J.: Structure of sickled erythrocytes and of sickle-cell hemoglobin fibers. Proc. Natl. Acad. Sci. USA *70*:718, 1973.
Finne, P. H., and Halvorsen, S.: Regulation of erythropoiesis in the fetus and newborn. Arch. Dis. Child. *47*:683, 1972.
Finney, R. A., Jr., and Hatch, F. E., Jr.: Effect of a carbonic anhydrase inhibitor (dichlorphenamide) on sickle cell anemia. Am. J. Med. Sci. *250*:154, 1965.

Fischer, S., Nagel, R., Bookchin, R., et al.: The binding of hemoglobin to membranes of normal and sickled erythrocytes. Biochim. Biophys. Acta *375*:422, 1975.

Fitch, W. M.: A comparison between evolutionary substitutions and variants in human hemoglobins. Ann. NY Acad. Sci. *241*:439, 1974.

Flatz, G., Kinderlerer, J. L., Kilmartin, J. V., et al.: Haemoglobin Tak: a variant with additional residues at the end of the β-chains. Lancet *1*:732, 1971.

Flye, M. W., and Silver, D.: The role of surgery in sickle cell disease. Surg. Gynecol. Obstet. *137*:115, 1973.

Forget, B. G.: The molecular basis of thalassemia. CRC Crit. Rev. Biochem. *2*:311, 1974.

Forget, B. G., and Nathan, D. G.: Molecular pathology of the thalassemias. Adv. Intern. Med. *21*:97, 1975.

Forget, B. G., Baltimore, D., Benz, E. J., Jr., et al.: Globin messenger RNA in the thalassemia syndromes. Ann. NY Acad. Sci. *232*:76, 1974a.

Forget, B. G., Marotta, C. A., Weissman, S. M., et al.: Nucleotide sequences of human globin messenger RNA. Ann NY Acad. Sci. *241*:290, 1974b.

Forget, B. G., Benz, E. J., Jr., Skoultchi, A., et al.: Absence of messenger RNA for beta globin chain in β^0-thalassemia. Nature *247*:379, 1974c.

Forget, B. G., Housman, D., Benz, E. J., Jr., et al.: Synthesis of DNA complementary to separated human alpha and beta globin messenger RNA's. Proc. Natl. Acad. Sci. USA *72*:984, 1975a.

Forget, B. G., Marotta, C. A., Weissman, S. M., et al.: Nucleotide sequences of the 3'-terminal untranslated region of messenger RNA for human beta globin chain. Proc. Natl. Acad. Sci. USA *72*:3614, 1975b.

Forget, B. G., Glass, J., and Housman, D.: Erythroid cell differentiation. In Neth, R., and Moloney, W. C. (eds.): Modern Trends in Human Leukemia II. Munich, Lehmanns Verlag, in press, 1976a.

Forget, B. G., Hillman, D. G., Lazarus, H., et al.: Absence of messenger RNA and gene DNA for β-globin chains in hereditary persistence of fetal hemoglobin. Cell *7*:323, 1976b.

Forget, B. G., Hillman, D. G., Cohen-Solal, M., et al.: Beta globin messenger RNA in beta^0 thalassemia. Blood *48*:998, 1976c.

Fraser, I. D.: Adult and foetal haemoglobin in Rh haemolytic disease. Br. J. Haematol. *23*:269, 1972.

Frazer, G. R., Kitsos, C., Motulsky, A. G., et al.: Thalassemias, abnormal hemoglobins, and glucose-6-phosphate dehydrogenase deficiency in the Arta area of Greece: diagnostic and genetic aspects of complete village studies. Ann NY Acad. Sci. *119*:415, 1964.

Freedman, M. L., and Karpatkin, S.: Short communication: elevated platelet count and megathrombocyte number in sickle cell anemia. Blood *46*:579, 1975.

Freedman, M. L., Geraghty, M., and Rosman, J.: Hemin control of globin synthesis: isolation of a hemin reversible translational repressor from human mature erythrocytes. J. Biol. Chem. *249*:7290, 1974.

Frick, P. G., Hitzig, W. H., and Betke, K.: Hemoglobin Zürich. A new hemoglobin anomaly associated with acute hemolytic episodes with inclusion bodies after sulfonamide therapy. Blood *20*:261, 1962.

Friedman, E. A., Sreepada Rao, T. K., Sprung, C. L., et al.: Uremia in sickle-cell anemia treated by maintenance hemodialysis. N. Engl. J. Med. *291*:431, 1974.

Friedman, S., and Schwartz, E.: Hereditary persistence of foetal haemoglobin with β-chain synthesis in cis position ($^G\gamma$-β^+-HPFH) in a Negro family. Nature *259*:138, 1976.

Friedman, S., Oski, F. A., and Schwartz, E.: Bone marrow and peripheral blood globin synthesis in an American Black family with beta thalassemia. Blood *39*:785, 1972.

Friedman, S., Hamilton, R. W., and Schwartz, E.: β-thalassemia in the American Negro. J. Clin. Invest. *52*:1453, 1973.

Friedman, S., Özsoylu, S., Luddy, R., et al.: Heterozygous beta thalassaemia of unusual severity. Br. J. Haematol. *32*:65, 1976a.

Friedman, S., Schwartz, E., Ahern, E., et al.: Variations in globin chain synthesis in hereditary persistence of fetal haemoglobin. Br. J. Haematol. *32*:357, 1976b.

Frischer, H., and Bowman, J.: Hemoglobin E, an oxidatively unstable mutation. J. Lab. Clin. Med. *85*:531, 1975.

Fuhr, J. E., Natta, C., Marks, P. A., and Bank, A.: Protein synthesis in cell-free systems from reticulocytes of thalassemic patients. Nature *224*:1305, 1969.

Fung, L. W., and Ho., C.: A proton nuclear magnetic resonance study of the quaternary structure of human hemoglobins in water. Biochemistry *14*:2526, 1975.

Gaburro, D., Volpato, S., and Vigi, V.: Diagnosis of beta thalassemia in the newborn by means of hemoglobin synthesis. Acta Pediatr. Scand. *59*:523, 1970.

Gabuzda, T. G., Nathan, D. G., and Gardner, F. H.: The turnover of hemoglobins A, F, and A_2 in the peripheral blood of three patients with thalassemia. J. Clin. Invest. *42*:1678, 1963.

Gabuzda, T. G., Nathan, D. G., and Gardner, F. H.: The metabolism of the individual C.[14] Labelled hemoglobin in patients with H-thalassemia; with observations on radiochromate binding to the hemoglobins during red cell survival. J. Clin. Invest. *44*:315, 1965.

Gacon, G., Wajcman, H., and Labie, D.: Hemoglobin E: Its oxygen affinity in relation with the ionic environment. FEBS Lett. *41*:147, 1974.

Gambino, R., Kacian, D., O'Donnel, J., et al.: A limited number of globin genes in human DNA. Proc. Natl. Acad. Sci USA *71*:3966, 1974.

Garby, L., Sjolin, S., and Vuille, J. C.: Studies on erythrokinetics in infancy. II. The relative rate of synthesis of haemoglobin F and haemoglobin A during the first months of life. Acta Paediatr. (Stockholm) *51*:245, 1962.

Garel, M. C., Cohen-Solal, M., Bluoquit, Y., et al.: A method for isolation of abnormal haemoglobins with high oxygen affinity due to a frozen quaternary R-structure: Application to Hb Creteil $\alpha_2{}^A\beta_2$ (F5) 89 Asn. FEBS Lett. *43*:93, 1974.

Garrick, M. D., Reichlin, M., Mattioli, M., and Manning, R.: The anemia-induced reversible switch from hemoglobin A to hemoglobin C in Caprine ruminants: immunochemical evidence that both hemoglobins are found in the same cell. Dev. Biol. *30*:1, 1973.

Gau, G. T., Fairbanks, V. F., Maldonado, J. E., *et al.*: Cardiac dysfunction in a patient with hemoglobin Malmö treated with repeated transfusions. Clin. Research *22*:276A, 1974.

Gerald, P. S.: The electrophoretic and spectroscopic characterization of Hgb M. Blood *13*:936, 1958.

Gerald, P. S., and Diamond, L. K.: The diagnosis of thalassemia trait by starch block electrophoresis of the hemoglobin. Blood *13*:61, 1958.

Gerald, P. S., and Efron, M. L.: Chemical studies of several varieties of Hb M. Proc. Natl. Acad. Sci. USA *47*:1758, 1961.

Gerald, P. S., Cook, C. D., and Diamond, L. K.: Hemoglobin M. Science *126*:300, 1957.

Gibson, Q. H., and Nagel, R. L.: Allosteric transition and ligand binding in hemoglobin Chesapeake. J. Biol. Chem. *249*:7255, 1974.

Gilbert, J. M., Thornton, A. G., Nienhuis, A., et al.: Cell-free hemoglobin synthesis in beta thalassemia. Proc. Natl. Acad. Sci. USA *67*:1854, 1970.

Gill, F., and Schwartz, E.: Free α globin pool in human bone marrow. J. Clin. Invest. *52*:3057, 1973.

Gill, F., Atwater, J., and Schwartz, E.: Hemoglobin Lepore trait: Globin synthesis in bone marrow and peripheral blood. Science *178*:623, 1972.

Gillette, P. N., Lu, Y. S., and Peterson, C. M.: The pharmacology of cyanate with a summary of its initial usage in sickle cell disease. Progr. Hematol. *8*:181, 1973.

Glader, B. E., Lux, S. E., Muller, A., et al.: Cation water and ATP content of irrerversibly sickled RBC's (ISC's) *in vivo*. Clin. Res. *24*:309, 1976.

Glynn, K. P., Penner, J. A., Smith, J. R., et al.: Familial erythrocytosis: description of three families, one with Hemoglobin Ypsilanti. Ann. Intern. Med. *69*:769, 1968.

Goldberg, M. A., Bunn, H. F., and Harkness, D. R.: The use of centrifugation in studying the interaction of sickle and non-sickle hemoglobins. Clin. Res. *23*:581A, 1975.

Goldberg, M. F.: Treatment of proliferative sickle retinopathy. Trans. Am. Acad. Ophthalmol. Otolaryngol. *75*:532, 1971.

Goldstein, G. W., Hammaker, L., and Schmid, R.: The catabolism of Heinz bodies: An experimental model demonstrating conversion to non-bilirubin catabolites. Blood *31*:388, 1968.

Gordon, P. A., Breeze, G. R., Mann, J. R., et al.: Coagulation fibrinolysis in sickle cell disease. J. Clin. Pathol. *27*:485, 1974.

Gordon-Smith, E. C., Dacie, J. V., Blecher, T. E., et al.: Haemoglobin Nottingham β FG5 (98) Val→Gly: A new unstable haemoglobin producing severe haemolysis. Proc. Roy. Soc. Med. *66*:507, 1973.
Gorski, J., Morrison, M. R., Merkel, C. G., and Lingrel, J. B.: Poly (A) size class distribution in globin mRNAs as a function of time. Nature *253*:749, 1975.
Grace, D. A., and Winter, C. C.: Priapism: an appraisal of management of twenty-three patients. J. Urol. *99*:301, 1968.
Graziano, J. H., Grady, R. W., and Cerami, A.: The identification of 2,3-dihydroxybenzoic acid as a potentially useful iron-chelating drug. J. Pharmacol. Exp. Ther. *190*:570, 1974.
Graziano, J. H., Miller, D. R., Grady, R. W., et al.: Inhibition of membrane peroxidation in thalassaemic erythrocytes by 2,3-dihydroxybenzoic acid. Br. J. Haematol. *32*:351, 1976.
Green, T. W., Conley, C. L., and Berthrong, M.: The liver in sickle cell anemias. Bull, Johns Hopkins Hosp. *92*:99, 1953.
Greenberg, M. S., and Kass, E. H.: Studies on the destruction of red blood cells. XIII. Observation on the role of pH in the pathogenesis and treatment of painful crisis in sickle cell disease. Arch. Intern. Med. *101*:355, 1958.
Greer, J.: Three-dimensional structure of abnormal human haemoglobins Kansas and Richmond. J. Mol. Biol. *59*:99, 1971a.
Greer, J.: Three-dimensional structure of abnormal human haemoglobins M Hyde Park and M Iwate. J. Mol. Biol. *59* 107, 1971b.
Greer, J.: Three-dimensional structure of abnormal human haemoglobins Chesapeake and J-Capetown. J. Mol. Biol. *62*:241, 1971c.
Greer, J., and Perutz, M. F.: Three-dimensional structure and haemoglobin Rainier. Nature [New Biol.] *230*:261, 1971.
Griggs, R. C., and Harris, J. W.: Biophysics of the variants of sickle cell disease. Arch. Intern. Med. *97*:315, 1956.
Grimes, A. J., and Meisler, A.: Possible cause of Heinz bodies in congenital Heinz-body anaemia. Nature *194*:190, 1962.
Grimes, A. J., Meisler, A., and Dacie, J. V.: Congenital Heinz-body anaemia: Further evidence on the cause of Heinz-body production in red cells. Br. J. Haematol. *10*:281, 1964.
Gross, R. T., Kriss, J. P., and Spaet, T. H.: The hematopoietic and goitrogenic effects of cobaltous chloride in patients with sickle cell anemia. Pediatrics *15*:284, 1955.
Grossbard, E., Terada, M., Dow, L. W., and Bank, A.: Decreased α globin messenger RNA activity associated with polyribosomes in α thalassemia. Nature [New Biol.] *241*:209, 1973.
Guidotti, G.: Thalassemia. In "Conference on Hemoglobin," Arden House, Columbia University, New York, 1962.
Gunn, R. B., Silvers, D. N., and Rosse, W. F.: Potassium permeability in β-thalassemia minor red blood cells. J. Clin. Invest. *51*:1043, 1972.
Hahn, E. V., and Gillespie, E. B.: Sickle cell anemia. Arch. Intern. Med. *39*:233, 1927.
Halbrecht, I., Isaacs, W. A., Lehmann, H., and Ben-Porat, F.: Hemoglobin Hasharon (α47 aspartic acid-histidine). Isr. J. Med. Sci. *3*:827, 1967.
Hall-Craggs, M., Marsden, P. D., Raper, A. B., et al.: Homozygous sickle-cell anaemia arising from two different haemoglobins S. Interaction of haemoglobins S and Stanleyville-II. Br. Med. J. *2*:87, 1964.
Ham, T. H., and Castle, W. B.: Relation of increased hypotonic fragility and of erythrostasis to the mechanism of hemolysis in certain anemias. Trans. Assn. Am. Physicians *55*:127, 1940.
Hamilton, H. B., Iuchi, I., Miyaji, T., et al.: Hemoglobin Hiroshima (β^{143} Histidine→ Aspartic acid): a newly identified fast moving beta chain variant associated with increased oxygen affinity and compensatory erythremia. J. Clin. Invest. *48*:525, 1969.
Hamilton, R. W., Schwartz, E., Atwater, J., et al.: Acquired hemoglobin H disease. N. Engl. J. Med. *285*:1217, 1971.
Harkness, D. R., and Roth, S.: Clinical evaluation of cyanate in sickle cell anemia. Progr. Hematol. 9:157, 1975.
Harris, J. W.: Studies on the destruction of red blood cells. VIII. Molecular orientation in sickle cell hemoglobin solution. Proc. Soc. Exp. Biol. Med. *75*:197, 1950.

Harris, J. W., and Bensusan, H. B.: The kinetics of the sol-gel transformation of deoxyhemoglobin S by continuous monitoring of viscosity. J. Lab. Clin. Med. *86*:564, 1975.

Harris, J. W., and Kellermeyer, R. W.: The Red Cell. Cambridge, Mass., Harvard University Press, 1970, p. 170.

Harris, J. W., Brewster, H. H., Ham, T. H., and Castle W. B.: Studies on the destruction of red blood cells. The biophysics and biology of sickle cell disease. Arch. Intern. Med. *97*:145, 1956.

Hartz, W. H., and Schwartz, S. O.: Hemoglobin C disease, report of four cases. Blood *10*:235, 1955.

Hasen, H. B., and Raines, S. L.: Priapism associated with sickle cell disease. J. Urol. *88*:71, 1962.

Hathorn, M., and Lewis, R. A.: Inhibition of sickling by phenothiazines. Effect on red cell survival. Br. J. Haematol. *12*:195, 1966.

Haut, M. J., Cowan, D. H., and Harris, J. W.: Platelet function and survival in sickle cell disease. J. Lab. Clin. Med. *82*:44, 1973.

Hayashi, A., Shimizu, A., Yamamura, Y., and Watari, H.: Hemoglobins M: Identification of Iwate, Boston and Saskatoon variants. Science *152*:207, 1966.

Hayashi, A., Shimizu, A., Suzuki, T., and Yamamura, Y.: The properties of hemoglobin M. Reactivity of methemoglobin M to cyanide, azide and fluoride. Biochim. Biophys. Acta *140*:251, 1967.

Hayashi, A., Suzuki, T., Shimizu, A., et al.: Properties of hemoglobin M. Unequivalent nature of the α and β subunits in the hemoglobin molecule. Biochim. Biophys. Acta *168*:262, 1968a.

Hayashi, A., Suzuki, T., Shimizu, A., et al.: Some observations on the physicochemical properties of hemoglobin $M_{Hyde\ Park}$. Arch. Biochem. Biophys. *125*:895, 1968b.

Hayashi, A., Stamatoyannopoulos, G., Yoshida, A., et al.: Haemoglobin Rainier: β145 (HC2) Tyrosine→Cysteine and Haemoglobin Bethesda: β145 (HC2) Tyrosine→Histidine. Nature [New Biol.] *230*:264, 1971.

Hecht, F., Motulsky, A. G., Lemire, R. J., and Shepard, T. E.: Predominance of hemoglobin Gower 1 in early human embryonic development. Science *152*:91, 1966.

Hecht, F., Jones, R. T., and Koler, R. D.: Newborn infants with Hb Portland 1; an indicator of α-chain deficiency. Ann. Hum. Genet. *31*:215, 1967.

Heinemann, H. O., and Cheung, M. W.: Renal concentrating mechanism in sickle cell anemia. J. Lab. Clin. Med. *49*:923, 1957.

Heinrich, H. C., Gabbe, E. E., Oppitz, K. H., et al.: Absorption of inorganic and food iron in children with heterozygous and homozygous β-thalassemia. Z. Kinderheilkd. *115*:1, 1973.

Heller, P.: Hemoglobin M—An early chapter in the saga of molecular pathology. Ann. Intern. Med. *70*:1038, 1969.

Heller, P.: Does the sickle cell trait have pathogenic significance? In Hercules, J. I., Schechter, A. N., Eaton, W. A., et al. (eds.): Proceedings of First National Symposium on Sickle Cell Disease, Washington, D.C. DHEW Pub. No. 75–723, (NIH), Bethesda, Md., 1974, p. 293.

Heller, P., and Yakulis, V.: The distribution of hemoglobin A_2. Ann. NY Acad. Sci. *165*:54, 1969.

Heller, P., Henderson, W., and Yakulis, V.: Autosomal inactivation in the sickle-cell trait. Lancet *2*:197, 1963a.

Heller, P., Yakulis, V., Epstein, R., and Friedland, S.: Variation in the amount of hemoglobin S in a patient with sickle cell trait and megaloblastic anemia. Blood *21*:479, 1963b.

Heller, P., Coleman, R. D., and Yakulis, V.: Structural studies of haemoglobin M—Hyde Park. Proceedings of the XI Congress of the International Society of Haematology, Sydney, 1966, pp. 427–434.

Hercules, J. I., Schechter, A. N., Eaton, W. A., et al. (eds.): Proceedings of First National Symposium on Sickle Cell Disease, Washington, D.C. DHEW Pub. No. 75–723 (NIH), Bethesda, Md., 1974.

Herrick, J. B.: Peculiar elongated and sickle-shaped red blood corpuscles in a case of severe anemia. Arch. Intern. Med. *6*:517, 1910.

Heywood, J. D., Karon, M., and Weissman, S.: Amino acids: incorporation into alpha- and beta-chains of hemoglobin by normal and thalassemic reticulocytes. Science *146*:530, 1964.

Heywood, J. D., Karon, M., and Weissman, S.: Asymmetrical incorporation of amino acids into the alpha- and beta-chains of hemoglobin synthesized in thalassemic reticulocytes. J. Lab. Clin. Med. *66*:476, 1965.

Hilkovitz, G.: Sickle cell disease: New method of treatment. Preliminary report. Br. Med. J. *2*:266, 1957.

Hill, R. L., Swenson, R. T., and Schwartz, H. C.: The chemical and genetic relationships between hemoglobins S and $G_{San\ Jose}$. Blood *19*:573, 1962.

Ho, C., and Lindstrom, T. R.: Functional non-equivalence of α and β hemes in human hemoglobins. Adv. Exp. Med. Biol. *28*:65, 1972.

Hobbins, J. C., and Mahoney, M. J.: In utero diagnosis of hemoglobinopathies. I. Technique for obtaining fetal blood. N. Engl. J. Med. *290*:1065, 1974.

Hobbins, J. C., and Mahoney, M. J.: Fetal blood drawing. Lancet *2*:107, 1975.

Hobolth, N.: Haemoglobin $M_{Århus}$. I. Clinical family study. Acta Paediatr. Scand. *54*:357, 1965a.

Hobolth, N.: Haemoglobin $M_{Århus}$. II. Studies on a new haemoglobin which causes congenital methaemoglobinaemia. Acta Paediatr. Scand. *54*:357, 1965b.

Hofrichter, J., Hendricker, D., and Eaton, W. A.: Structure of hemoglobin S fibers: optical determination of the molecular orientation in sickled erythrocytes. Proc. Natl. Acad. Sci. USA *70*:3604, 1973.

Hofrichter, J., Ross, P. D., and Eaton, W. A.: Kinetics and mechanism of deoxyhemoglobin S gelatin: a new approach to understanding sickle cell disease. Proc. Natl. Acad. Sci. USA *71*:4864, 1974.

Hollan, S. R., Szelenyi, J. G., Brimhall, B., et al.: Multiple alpha chain loci for human haemoglobins: Hb J-Buda and Hb G-Pest. Nature *235*:47, 1972.

Hollenberg, M. D., Kalback, M. M., and Kazazian, H. H., Jr.: Adult hemoglobin synthesis by reticulocytes from the human fetus at midtrimester. Science *174*:698, 1971.

Hollender, A., Lorkin, P. A., Lehmann, H., and Svensson, B.: New unstable haemoglobin Boräs, β88 (F4) Leucine→Arginine. Nature (London) *222*:953, 1969.

Honig, G. R., Green, D., Shamsuddin, M., et al.: Hemoglobin Abraham Lincoln, β32 (B14) leucine→proline, an unstable variant producing severe hemolytic disease. J. Clin. Invest. *52*:1746, 1973.

Honig, G. R., Mason, R. G., Vida, L. N., and Shamsuddin, M.: Synthesis of Hemoglobin Abraham Lincoln (β32 Leu→Pro). Blood *43*:657, 1974.

Hörlein, H., and Weber, G.: Über chronische familiäre Methämoglobinämie und eine neue Modifikation des Methämoglobins. Dtsch. Med. Wochenschr. *73*:476, 1948.

Hosoi, T.: Studies on hemoglobin F within a single erythrocyte by fluorescent antibody technique. Exp. Cell Res. *37*:680, 1965.

Housman, D., Forget, B. G., Skoutchi, A., and Benz, E. J., Jr.: Quantitative deficiency of chain specific globin mRNA in the thalassemia syndromes. Proc. Natl. Acad. Sci. USA *70*:1809, 1973.

Housman, D., Skoultchi, A., Forget, B. G., et al.: Use of globin cDNA as a hybridization probe for globin mRNA. Ann. NY Acad. Sci. *241*:280, 1974.

Huehns, E. R.: The unstable hemoglobins. Bull. Soc. Chim. Biol. *52*:1131, 1970.

Huehns, E. R., and Farooqui, A. M.: Oxygen dissociation properties of human embryonic red cells. Nature *254*:335, 1975.

Huehns, E. R., Flynn, F. V., Butler, E. A., and Beaven, G. H.: Two new haemoglobin variants in a very young human embryo. Nature *189*:496, 1961.

Huehns, E. R., Dance, N., Beaven, G. H., et al.: Human embryonic hemoglobins. Cold Spring Harbor Symp. Quant. Biol. *21*:327, 1964.

Huehns, E. R., Hecht, F., Yoshida, A., et al.: Hemoglobin Seattle ($\alpha_2{}^A\beta_2{}^{76}$): An unstable hemoglobin causing chronic hemolytic anemia. Blood *36*:209, 1970.

Huestis, W. H., and Raftery, M. A.: ^{31}P-NMR studies of the release of diphosphoglyceric acid on carbon monoxide binding to hemoglobin. Biochem. Biophys. Res. Commun. *49*:428, 1972.

Hugh-Jones, K., Lehmann, H., and McAlister, J. M.: Some experiences in managing sickle-cell anaemia in children and young adults, using alkalis and magnesium. Br. Med. J. *2*:226, 1964.

Huisman, T. H. J.: Chromatographic separation of hemoglobins A_2 and C. The quantities of hemoglobin A_2 in patients with AC trait, CC disease and C–β-thalassemia. Clin. Chim. Acta *40*:159, 1972.

Huisman, T. H. J., Boyd, E. M., Kitchens, J., et al.: Oxygen equilibria and biochemical changes of whole blood stored in different preservation media. Transfusion *9*:180, 1969.

Huisman, T. H. J., Schroeder, W. A., et al.: Nature of fetal hemoglobin in the Greek type of hereditary persistence of fetal hemoglobin, with and without concurrent β-thalassemia. J. Clin. Invest. *49*:1035, 1970.

Huisman, T. H. J., Brown, A. K., Efremov, G. D., et al.: Hemoglobin Savannah (B6[24] β-glycine→valine): an unstable variant causing anemia with inclusion bodies. J. Clin. Invest. *50*:650, 1971a.
Huisman, T. H. J., Schroeder, W. A., et al.: Evidence for four nonallelic structural genes for the γ chain of human fetal hemoglobin. Biochem. Genet. *7*:131, 1972a.
Huisman, T. H. J., Wrightstone, R. N., Wilson, J. B., et al.: Hemoglobin Kenya, the product of fusion of γ and β polypeptide chains. Arch. Biochem. Biophys. *153*:850, 1972b.
Huisman, T. H. J., Wilson, J. B., Gravely, M., et al.: Hemoglobin Grady: the first example of a variant with elongated chains due to an insertion of residues. Proc. Natl. Acad. Sci. USA *71*:3270, 1974.
Huisman, T. H. J., Miller, A., and Schroeder, W. A.: $A^{G}\gamma$ type of hereditary persistence of fetal hemoglobin with β chain production *in cis.* Am. J. Hum. Genet. *27*:765, 1975.
Hultquist, D. E., Dean, R. T., and Douglas, R. H.: Homogeneous cytochrome b_5 from human erythrocytes. Biochem. Biophys. Res. Commun. *60*:28, 1974.
Humpeler, E., Amor, H., and Braunsteiner, H.: Unterschedliche Sauerstoffaffinitât des Hämoglobins bei Anämien verschiedener Åtiologie. Blut *29*:382, 1974.
Hunt, J. T., and Ingram, V. M.: Abnormal human haemoglobins. IV. The chemical difference between normal human haemoglobin and haemoglobin C. Biochim. Biophys. Acta *42*:409, 1960.
Huntsman, R. G., and Lehmann, H.: The hemoglobinopathies. In Stanbury, J. B., et al. (eds.): Metabolic Basis of Inherited Diseases. New York, McGraw-Hill Book Co., 3rd ed. 1972, pp. 297–369.
Hutchison, H. E., Pinkerton, P. H., Waters, P., et al.: Hereditary Heinz body anaemia, thrombocytopenia and haemoglobinopathy (Hb Köln) in a Glasgow family. Br. Med. J. *2*:1099, 1964.
Idelson, L. I., Didkowsky, N. A., Casey, R., et al.: New unstable haemoglobin (Hb Moscva, β24(B4)Gly→Asp) found in the USSR. Nature *249*:768, 1974.
Imai, K., Morimoto, H., Kotan, M., et al.: Studies on the function of abnormal hemoglobins. II. Oxygen equilibrium of abnormal hemoglobins: Shimonosecki, Ube II, Hikari, Gifu and Agenogi. Biochim. Biophys. Acta *200*:197, 1970.
Imamura, T., Fujita, S., and Ohta, Y.: Hemoglobin Yoshizuka (G10[108] β asparagine→aspartic acid): A new variant with a reduced oxygen affinity from a Japanese family. J. Clin. Invest. *48*:2341, 1969.
Ingram, V. M.: Abnormal human haemoglobins. II. The chemical difference between normal and sickle cell haemoglobins. Biochim. Biophys. Acta *36*:402, 1959.
Ingram, V. M.: A molecular model for thalassemia. Ann. NY Acad. Sci. *119*:485, 1964.
Isaacs, W. A., and Hayhoe, F. G. J.: Steroid hormones in sickle-cell disease. Nature *215*:1139, 1967.
Itano, H. A.: A third abnormal hemoglobin associated with hereditary hemolytic anemia. Proc. Natl. Acad. Sci. USA *37*:775, 1951.
Itano, H. A.: The synthesis and structure of normal and abnormal hemoglobins. In Jonxis, J. H. P. (ed.): Abnormal Haemoglobins in Africa. Oxford, Blackwell Scientific Publications, 1965, p. 3.
Itano, H. A., and Neel, J. V.: A new inherited abnormality of human hemoglobin. Proc. Natl. Acad. Sci. USA *36*:613, 1950.
Jackson, J. F., Odom, J. L., and Bell, W. N.: Amelioration of sickle cell disease by persistent fetal hemoglobin. JAMA *177*:867, 1961.
Jackson, J. M., Yates, A., and Huehns, E. R.: Haemoglobin Perth: β32 (B14) leu→pro, an unstable haemoglobin causing haemolysis. Br. J. Haematol. *25*:607, 1973.
Jacob, H. S., and Amsden, T.: Acute hemolytic anemia with rigid red cells in hypophosphatemia. N. Engl. J. Med. *285*:1446, 1971.
Jacob, H. S., and Winterhalter, K. H.: The role of hemoglobin heme loss in Heinz body formation: Studies with a partially heme-deficient hemoglobin and with genetically unstable hemoglobin. J. Clin. Invest. *49*:2008, 1970a.
Jacob, H. S., and Winterhalter, K. H.: Unstable hemoglobins: The role of heme loss in Heinz body formation. Proc. Natl. Acad. Sci. USA *65*:697, 1970b.

Jacob, H. S., Brain, M. C., and Dacie, J. V.: Altered sulfhydryl reactivity of hemoglobins and red blood cell membranes in congenital Heinz body hemolytic anemia. J. Clin. Invest. *47*:2664, 1968a.

Jacob, H. S., Brain, M. C., Dacie, J. V., et al.: Abnormal haem binding and globin SH group blockade in unstable haemoglobins. Nature *218*:1214, 1968b.

Jacobs-Lorena, M., and Baglioni, C.: Synthesis of rabbit globin by reticulocyte postribosomal supernatant and heterologous ribosomes. Eur. J. Biochem. *35*:559, 1973.

Jacon, G., Wajcman, H., and Labie, D.: Structural and functional study of Hb Nancy, β145 (HC2) Tyr→Asp. A high oxygen affinity hemoglobin. FEBS Lett. *56*:39, 1975.

Jandl, J. H., and Greenberg, M. S.: Bone marrow failure due to relative nutritional deficiency in Cooley's hemolytic anemia. N. Engl. J. Med. *280*:461, 1959.

Jandl, J. H., Simmons, R. L., and Castle, W. B.: Red cell filtration and the pathogenesis of certain hemolytic anemias. Blood *18*:133, 1961.

Jenkins, M. E., Scott, R. B., and Baird, R. L.: Studies in sickle cell anemia. XVI. Sudden death during sickle cell anemia crises in young children. J. Pediatr. *56*:30, 1960.

Jensen, M., Bunn, H. F., Halikas, G., et al.: Effect of cyanate and 2,3-diphosphoglycerate on sickling. J. Clin. Invest. *52*:2542, 1973a.

Jensen, M., Shohet, S. B., and Nathan, D. G.: The role of red cell energy metabolism in the generation of irreversibly sickled cells in vitro. Blood *42*:835, 1973c.

Jensen, M., Oski, F. A., Nathan, D. G., and Bunn, H. F.: Hemoglobin Syracuse (α_2 $\beta_2^{143\ [H21]\ His \rightarrow Pro}$). A new high-affinity variant detected by special electrophoretic methods. J. Clin. Invest. *55*:469, 1975.

Jensen, W. N., Schofield, R. A., and Agner, R.: Clinical and necropsy findings in hemoglobin C disease. Blood *12*:74, 1957.

Jensen, W. N., Ricknagel, D. L., and Taylor, W. J.: In vivo study of the sickle cell phenomenon. J. Lab. Clin. Med. *56*:854, 1960.

Jensen, W. N., Bromberg, P. A., and Barefield, K.: Membrane deformation: A cause of the irreversibly sickled cell (ISC). Clin. Res. *17*:464, 1969.

Jeppson, J. O., and Berglund, S.: Thin layer isoelectric focusing and its application to haemoglobin Malmö. Clin. Chim. Acta *40*:153, 1972.

Johnston, F. E., Hertzog, K. P., and Malina, R. M.: Longitudinal growth in thalassemia major. Am. J. Dis. Child. *112*:396, 1966.

Johnston, R. B.: Increased susceptibility to infection in sickle cell disease: Review of its occurrence and possible causes. South. Med. J. *67*:1342, 1974.

Johnston, R. B., Newman, S. L., and Struth, A. G.: An abnormality of the alternate pathway of complement activation in sickle-cell disease. N. Engl. J. Med. *288*:803, 1973.

Jones, R. L., Peterson, C. M., Graziano, J. R., et al.: 2,3-Dihydroxybenzoic acid and iron overload. Blood *46*:1027(Abst.), 1975.

Jones, R. T., and Schroeder, W. A.: Chemical characterization and subunit hybridization of human hemoglobin H and associated compounds. Biochemistry *2*:1357, 1963.

Jones, R. T., Brimhall, B., Huisman, T. H. J., et al.: Hemoglobin Freiburg: Abnormal hemoglobin due to deletion of a single amino acid residue. Science *154*:1024, 1966.

Jones, R. T., Osgood, E. E., Brimhall, B., and Koler, R. D.: Hemoglobin Yakima. I. Clinical and biochemical studies. J. Clin. Invest. *46*:1840, 1967.

Jones, S. R., Binder, R. A., and Donowho, E. M.: Sudden death in sickle-cell trait. N. Engl. J. Med. *282*:323, 1970.

Jonxis, J. H. P., and Visser, H. K. A.: Determination of low percentages of fetal hemoglobin in blood of normal children. Am. J. Dis. Child. *92*:588, 1956.

Josephs, R., Jarosch, H. S., and Edelstein, S. J.: Polymorphism of sickle cell hemoglobin fibers. J. Mol. Biol. *102*:409, 1976.

Josephson, A. M., Masri, M. S., Singer, L., et al.: Starch block electrophoretic studies of human hemoglobin solutions. II. Results in cord blood, thalassemia and other hematologic disorders: comparison with Tiselius electrophoresis. Blood *13*:543, 1958.

Josephson, A. M., Weinstein, H. G., Yakulis, B. S., et al.: A new variant of hemoglobin M disease: Hemoglobin $M_{Chicago}$. J. Lab. Clin. Med. *59*:918, 1962.

Jurkiewicz, M. J., Pearson, H. A., and Furlow, L. T.: Reconstruction of the maxilla in thalassemia. Ann. NY Acad. Sci. *165*:437, 1969.

Kabat, D.: The switch from fetal to adult hemoglobin in humans: evidence suggesting a role for γ-β gene linkage. Ann. NY Acad. Sci. *241*:119, 1974.

Kacian, D. L., Gambino, R., Dow, L. W., et al.: Decreased globin messenger RNA in thalassemia detected by molecular hybridization. Proc. Natl. Acad. Sci. USA *70*:1886, 1973.

Kamuzora, H., and Lehmann, H.: A new haemoglobin variant—Haemoglobin J Birmingham, α120 (H3) Ala→Glu. Ann. Clin. Biochem. *11*:53, 1974.

Kamuzora, H., and Lehmann, H.: Human embryonic haemoglobins including a comparison by homology of the human ζ and α chains. Nature *256*:511, 1975.

Kamuzora, H., Jones, R. T., and Lehmann, H.: The ζ chain, an α-like chain of human embryonic haemoglobin. FEBS Lett. *46*:195, 1974.

Kan, Y. W., and Golbus, M. S.: Prenatal diagnosis of hereditary hemoglobin disorders: current developments. Pediatr. Res. *10*:367(Abstr. 397), 1976.

Kan, Y. W., and Nathan, D. G.: Mild thalassemia: the result of interaction of alpha and beta thalassemia genes. J. Clin. Invest. *49*:635, 1970.

Kan, Y. W., Allen, A., and Lowenstein, L.: Hydrops fetalis with alpha thalassemia. N. Engl. J. Med. *276*:18, 1967.

Kan, Y. W., Schwartz, E., and Nathan, D. G.: Globin chain synthesis in the alpha thalassemia syndromes. J. Clin. Invest. *47*:2515, 1968.

Kan, Y. W., Dozy, A. M., Alter, B. P., et al.: Detection of the sickle gene in the human fetus. Potential for intrauterine diagnosis of sickle cell anemia. N. Engl. J. Med. *287*:1, 1972a.

Kan, Y. W., Forget, B. G., and Nathan, D. G.: Gamma-beta thalassemia: a cause of hemolytic disease of newborns. N. Engl. J. Med. *286*:129, 1972b.

Kan, Y. W., Nathan, D. G., and Lodish, H. F.: Equal synthesis of α- and β-globin chains in erythroid precursors in heterozygous β-thalassemia. J. Clin. Invest. *51*:1906, 1972c.

Kan, Y. W., Todd, D., and Dozy, A. M.: Hemoglobin Constant Spring: possibly unstable mRNA and evidence for 2 locus theory for α chain production. Clin. Res. *20*:471, 1972d.

Kan, Y. W., Bellevue, R., Rieder, R., et al.: Prenatal diagnosis of α thalassemia. Clin. Res. *22*:374A, 1974a.

Kan, Y. W., Nathan, D. G., Cividalli, G., et al.: Concentration of fetal red blood cells from a mixture of maternal and fetal blood by anti-i serum: an aid to prenatal diagnosis of hemoglobinopathies. Blood *43*:411, 1974b.

Kan, Y. W., Todd, D., and Dozy, A. M.: Haemoglobin Constant Spring synthesis in red cell precursors. Br. J. Haematol. *28*:103, 1974c.

Kan, Y. W., Valenti, C., Guidotti, R., et al.: Fetal blood-sampling *in utero*. Lancet *1*:79, 1974d.

Kan, Y. W., Dozy, A. M., Varmus, H. E., et al.: Deletion of α-globin genes in haemoglobin-H disease demonstrates multiple α-globin structural loci. Nature *255*:255, 1975a.

Kan, Y. W., Globus, M. S., Klein, P., et al.: Successful application of prenatal diagnosis in a pregnancy at risk for homozygous β-thalassemia N. Engl. J. Med. *292*:1096, 1975b.

Kan, Y. W., Golbus, M. S., Trecartin, R., et al.: Prenatal diagnosis of homozygous β-thalassaemia. Lancet *2*:790, 1975c.

Kan, Y. W., Holland, J. P., Dozy, A. M., et al.: Deletion of the β-globin structure gene in hereditary persistence of foetal hemoglobin. Nature *258*:162, 1975d.

Kan, Y. W., Holland, J. P., Dozy, A. M., et al.: Demonstration of non-functional β-globin mRNA in homozygous β°-thalassemia. Proc. Natl. Acad. Sci. USA *72*:5140, 1975e.

Kan, Y. W., Golbus, M. S., and Dozy, A. M.: Application of molecular hybridization to prenatal diagnosis of α thalassemia. Clin. Res. *24*:435(Abst.), 1976a.

Kan, Y. W., Golbus, M. S., and Trecartin, R.: Prenatal diagnosis of sickle-cell anemia. N. Engl. J. Med. *294*:1039, 1976b.

Kaplan, E., Zuelzer, W. W., and Neel, J. V.: A new inherited abnormality of hemoglobin and its interaction with sickle cell hemoglobin. Blood *6*:1240, 1951.

Karayalcin, G., Imran, M., and Rosner, F.: Priapism in sickle cell disease: report of five cases. Am. J. Med. Sci. *264*:289, 1972.

Kattamis, C., and Lehmann, H.: Duplication of alpha thalassaemia gene in three Greek families with haemoglobin H disease. Lancet *2*:635, 1970.

Kattamis, C., Touliatos, N., Haidas, S., and Matsaniotis, N.: Growth of children with thalassemia: effect of different transfusion regimens. Arch. Dis. Child. *45*:502, 1970.

Kattamis, C., Lagos, P., Metaxotou-Mavromati, A., et al.: Serum iron and unsaturated iron-binding capacity in the β-thalassemia trait: their relation to the levels of haemoglobins A, A_2, and F. J. Med. Genet. *9*:154, 1972.

Kattamis, C., Metaxotou-Mavromati, A., Karamboula, K., et al.: The clinical and haematological findings in children inheriting two types of thalassaemia: high-A_2 type β-thalassaemia, and high-F type of $\delta\beta$-thalassaemia. Br. J. Haematol. *25*:375, 1973.

Kazazian, H. H., Jr., and Woodhead, A. P.: Hemoglobin A synthesis in the developing fetus. N. Engl. J. Med., *289*:58, 1973.

Kazazian, H. H., Jr., Ginder, G. D., Snyder, P. G., et al.: Further evidence of a quantitative deficiency of chain-specific globin mRNA in the thalassemia syndromes. Proc. Natl. Acad. Sci. USA *72*:567, 1975.

Kazazian, H. H., Jr., Silverstein, A. M., Snyder, P. G., et al.: Increasing haemoglobin β-chain synthesis in foetal development is associated with a declining γ- to α-mRNA ratio. Nature *260*:67, 1976.

Keberle, H.: The biochemistry of desferrioxamine and its relation to iron metabolism. Ann. NY Acad. Sci. *119*:758, 1964.

Keeling, M. M., Ogden, L. L., Wrightstone, R. N., et al.: Hemoglobin Louisville (β42 [CD1] Phe→Leu): an unstable variant causing mild hemolytic anemia. J. Clin. Invest. *50*:2395, 1971.

Keitel, A. G., Thompson, D., and Itano, H. A.: Hyposthenuria in sickle cell anemia: a reversible renal defect. J. Clin. Invest. *35*:998, 1958.

Keitt, A. S., Smith, T. W., and Jandl, J. H.: Red-cell "pseudo-mosaicism" in congenital methaemoglobinemia. N. Engl. J. Med. *275*:397, 1966.

Kendall, A. G., Ojwang, P. J., et al.: Hemoglobin Kenya, the product of a γ-β fusion gene: studies of the family. Am. J. Hum. Genet. *25*:548, 1973.

Kendrew, J. C.: The three-dimensional structure of a protein molecule. Sci. Am. *205*:104, 1961.

Kennedy, D. S., Bester, A. J., and Heywood, S. M.: The regulation of protein synthesis by translational control RNA. Biochem. Biophys. Res. Commun. *61*:415, 1974.

Kiese, M., Kurz, H., and Schneider, C.: Chronische Hämoglobinämie durch pathologischen Blutfarbstoff. Klin. Wochenschr. *34*:957, 1956.

Kikuchi, G., Hayashi, N., and Tamura, A.: Oxygen equilibrium of hemoglobin M_{Iwate}. Biochim. Biophys. Acta *90*:199, 1964.

Kilmartin, J. V., and Rossi-Bernardi, L.: Inhibition of CO_2 combination and reduction of the Bohr effect in haemoglobin chemically modified at its α-amino groups. Nature *222*:1243, 1969.

Kilmartin, J. V., Breen, J. J., Roberts, G. C. K., and Ho, C.: Direct measurement of the pK values of an alkaline Bohr group in human hemoglobin. Proc. Natl. Acad. Sci. USA *70*:1246, 1973a.

Kim, H. C., Marks, P. A., Rifkind, R. A., et al.: Isolation and *in vitro* differentiation of human erythroid precursor cells. Blood *47*:767, 1976.

King, M. A. R., Wiltshire, B. G., Lehmann, H., and Morimoto, H.: An unstable haemoglobin with reduced oxygen affinity: Haemoglobin Peterborough, β 111 (C13) valine→phenylalanine, its interaction with normal haemoglobin and with haemoglobin Lepore. Br. J. Haematol. 22:125, 1972.

Kleckner, H. B., Wilson, J. B., Lindeman, J. G., et al.: Hemoglobin Fort-Gordon or $\alpha_2\beta_2^{145\ Tyr\rightarrow Asp}$, a new high-affinity variant. Biochim. Biophys. Acta *400*(2):343, 1975.

Kleihauer, E. F., Reynolds, C. A., Dozy, A. M., et al.: Hemoglobin Bibba or $\alpha_2^{136\ Pro}\ \beta_2$, an unstable α chain abnormal hemoglobin. Biochim. Biophys. Acta *154*:220, 1968.

Klinefelter, H. F.: The heart in sickle cell anemia. Am. J. Med. Sci. *203*:34, 1942.

Klion, F. M., Weiner, M. J., and Schaffner, F.: Cholestasis in sickle cell anemia. Am. J. Med. *37*:829, 1964.

Klocke, R. A.: Oxygen transport and 2,3-diphosphoglycerate. Chest *62*:795, 1972.

Knöchel, W., and Tiedemann, H.: Size distribution and cell-free translation of globin-coding HnRNA from avian erythroblasts. Biochim. Biophys. Acta *378*:383, 1975.

Knox-Macauley, H. H. M., Weatherall, D. J., Clegg, J. B., et al.: The clinical and biosynthetic characterization of $\alpha\beta$-thalassemia. Br. J. Haematol. *22*:497, 1972.

Koenig, R. J., Peterson, C. M., Jones, R. L., et al.: Correlation of glucose regulation and hemoglobin A_{IC} in diabetes mellitus. N. Engl. J. Med. 295:417, 1976.

Kohne, E., Grosse, H. P., Versmold, K., et al.: Hb M Erlangen: $\alpha_2\beta_2^{63(E7)\ Tyr}$: Eine neue Mutation mit Hämolyse und Diaphorasemangel. Z. Kinderheilkd. *120*:69, 1975.

Kolatat, T.: Oxygen affinity of hemoglobin E. Siriraj Hosp. Gaz. *16*:205, 1964.

Koler, R. D., and Rigas, D. A.: Genetics of haemoglobin H. Ann. Hum. Genet. *25*:95, 1961.

Koler, R. D., Jones, R. T., Wasi, P., and Pootrakul, S.: Genetics of haemoglobin H and α-thalassaemia. Ann. Hum. Genet. *34*:371, 1971.

Koler, R. D., Jones, R. T., Bigley, R. H., et al.: Hemoglobin Casper β106 (G8) Leu→Pro, a contemporary mutation. Am. J. Med. *55*:549, 1973.

Konotey-Ahulu, F. I. D.: Effect of environment on sickle cell disease in West Africa: Epidemiologic and clinical considerations. In Abramson, H., Bertles, J. F., and Wethers, D. L. (eds.): Sickle Cell Disease: Diagnosis, Management, Education and Research. St. Louis, The C. V. Mosby Co., 1973, p. 20.

Konotey-Ahulu, F. I. D.: The sickle cell diseases. Arch. Intern. Med. *133*:611, 1974.

Konotey-Ahulu, F. I. D., Gallo, E., Lehmann, H., et al.: Haemoglobin Korle-Bu (β^{73} Aspartic acid→Asparagine) showing one of the two amino acids substitutions of haemoglobin C Harlem. J. Med. Genet. *5*:107, 1968.

Konotey-Ahulu, F. I. D., Kinderlerer, J. L., Lehmann, H., et al.: Haemoglobin Osu-Christiansborg: A new β-chain variant of haemoglobin A (β^{52} [D3] Aspartic acid→Asparagine) in combination with haemoglobin S. J. Med. Genet. *8*:302, 1971.

Koutras, G. A., Hattori, M., Schneider, A. S., et al.: Studies on chromated erythrocytes. Effect of sodium chromate on erythrocyte glutathione reductase. J. Clin. Invest. *43*:323, 1964.

Kraus, A. P., and Diggs, L. W.: In vitro crystallization of hemoglobin occurring in citrated blood from patients with hemoglobin C. J. Lab. Clin. Med. *47*:700, 1956.

Kraus, L. M., Miyaji, T., Iuchi, I., and Kraus, A. P.: Characterization of α^{23}GluNH_2 in hemoglobin Memphis. Hemoglobin Memphis/S, a new variant of molecular disease. Biochemistry *5*:3701, 1966.

Kreimer-Birnbaum, M., Pinkerton, P. H., Bannerman, R. M., et al.: Dipyrrolic urinary pigments in congenital Heinz-body anaemia due to Hb Köln and in thalassaemia. Br. Med. J. *2*:396, 1966a.

Kreimer-Birnbaum, M., Pinkerton, P. H., Bannerman, R. M., et al.: Urinary "dipyrroles"; their occurrence and significance in thalassemia and other disorders. Blood *28*:993, 1966b.

Lassman, M. N., Genel, M., and Wise, J. K.: Carbohydrate homeostasis and pancreatic islet cell function in thalassemia. Ann. Intern. Med. *80*:65, 1974.

Laux, B., Dennis, D., and White, H. B., III: Human α-chain globin messenger: prediction of a nucleotide sequence. Biochem. Biophys. Res. Commun. *54*:894, 1973.

Laver, M. B., Tung, C., Jackson, E., et al.: Effect of benzoic acid derivatives of O_2 affinity of hemoglobin solutions, intact RBCs in vitro and in vivo. Fed. Proc. *33*:335, 1974.

Lee-Potter, J. P., Deacon-Smith, R. A., Simpkiss, M. J., et al.: A new cause of haemolytic anaemia in the newborn. A description of an unstable fetal haemoglobin: F Poole, $\alpha_2{}^G\gamma_2{}^{130\ Trp \rightarrow Gly}$. J. Clin. Pathol. *28*:317, 1975.

Lehmann, H.: Different types of alpha thalassaemia and significance of haemoglobin Bart's in neonates. Lancet *2*:78, 1970.

Lehmann, H., and Carrell, R. W.: Differences between α and β chain mutants of human hemoglobin and between α and β thalassaemia. Possible duplication of the α-chain gene. Br. Med. J. *4*:748, 1968.

Lehmann, H., and Carrell, R. W.: Variations in the structure of human haemoglobin with particular reference to the unstable haemoglobins. Br. Med. Bull. *25*:14, 1969.

Lehmann, H., and Charlesworth, D.: Observations on hemoglobin P (Congo type). Biochem. J. *119*:43, 1970.

Lehmann, H., and Huntsman, R. G.: Man's Haemoglobins. Philadelphia, J. B. Lippincott Co., 1966.

Lehmann, H., Story, P., and Thien, H.: Hemoglobin E in Burmese. Br. Med. J. *1*:544, 1956.

Lehmann, H., Casey, R., Lang, A., et al.: Haemoglobin Tak: a β-chain elongation. Br. J. Haematol. *31*(Suppl.):119, 1975.

Lessin, L. S., Jensen, W. N., and Ponder, E.: Molecular mechanism of hemolytic anemia in homozygous hemoglobin C disease. J. Exp. Med. *130*:443, 1969.

Levere, R. D., Lichtman, H. C., and Levine, J.: Effect of iron deficiency anaemia on the metabolism of the heterogenic haemoglobins in sickle cell trait. Nature *202*:499, 1964.

Libnoch, J. A., Taketa, F., Mauk, A. G., et al.: Hemoglobin Wood β97 (FG4) His→Leu. Cause of familial erythrocytosis and drug-induced methemoglobinemia. Blood *46*:1030, 1975.
Lichtman, M. A., Miller, D. R., Cohen, J., et al.: Reduced red cell glycolysis, 2,3-diphosphoglycerate and adenosine triphosphate concentration and increased hemoglobin-oxygen affinity caused by hypophosphatemia. Ann. Intern. Med. *74*:562, 1971.
Lichtman, M. A., Whitbeck, A. A., and Murphy, M.: Fictitious changes in binding of oxygen to hemoglobin when based on extracellular pH in the presence of certain blood additives like radiographic contrast media. Invest. Radiol. *10*:225, 1975.
Liebman, J., Lucas, R., Moss, A., et al.: Airline travel for children with chronic pulmonary disease. Pediatrics *57*:408, 1976.
Lief, P. D., Sullivan, A., and Goldberg, M.: Physiological contributions of thin and thick loops of Henle to the renal concentrating mechanism. J. Clin. Invest. *48*:52(Abst.), 1969.
Lie-Injo, L. E.: Alpha-chain thalassemia and hydrops fetalis in Malaya: report of five cases. Blood *20*:581, 1962.
Lie-Injö, L. E., and Jo, B. H.: A fast-moving haemoglobin in hydrops fetalis. Nature *185*:698, 1960.
Lie-Injo, L. E., Ganesan, J., Clegg, J. B., and Weatherall, D. J.: The homozygous state for Hb Constant Spring. Blood *43*:251, 1974.
Lindsay, J., Meshel, J. C., and Patterson, R. M.: The cardiovascular manifestations of sickle cell disease. Arch. Intern. Med. *133*:643, 1974.
Lindstrom, T. R., Ho, C., and Pisciotta, A. V.: Nuclear magnetic resonance studies of haemoglobin M Milwaukee. Nature [New Biol.] *237*:263, 1972a.
Lindstrom, T. R., Noren, I. B. E., Charache, S., et al.: Nuclear magnetic resonance studies of hemoglobins. VII. Tertiary structure around ligand binding site in carbonmonoxy-hemoglobin. Biochemistry *11*:1677, 1972b.
Lindstrom, T. R., Baldassare, J. J., Bunn, H. F., and Ho., C.: Nuclear magnetic resonance and spin-label studies of hemoglobin Kempsey. Biochemistry. *12*:4212, 1973.
Lindstrom, T. R., Koenig, S. H., Boussios, T., et al.: Intermolecular interactions of oxygenated sickle hemoglobin molecules in cells and cell-free solutions. Biophys. J. *16*:679, 1976.
Lines, J. G., and McIntosh, R.: Oxygen binding by haemoglobin J-Cape Town ($\alpha_2{}^{92}{}_{\mathrm{Arg \rightarrow Gln}}$). Nature *215*:297, 1967.
Lipschitz, D. A., Dugard, J., Simon, M. O., et al.: The site of action of desferrioxamine. Br. J. Haematol. *20*:395, 1971.
Logothetis, J., Economidou, J., Constantoulakis, M., et al.: Cephalofacial deformities in thalassemia major (Cooley's anemia). Am. J. Dis. Child. *121*:300, 1971.
Logothetis, J., Loewenson, R. B., Augoustaki, O., et al.: Body growth in Cooley's anemia (homozygous beta-thalassemia) with a correlative study as to other aspects of the illness in 138 cases. Pediatrics *50*:92, 1972.
Lokich, J. J., Maloney, W. C., Bunn, H. F., et al.: Hemoglobin Brigham ($\alpha_2{}^{A}\beta_2{}^{100}{}_{\mathrm{Pro \rightarrow Leu}}$), hemoglobin variant associated with familial erythrocytosis. J. Clin. Invest. *52*:2060, 1973.
Lorkin, P. A.: Fetal and embryonic haemoglobins. J. Med. Genet. *10*:50, 1973.
Lorkin, P. A., and Lehmann, H.: Fetal and embryonic haemoglobins. J. Med. Genet. *10*:50, 1973.
Lorkin, P. A., Lehmann, H., Fairbanks, V. P., et al.: Two new pathological haemoglobins: Olmsted β141 (H19) Leu→Arg and Malmö β97 (FG4) His→Gln. Biochem. J. *119*:68, 1970.
Lorkin, P. A., Stephens, A. D., Beard, M. E. J., et al.: Haemoglobin Rahere (β82 Lys→Thr): a new high affinity haemoglobin associated with decreased 2,3-diphosphoglycerate binding and relative polycythaemia. Br. Med. J. *4*:200, 1975.
Loukopoulos, D., and Fessas, P.: The distribution of hemoglobin types in thalassemic erythrocytes. J. Clin. Invest. *44*:231, 1965.
Lubin, A., and Desforges, J.: Effect of Heinz bodies on red cell deformability. Blood *39*:658, 1972.
Lubin, B. H., Pena, V., Mentzer, W. C., et al.: Dimethyl adipimidate: a new anti-sickling agent. Proc. Natl. Acad. Sci. USA *72*:43, 1975.
Lucas, W. M., and Bullock, W.: Hematuria in sickle cell disease. J. Urol. *83*:733, 1960.

Luhby, A. L., and Cooperman, J. M.: Folic acid deficiency in thalassaemia major. Lancet *2*:490, 1961.
Luhby, A. L., Cooperman, J. M., Feldman, R., et al.: Folic acid deficiency as a limiting factor in the anemias of thalassemia major. Blood *18*:786, 1961.
Lukens, J. N., and Neuman, L. A.: Excretion and distribution of iron during chronic deferoxamine therapy. Blood *38*:614, 1971.
Lundh, B., and Gardner, F. H.: The haematological response to androgens in sickle cell anemia. Scand. J. Haematol. *7*:389, 1970.
Lutcher, C. L., Wilson, J. B., Gravely, M. E., et al.: Hb Leslie, an unstable hemoglobin due to deletion of glutaminyl residue β131 (H9) occurring in association with β^0-thalassemia, Hb C and Hb S. Blood *47*:99, 1976.
Lux, S. E., and John, K. M.: The membrane defect in irreversibly sickled red cells (ISC's). Irreversible deformation of the spectrin-actin lattice. Blood *46*:1052, 1975.
Luzzato, L., Nwachuku-Jarrett, E. S., and Reddy, S.: Increased sickling of parasitized erythrocytes as mechanism of resistance against malaria in sickle-cell trait. Lancet *1*:319, 1970.
Magdoff-Fairchild, B., Swerdlow, P. H., and Bertles, J. F.: Intermolecular organization of deoxygenated sickle haemoglobin determined by X-ray diffraction. Nature *239*:217, 1972.
Malfa, R., and Steinhardt, J.: A temperature-dependent latent-period in the aggregation of sickle-cell deoxyhemoglobin. Biochem. Biophys. Res. Commun. *59*:887, 1974.
Mann, J. R., and Stuart, J.: Sodium bicarbonate prophylaxis of sickle cell crisis. Pediatrics *53*:414, 1974.
Mann, J. R., MacNeish, A. S., Bannister, D., et al.: $\delta\beta$-Thalassemia in a Chinese family. Br. J. Haematol. *23*:393, 1972.
Marotta, C. A., Forget, B. G., Weissman, S. M., et al.: Nucleotide sequences of human globin messenger RNA. Proc. Natl. Acad. Sci. USA *71*:2300, 1974.
Marotta, C. A., Forget, B. G., Cohen-Solal, M., et al.: Nucleotide sequence analysis of coding and noncoding regions of human β-globin mRNA. *In* Cohn, W. E. (ed.): Progress in Nucleic Acid Research and Molecular Biology, New York, Academic Press, Vol. 19, p. 165, 1977.
Marti, H. R.: Normale und Anormale Menschliche Hämoglobine. Berlin, Springer Verlag, 1963, p. 81.
Martinez, G., and Colombo, B.: A new type of hereditary persistence of foetal haemoglobin: is a diffusible factor regulating γ-chain synthesis? Nature *252*:735, 1974.
Masys, D. R., Bromberg, P. A., and Balcerzak, S. P.: Red cells shrink during sickling. Blood *44*:885, 1974.
Mattii, R., Weinger, R., and Sise, H. S.: Coagulation, fibrinogen survival and fibrin split products in sickle cell disease. Blood *42*:1004 (Abst.), 1973.
Maurer, H. S., Behrman, R. E., and Honig, G. R.: Dependence of the oxygen affinity of blood on the presence of foetal or adult hemoglobin. Nature *227*:388, 1970.
Maurer, H. S., Vida, L. N., and Honig, G. R.: Similarities of the erythocytes in juvenile chronic myelogenic leukemia to fetal erythrocytes. Blood *39*:778, 1972.
May, A., and Huehns, E. R.: The control of oxygen affinity of red cells with Hb Shepherds Bush. Br. J. Haematol. *22*:599, 1972a.
May, A., and Huehns, E. R.: The mechanism of the low oxygen affinity of red cells in sickle cell disease. Haematol. Bluttransfus. *10*:279, 1972b.
McCarthy, G. M., Temperley, I. J., Clegg, J. B., and Weatherall, D. J.: Thalassemia in an Irish family. Ir. J. Med. Sci. (7th Series) *1*:303, 1968.
McConn, R.: The oxyhemoglobin dissociation curve in acute disease. Surg. Clin. N. Am. *55*:627, 1975.
McCoy, R. C.: Ultrastructural alterations in the kidney of patients with sickle cell disease and the nephrotic syndrome. Lab. Invest. *21*:85, 1969.
McCurdy, P. R.: Clinical and physiological studies in a Negro with sickle cell hemoglobin D disease. N. Engl. J. Med. *262*:961, 1960.
McCurdy, P. R., Lorkin, P. A., Casey, R., et al.: Hemoglobin S-G (S-D) syndrome. Am. J. Med. *57*:665, 1974.
McCurdy, P. R., Sherman, A. S., Kamuzora, H., et al.: Globin synthesis in subjects doubly heterozygous for hemoglobin G Philadelphia and hemoglobin S or C. J. Lab. Clin. Med. *85*:891, 1975.

McDonald, M. J., Noble, R. W., Sharma, V. S., and Ranney, H. M.: Equilibrium and kinetic studies of hemoglobin I: a functionally silent amino acid substitution at an invariant residue. J. Mol. Biol. *89*:245, 1974.

McKeehan, W. L.: Regulation of hemoglobin synthesis. J. Biol. Chem. *249*:6517, 1974.

Melderis, H., Steinheider, G., and Ostertag, W.: Evidence for a unique kind of α-type globin chains in early mammalian embryos. Nature *250*:774, 1974.

Mentzer, W. C.: Differentiation of iron deficiency from thalassaemia trait. Lancet *1*:882, 1973.

Messer, M. J., and Harris, J. W.: Filtration characteristics of sickle cells: Rates of alteration of filterability after deoxygenation, reoxygenation and correlations with sickling and unsickling. J. Lab. Clin. Med. *76*:537, 1970.

Messer, M. J., Hahn, J. A., and Bradley, T. B.: The kinetics of sickling and unsickling of red cells under physiologic conditions: rheologic and ultrastructural correlations. Presented at Symposium on Molecular and Cellular Aspects of Sickle Cell Disease, December 10, 1975. DHEW Publ. No. (NIH)76-1007.

Miller, D. R., Weed, R. I., Stamatoyannopoulos, G., and Yoshida, A.: Hemoglobin Köln disease occurring as a fresh mutation: Erythrocyte metabolism and survival. Blood *38*:715, 1971.

Mills, G. C., Levin, W. C., and Alperin, J. B.: Hemolytic anemia associated with low erythrocyte ATP. Blood *32*:15, 1968.

Milner, P. F.: The sickling disorders. Clin. Haematol. *3*:289, 1974.

Milner, P. F., Miller, C., Grey, R., et al.: Hemoglobin O Arab in four Negro families and its interaction with hemoglobin S and hemoglobin C. N. Engl. J. Med. *283*:1417, 1970.

Milner, P. F., Clegg, J. B., and Weatherall, D. J.: Haemoglobin H disease due to a unique haemoglobin variant with an elongated α-chain. Lancet *1*:729, 1971.

Milosz, A., and Settle, W.: A new approach to the treatment of sickle cell anemia. Res. Commun. Chem. Pathol. Pharmacol. *12*:137, 1975.

Minnich, V., Hill, R. J., Khuri, P. D., and Anderson, M. E.: Hemoglobin Hope: A beta chain variant. Blood *25*:830, 1965.

Modell, C. B., and Beck, J.: Long-term desferrioxamine therapy in thalassemia. Ann. NY Acad. Sci. *232*:201, 1974.

Modell, C. B., Latter, A., Steadman, J. H., et al.: Haemoglobin synthesis in β-thalassaemia. Br. J. Haematol. *17*:485, 1969.

Moffat, K.: Gelation of sickle cell hemoglobin: effects of hybrid tetramer formation in hemoglobin mixtures. Science *185*:274, 1974.

Moffat, K., and Gibson, Q. H.: The rates of polymerization and depolymerization of sickle cell hemoglobin. Biochem. Biophys. Res. Commun. *61*:237, 1974.

Monn, E., and Bjark, P.: Hb Sögn (β14 arginine). Haematological and genetical studies. Scand. J. Haematol. *7*:455, 1970.

Monn, E., Gaffney, P. J., Jr., and Lehmann, H.: Haemoglobin Sögn (β14 arginine). A new haemoglobin variant. Scand. J. Haematol. *5*:353, 1968.

Monte, M., Beuzard, Y., and Rosa, J.: Mapping of several abnormal hemoglobins by horizontal polyacrylamide gel isoelectric focusing. Am. J. Clin. Path. *66*:753, 1976.

Moo-Penn, W., Bechtel, K. C., Jue, M. S., et al.: The presence of hemoglobin S and C-Harlem in an individual in the United States. Blood *46*:363, 1975.

Morimoto, H., Lehmann, H., and Perutz, M. F.: Molecular pathology of human haemoglobin: Stereochemical interpretation of abnormal oxygen affinities. Nature *232*:408, 1971.

Moser, K. M., and Shea, J. C. L.: The relationship between pulmonary infarction, cor pulmonale and sickle states. Am. J. Med. *22*:561, 1957.

Mostofi, F. K., and Bruegge, C. F.V.: Lesions in kidneys removed for unilateral hematuria in sickle cell disease. Arch. Pathol. *63*:336, 1957.

Motulsky, A. G.: Frequency of sickling disorders in U.S. Blacks. N. Engl. J. Med. *288*:31, 1973.

Muirhead, H., et al.: Structure and function of haemoglobin. III. A three-dimensional Fourier synthesis of human deoxyhaemoglobin at 5.5 Ångström resolution. J. Mol. Biol. *28*:117, 1967.

Muller, C. J., and Kingma, S.: Haemoglobin Zürich, $\alpha_2{}^{A}\beta_2{}^{63\ Arg}$. Biochim. Biophys. Acta *50*:595, 1961.

Murayama, M.: Molecular mechanism of red cell "sickling." Science *153*:145, 1966.

Murayama, M., in Nalbandian, R. M. (ed.): Molecular Aspects of Sickle Cell Hemoglobin. Springfield, Illinois, Charles C Thomas, 1971.
Murphy, J. R.: Hemoglobin CC disease: rheological properties of erythrocytes and abnormalities in cell water. J. Clin. Invest. *47*:1483, 1968.
Murphy, J. R.: Sickle cell hemoglobin (Hb AS) in black football players. JAMA *225*:981, 1973.
Nagel, R. L., and Bookchin, R. M.: The effect of 2,3-diphosphoglycerate on gelation of hemoglobin S and its molecular mechanism. Clin. Res. *22*:399A, 1974a.
Nagel, R. L., and Bookchin, R. M.: Human hemoglobin mutants with abnormal oxygen binding. Semin. Hematol. *11*:385, 1974b.
Nagel, R. L., and Gibson, Q. H.: Kinetics and mechanism of the complex formation between hemoglobin and haptoglobin. J. Biol. Chem. *242*:3428, 1967.
Nagel, R. L., and Gibson, Q. H.: The hemoglobin-haptoglobin reaction as a probe of hemoglobin conformation. Biochem. Biophys. Res. Commun. *48*:959, 1972.
Nagel, R. L., Gibson, Q. H., and Charache, S.: Relation between structure and function in hemoglobin Chesapeake. Biochemistry *6*:2395, 1967.
Nagel, R. L., Ranney, H. M., Bradley, T. B., Jr., et al.: Hemoglobin L Ferrara trait in a Jewish family associated with a hemolytic state in the propositus. Blood *34*:157, 1969.
Nagel, R. L., Rieder, R. F., Bookchin, R. M., et al.: Some functional properties of hemoglobin Leiden. Biochem. Biophys. Res. Commun. *53*:1240, 1973.
Nagel, R. L., Lynfield, J., Johnson, J., et al.: Hemoglobin Beth Israel: A mutant causing clinically apparent cyanosis. N. Engl. J. Med. *295*:125, 1976.
Najman, A., Duhamel, G., Andre, R., et al.: Hemolytic anemia due to unstable hemoglobin with deletion. Study of 2 new cases—Hb Tours (Thr β87 deleted) and Hb St. Antoine (Gly→Leu β74, 75 deleted). Nouv. Rev. Fr. Hematol. *13*:803, 1973.
Na-Nakorn, S., and Wasi, P.: Alpha-thalassemia in Northern Thailand. Am. J. Hum. Genet. *22*:645, 1970.
Na-Nakorn, S., Wasi, P., Pornpatkul, M., et al.: Further evidence for a genetic basis of haemoglobin H disease from newborn offspring of patients. Nature *223*:59, 1969.
Nance, W. E., Conneally, M., Kang, K. W., et al.: Genetic linkage analysis of human hemoglobin variants. Am. J. Hum. Genet. *22*:453, 1970.
Nathan, D. G.: Thalassemia. N. Engl. J. Med. *286*:586, 1972.
Nathan, D. G.: Thalassemia: a progress report in applied molecular biology. N. Engl. J. Med. *288*:1122, 1973.
Nathan, D. G., and Alter, B. P.: Antenatal diagnosis of the haemoglobinopathies. Br. J. Haematol. *31*(Suppl.):143, 1975.
Nathan, D. G., and Gunn, R. B.: Thalassemia: the consequences of unbalanced hemoglobin synthesis. Am. J. Med. *41*:815, 1966.
Nathan, D. G., and Oski, F. A. (eds.): Hematology of Infancy and Childhood. Philadelphia, W. B. Saunders Co., 1971.
Nathan, D. G., Stossel, T. B., Gunn, R. B., et al.: Influence of hemoglobin precipitation on erythrocyte metabolism in alpha and beta thalassemia. J. Clin. Invest. *48*:33, 1969.
Nathan, D. G., Lodish, H., Kan, Y. M., and Housman, D.: Beta thalassemia and translation of globin messenger RNA. Proc. Natl. Acad. Sci. USA *68*:2514, 1971.
Natta, C. L., Banks, J., Niazi, G., et al.: Decreased β-globin mRNA activity in bone marrow cells in homozygous and heterozygous β-thalassaemia. Nature [New Biol.] *244*:280, 1973a.
Natta, C. L., Niazi, G., Ford, S., et al.: Balanced globin chain synthesis in hereditary persistence of fetal hemoglobin (HPFH). Blood *42*:991, 1973b.
Necheles, T. F., Allen, D. M., and Finkel, H. E.: Clinical Disorders of Hemoglobin Structure and Synthesis. New York, Appleton-Century-Crofts, 1969a.
Necheles, T. F., Beard, M. E. J., and Allen, D. M.: Myocardial hemosiderosis in hypoxic mice. Ann NY Acad. Sci. *165*:167, 1969b.
Necheles, T. F., Sabbah, R., and Chung, S., et al.: Intensive transfusion therapy in thalassemia major. An eight year follow-up. Ann NY Acad. Sci. *232*:179, 1974.
Neel, J. V.: The clinical detection of the genetic carriers of inherited disease. Medicine (Baltimore) *26*:115, 1947.
Neel, J. V.: The inheritance of sickle cell anemia. Science *110*:64, 1949.
Neel, J. V.: The inheritance of the sickling phenomenon, with particular reference to sickle cell disease. Blood *6*:389, 1951.

Nienhuis, A. W., and Anderson, W. F.: Isolation and translation of hemoglobin messenger RNA from thalassemia, sickle cell anemia and normal human reticulocytes. J. Clin. Invest. *50*:2458, 1971.

Nienhuis, A. W., and Bunn, H. F.: Hemoglobin switching in sheep and goats: Occurrence of hemoglobins A and C in the same red cell. Science *185*:946, 1974.

Nienhuis, A. W., Laycock, D. G., and Anderson, W. F.: Translation of rabbit haemoglobin messenger RNA by thalassaemic and non-thalassaemic ribosomes. Nature [New Biol.] *231*:205, 1971.

Nienhuis, A. W., Canfield, P. H., and Anderson, W. F.: Hemoglobin messenger RNA from human bone marrow: isolation and translation in homozygous and heterozygous β-thalassemia. J. Clin. Invest. *52*:1735, 1973.

Nienhuis, A. W., Delea, C., Aamodt, R., et al.: Potential role for desferrioxamine and ascorbic acid in the treatment of chronic iron overload. Blood *46*:1026(Abst.), 1975.

Nigen, A. M., Njikam, N., Lee, C. K., and Manning, J. M.: Studies on mechanism of action of cyanate in sickle cell disease. Oxygen affinity and gelling properties of hemoglobin S carbamylated on specific chains. J. Biol. Chem. *249*:6611, 1974.

Nishikura, K., Sugita, Y., Nagai, M., et al.: High cooperativity of haemoglobin M Boston in the completely reduced state. Nature *254*:727, 1975.

Noble, R. W.: Relation between allosteric effects and changes in the energy of bonding between molecular subunits. J. Mol. Biol. *39*:479, 1969.

Novy, M. J., and Parer, J. T.: Absence of high blood oxygen affinity in the fetal cat. Respir. Physiol. *6*:144, 1969.

Novy, M. J., Edwards, M. J., and Metcalfe, J.: Hemoglobin Yakima. II. High blood oxygen affinity associated with compensatory erythrocytosis and normal hemodynamics. J. Clin. Invest. *46*:1848, 1967.

Nute, P. E., et al.: Multiple hemoglobin α-chain loci in monkeys, apes, and man. Ann. NY Acad. Sci. *241*:39, 1974a.

Nute, P. E., Stamatoyannopoulos, G., Hermodson, M. A., and Roth, D.: Hemoglobinopathic erythrocytosis due to a new electrophoretically silent variant, Hemoglobin San Diego (β109 (G11) Val$\rightarrow$Met). J. Clin. Invest. *53*:320, 1974b.

Nute, P. E., Wood, W. G., Stamatoyannopoulos, G., et al.: The Kenya form of hereditary persistence of fetal haemoglobin: structural studies and evidence for homogeneous distribution of haemoglobin F using fluorescent anti-haemoglobin F antibodies. Br. J. Haematol. *32*:55, 1976.

O'Brien, R. T.: The effect of iron deficiency on the expression of hemoglobin H. Blood *41*:853, 1973.

O'Brien, R. T.: Ascorbic acid enhancement of desferrioxamine-induced urinary iron excretion in thalassemia major. Ann. NY Acad. Sci. *232*:221, 1974.

O'Brien, R. T., and Pearson, H. A.: Splenic function and hematologic changes during the first year of life in sickle cell anemia. In Hercules, J. I., Schechter, A. N., Eaton, W. A., et al. (eds.): Proceedings of First National Symposium on Sickle Cell Disease, Washington, D.C. DHEW Pub. No. 75–723 (NIH), Bethesda, Md., 1974, p. 73.

O'Brien, R. T., Pearson, H. A., and Spencer, R. P.: Transfusion-induced decrease in spleen size in thalassemia major: documentation by radioisotopic scan. J. Pediatr. *81*:105, 1972.

Ogata, R. T., McConnell, H. M., and Jones, R. T.: Binding of triphosphate spin labels to hemoglobin Kempsey. Biochem. Biophys. Res. Commun. *47*:157, 1972.

Ogawa, S., Mayer, A., and Shulman, R. G.: High resolution proton magnetic resonance study of the two quaternary states in fully ligated hemoglobin Kansas. Biochem. Biophys. Res. Commun. *49*:1485, 1972.

O'Gorman, P., Allsopp, K. M., Lehmann, H., and Sukumaran, P. K.: Sickle-cell haemoglobin K disease. Br. Med. J. 2:1381, 1963.

Ohta, Y., Yamaoka, K., Sumida, I., et al.: Two unique structural and synthetic variants, Hb Miyada and homozygous δ-thalassemia, discovered in Japanese. XIII International Congress of Haematology, Munich. Abstracts, Munich, R. F. Lehmanns Verlag, 1970, p. 233.

Ohta, Y., Yamaoka, K., Sumida, I., et al.: Haemoglobin Miyada, a β-δ fusion peptide (anti-Lepore) type discovered in a Japanese family. Nature [New Biol.] *234*:218, 1971.

Olson, J. S., and Gibson, Q. H.: The functional properties of hemoglobin Bethesda ($\alpha_2\beta_2^{145\ His}$). J. Biol. Chem. *247*:3662, 1972.

Olson, J. S., Gibson, Q. H., Nagel, R. L., et al.: The ligand-binding properties of hemoglobin Hiroshima ($\alpha_2\beta_2^{146\,Asp}$). J. Biol. Chem. *247*:7485, 1972.

Opalinski, A., and Beutler, E.: Creatine, 2,3-diphosphoglycerate and anemia. N. Engl. J. Med. *285*:483, 1971.

Opfell, R. W., Lorkin, P. A., and Lehmann, H.: Hereditary non-spherocytic haemolytic anaemia with post-splenectomy inclusion bodies and pigmenturia caused by an unstable haemoglobin Santa Ana—β88 (F4) leucine→proline. J. Med. Genet. *5*:292, 1968.

Orkin, S. H., Swan, D., and Leder, P.: Differential expression of α- and β-globin genes during differentiation of cultured erythroleukemic cells. J. Biol. Chem. *250*:8753, 1975.

Oski, F. A., and Gottlieb, A. J.: The interrelationships between red blood cell metabolites, hemoglobin and the oxygen-equilibrium curve. Progr. Hematol. *7*:33, 1971.

Oski, F. A., Viner, E. D., Purugganan, H. B., and McElfresh, A. E.: Low molecular weight dextran in sickle cell crisis. JAMA *191*:43, 1965.

Oski, F. A., Call, F. L., and Lessen, L.: Failure of promazine HCl to prevent the painful episodes in sickle cell anemia. J. Pediatr. *73*:265, 1968.

Oski, F. A., Gottlieb, A. J., Miller, W. W., et al.: The effects of deoxygenation of adult and fetal hemoglobin on the synthesis of red cell 2,3-diphosphoglycerate and its in vivo consequences. J. Clin. Invest. *49*:400, 1970.

Oski, F. A., Marshall, B. E., Cohen, P. F., et al.: Exercise with anemia. The role of the left-shifted or right-shifted oxygen-hemoglobin equilibrium curve. Ann. Intern. Med. *74*:44, 1971a.

Oski, F. A., Travis, S. F., Miller, L. D., et al.: The in vitro restoration of red cell 2,3-diphosphoglycerate levels in banked blood. Blood *37*:52, 1971b.

Oster, J. R., Lee, S. M., Lespier, L. E., et al.: Renal acidification in sickle-cell trait. Arch. Intern. Med. *136*:30, 1976.

Ostertag, W., von Ehrenstein, G., and Charache, S.: Duplicated α-chain genes in Hopkins-2 haemoglobin of man and evidence for unequal crossing-over between them. Nature [New Biol.] *237*:90, 1972b.

Ottolenghi, S., Lanyon, W. G., Paul, J., et al.: The severe form of α-thalassaemia is caused by a haemoglobin gene deletion. Nature *251*:389, 1974.

Ottolenghi, S., Lanyon, W. G., Williamson, R., et al.: Human globin gene analysis for a patient with $\beta^0/\delta\beta^0$-thalassemia. Proc. Natl. Acad. Sci. USA *72*:2294, 1975.

Ottolenghi, S., Comi, P., Giglioni, B., et al.: δβ-thalassemia is due to a gene deletion. Cell *9*:71, 1976.

Overly, W. L., Rosenberg, A., and Harris, J. W.: Hemoglobin M Reserve: studies on identification and characterization. J. Lab. Clin. Med. *69*:62, 1967.

Özsoylu, S.: Homozygous hemoglobin D-Punjab. Acta Haematol. (Basel) *43*:353, 1970.

Padilla, F., Bromberg, P. A., and Jensen, W. N.: The sickle-unsickle cycle: a cause of fragmentation leading to permanently deformed cells. Blood *41*:653, 1973.

Pagnier, J., Labie, D., Kaplan, J. C., et al.: Étude biochimique d'un cas d'érythroleucémie. Nouv. Rev. Fr. Hematol. *12*:317, 1972.

Pagnier, J., Wajcman, H., and Labie, D.: Defect in hemoglobin synthesis possibly due to a disturbed association. FEBS Lett. *45*:252, 1974.

Palek, J.: Calcium accumulation during sickling of hemoglobin S (HbSS) red cells. Blood *42*:988, 1973.

Palek, J., Church, A., and Fairbanks, G.: Trans-membrane movements and distribution of calcium in normal and hemoglobin S erythrocytes. In Leaf, A.,Hoffman, J. F., and Bolis, L. (eds.): Membranes and Diseases. Proceedings of International Conference on Biological Membranes. Craus-sur-Sierre, Switzerland, 1975.

Paniker, N. V., Ben-Bassat, I., and Beutler, E.: Evaluation of sickle hemoglobin and desickling agents by falling ball viscometry. J. Lab. Clin. Med. *80*:282, 1972.

Pardo, V., Strauss, J., Kramer, H., et al.: Nephropathy associated with sickle cell anemia: an autologous immune complex nephritis. Am. J. Med. *59*:650, 1975.

Park, C. M.: Isoelectric focusing and the study of interacting protein systems: ligand binding, phosphate binding and subunit exchange in hemoglobin. Ann NY Acad. Sci. *209*:237, 1973.

Parker, J. P., Beirne, G. J., Desai, J. N., et al.: Androgen-induced increase in red-cell 2,3-diphosphoglycerate. N. Engl. J. Med. *287*:381, 1972.

Pataryas, H. A., and Stamatoyannopoulos, G.: Hemoglobins in human fetuses; evidence for adult hemoglobin production after the 11th gestational week. Blood *39*:688, 1972.
Pauling, L., Itano, H. A., Singer, S. J., and Wells, I. C.: Sickle cell anemia: A molecular disease. Science *110*:543, 1949.
Pearson, H. A.: Hemoglobin S–thalassemia syndrome in Negro children. Ann. NY Acad. Sci. *165*:83, 1969.
Pearson, H. A.: Progress in early diagnosis of sickle cell disease. Children *18*:222, 1971.
Pearson, H. A.: Sickle cell anemia: Clinical managment during the early years of life. In Abramson, H., Bertles, J. F., and Wethers, D. L. (eds.): Sickle Cell Disease, Diagnosis, Management, Education and Research. St. Louis, The C. V. Mosby Co., 1973, p. 244.
Pearson, H. A.: Routine screening of umbilical cord blood for sickle cell diseases. JAMA *227*:420, 1974.
Pearson, H. A.: O_2 dissociation and RBC 2,3-DPG in thalassemia. Blood *46*:1027, 1975.
Pearson, H. A., and Moore, M. M.: Human hemoglobin gene linkage: report of a family with hemoglobin β_2, hemoglobin S and β-thalassemia, including a probable crossover between thalassemia and the delta loci. Am. J. Hum. Genet. *17*:125, 1965.
Pearson, H. A., and Noyes, W. D.: Failure of phenothiazines in sickle cell anemia. JAMA *199*:33, 1967.
Pearson, H. A., Cornelius, E. A., Schwartz, A. D., et al.: Transfusion-reversible functional asplenia in young children with sickle-cell anemia. N. Engl. J. Med. *283*:334, 1970.
Pearson, H. A., O'Brien, R. T., and McIntosh, S.: Screening for thalassemia trait by electronic measurement of mean corpuscular volume (MCV). N. Engl. J. Med. *288*:351, 1973.
Pederson, P. R., McCurdy, P. R., Wrightstone, R. N., et al.: Hemoglobin Köln in a Black: Pre- and post-splenectomy red cell survival ($DF^{32}P$ and ^{51}Cr) and the pathogenesis of hemoglobin instability. Blood *42*:771, 1973.
Pembrey, M. E., Weatherall, D. J., and Clegg, J. B.: Maternal synthesis of haemoglobin F in pregnancy. Lancet *1*:1350, 1973.
Perillie, P. E., and Epstein, F. H.: Sickling phenomenon produced by hypertonic solutions: a possible explanation for the hyposthenuria of sicklemia. J. Clin. Invest. *42*:570, 1963.
Perrine, R. P.: Cholelithiasis in sickle cell anemia in a Caucasian population. Am. J. Med. *54*:327, 1973.
Perutz, M. F.: Stereochemistry of cooperative effects in haemoglobin. Nature *228*:726, 1970a.
Perutz, M. F.: The Bohr effect and combination with organic phosphates. Nature *228*:734, 1970b.
Perutz, M. F.: Sir Lawrence Bragg. N. Scient. Sci. J. July 8, 1971, p. 67.
Perutz, M. F.: Stereochemical interpretation of high oxygen affinity of haemoglobin Little Rock ($\alpha_2\beta_2$ 143 His→Glu). Nature [New Biol.] *243*:180, 1973.
Perutz, M. F., and Lehmann, H.: Molecular pathology of human haemoglobin. Nature *219*:902, 1968.
Perutz, M. F., and Mitchison, J. M.: State of haemoglobin in sickle cell anaemia. Nature *166*:677, 1950.
Perutz, M. F., Pulsinelli, P., Ten Eyck, L., et al.: Haemoglobin Hiroshima and the mechanism of the alkaline Bohr effect. Nature [New Biol.] *232*:147, 1971.
Perutz, M. F., Pulsinelli, P. D., and Ranney, H. M.: Structure and subunit interaction of haemoglobin M Milwaukee. Nature [New Biol.] *237*:259, 1972.
Perutz, M. F., Fersht, A. R., Simon, S. R., and Roberts, G. C. K.: Influence of globin structure on the state of the heme. II. Allosteric transitions in methemoglobin. Biochemistry *13*:2174, 1974b.
Peterson, C. M., Graziano, J. H., de Ciutiis, A., et al.: Metal metabolism, sickle cell disease and response to cyanate. Blood *44*:945(Abst.), 1974a.
Peterson, C. M., de Ciutiis, A. C., and Cerami, A.: Sodium cyanate and sickle cell disease: efficacy vs. toxicity. In Hercules, J. I., Schechter, A. N., Eaton, W. A., et al. (eds.): Proceedings of First National Symposium on Sickle Cell Disease, Washington, D.C. DHEW Pub. No. 75–723 (NIH), Bethesda, Md., 1974b, pp. 37–38.

Peterson, C. M., Tsairis, P., Ohnishi, A., et al.: Sodium cyanate induced polyneuropathy in patients with sickle cell disease. Ann. Intern. Med. *81*:152, 1974c.
Pietschmann, H., Kolarz, G., and Singer, F.: Zytochemische Untersuchungen bei einer neuen Hämoglobinopathie (Hämoglobin Wien). Wien Klin. Wochenschr. *83*:362, 1971.
Piomelli, S., Danoff, S. J., Becker, M. H., et al.: Prevention of bone malformations and cardiomegaly in Cooley's anemia by early hypertransfusion regimen. Ann. NY Acad. Sci. *165*:427, 1969.
Piomelli, S., Reindorf, C. A., Arzanian, M. T., et al.: Clinical and biochemical interactions of glucose-6-phosphate dehydrogenase deficiency and sickle-cell anemia. N. Engl. J. Med. *287*:213, 1972.
Piomelli, S., Becker, M., Arzanian, M. T., et al.: Early hypertransfusion regimen in patients with Cooley's anemia. Ann. NY Acad. Sci. *232*:186, 1974.
Pisciotta, A. V., Ebbe, S. N., and Hinz, J. E.: Clinical and laboratory features of two variants of methemoglobin M disease. J. Lab. Clin. Med. *54*:73, 1959.
Pitcock, J. A., Muirhead, E. E., Hatch, F. E., et al.: Early renal changes in sickle cell anemia. Arch. Pathol. *90*:403, 1970.
Pootrakul, S., Wasi, P., and Na-Nakorn, S.: Haemoglobin Bart's hydrops foetalis in Thailand. Ann. Hum. Genet. *30*:203, 1967a.
Pootrakul, S., Wasi, P., and Na-Nakorn, S.: Studies on haemoglobin Bart's (Hb-γ^4) in Thailand: the incidence and the mechanism of occurrence in cord blood. Ann. Hum. Genet. *31*:149, 1967b.
Pootrakul, S., Wasi, P., Pornpatkul, M., et al.: Incidence of alpha thalassemia in Bangkok. J. Med. Assn. Thai. *53*:250, 1970.
Pootrakul, S., Wasi, P., and Na-Nakorn, S., et al.: Haematological data in 312 cases of β-thalassaemia trait in Thailand. Br. J. Haematol. *24*:703, 1973.
Pootrakul, S., Pongsamart, S., Prawatmuang, P., et al.: Hb Constant Spring: degradation and Hb synthesis studies. Proceedings of the 16th International Congress of Hematology, Kyoto, Japan, 1976. Excerpta Medica (in press).
Portnoy, B. A., and Herion, J. C.: Neurological manifestations in sickle-cell disease; with a review of the literature and emphasis on the prevalence of hemiplegia. Ann. Inter. Med. *76*:643, 1972.
Powars, D. R.: The natural history of sickle cell disease—the first ten years. Semin. Hematol. *12*:267, 1975.
Power, H. W.: A model of how the sickle-cell gene produces malaria resistance. J. Theor. Biol. *50*:121, 1975.
Prankerd, T. A. J.: The spleen and anaemia. Br. Med. J. *2*:517, 1963.
Prato, V., Gallo, E., Ricco, G., et al.: Haemolytic anaemia due to haemoglobin Torino. Br. J. Haematol. *19*:105, 1970.
Prensky, W., and Holmquist, G.: Chromosomal localization of human haemoglobin structural genes: techniques queried. Nature *241*:44, 1973.
Pribilla, W., Klesse, P., Betke, K., et al.: Hämoglobin-Köln-Krankheit: Familiäre hypochrome hämolytische Anämie mit Hämoglobinanomalie. Klin. Wochenschr. *43*:1049, 1965.
Price, P. M., Conover, J. H., and Hirschhorn, K.: Chromosomal localization of human haemoglobin structural genes. Nature *237*:340, 1972.
Prichard, P. M., Gilbert, J. M., Shafritz, D. A., et al.: Factors for the initiation of haemoglobin synthesis by rabbit reticulocyte ribosomes. Nature *226*:511, 1970.
Prindle, K. M., and McCurdy, P. R.: Red cell life span in hemoglobin C disorders. Clin. Res. *17*:33, 1969.
Pritchard, J. A., Scott, D. E., and Whalley, P.: The effects of maternal sickle cell hemoglobinopathies and sickle cell trait on reproductive performance. Am. J. Obstet. Gynecol. *117*:662, 1971.
Pritchard, J., Hillman, D. G., Glass, J., et al.: Deficiency of β-globin chain messenger RNA (mRNA) in nucleated red cell precursors from heterozygous β-thalassemia (Hetero β-Thal) marrow. Blood *46*:1050, 1975.
Propper, R. D., Shurin, S. B., and Nathan, D. G.: Reassessment of the use of desferrioxamine B in iron overload. N. Engl. J. Med. *294*:1421, 1976.
Pugh, R. P., Monical, T. V., and Minnich, V.: Sickle cell anemia with two adult hemoglobins—Hb S and Hb G-Philadelphia/S. Blood *23*:206, 1964.
Pulsinelli, P. D.: Structure of deoxyhaemoglobin Yakima: a high affinity mutant form exhibiting oxy-like $\alpha_1\beta_2$ subunit interactions. J. Mol. Biol. *74*:57, 1973.

Pulsinelli, P. D., Perutz, M. F., and Nagel, R. L.: Structure of Hemoglobin M Boston, a variant with a five coordinated ferric heme. Proc. Natl. Acad. Sci. USA *70*:3870, 1973.

Purugganan, H. B., and McElfresh, A. E.: Failure of carbonmonoxy sickle-cell haemoglobin to alter the sickle state. Lancet *1*:79, 1964.

Rabinovitz, M., Freedman, M. L., Fisher, J. M., Maxwell, C. R.: Translational control in hemoglobin synthesis. Cold Spring Harbor Symp. Quant. Biol. *34*:567, 1969.

Rachmilewitz, E. A.: Denaturation of the normal and abnormal hemoglobin molecule. Semin. Hematol. *11*:441, 1974.

Rachmilewitz, E. A., and Harari, E.: Intermediate hemichrome formation after oxidation of three unstable hemoglobins (Freiburg, Riverdale-Bronx and Köln). Haematol. Bluttransfus. *10*:241, 1972.

Rachmilewitz, E. A., and Thorell, B.: Hemichromes in single inclusion bodies in red cells of beta thalassemia. Blood *39*:794, 1972.

Rachmilewitz, E. A., and White, J. M.: Haemichrome formation during the *in vitro* oxidation of haemoglobin Köln. Nature [New Biol.] *241*:115, 1973.

Rachmilewitz, E. A., Peisach, J., and Blumberg, W. E.: Studies on the stability of oxyhemoglobin A and its constituent chains and their derivatives. J. Biol. Chem. *246*:3356, 1971.

Rachmilewitz, E. A., Lubin, B. H., and Shohet, S. B.: Lipid membrane peroxidation in β-thalassemia major. Blood *47*:495, 1976.

Raffel, C., Stein, S., and Kaempfer, R.: Role for heme in mammalian protein synthesis: activation of an initiation factor. Proc. Natl. Acad. Sci. USA *71*:4020, 1974.

Raik, E., Hunter, E. G., and Lindsay, D. A.: Compensated hereditary haemolytic disease resulting from an unstable haemoglobin fraction. Med. J. Aust. *1*:955, 1967.

Ramirez, F., Natta, C., O'Donnell, J. V., et al.: Relative numbers of human globin genes assayed with purified α and β complementary human DNA. Proc. Natl. Acad. Sci. USA *72*:1550, 1975b.

Ramirez, F., O'Donnell, J. V., Marks, P. A., et al.: Abnormal or absent βmRNA in β^0 Ferrara and gene deletion in $\delta\beta$ thalassaemia. Nature *263*:471, 1976.

Rampling, M. W., and Sirs, J. A.: The rate of sickling of cells containing sickle-cell haemoglobin. Clin. Sci. Mol. Med. *45*:655, 1973.

Ranney, H. M., Larson, D. L., and McCormack, G. H.: Some clinical, biochemical and genetic observations on hemoglobin C. J. Clin. Invest. *32*:1277, 1953.

Ranney, H. M., Jacobs, A. S., Udem, L., and Zalusky, R.: Hemoglobin Riverdale-Bronx, an unstable hemoglobin resulting from the substitution of arginine for glycine at helical residue B6 of the β polypeptide chain. Biochem. Biophys. Res. Commun. *33*:1004, 1968a.

Ranney, H. M., Nagel, R. L., Heller, P., and Udem, L.: Oxygen equilibrium of hemoglobin M-Hyde Park. Biochim. Biophys. Acta *160*:112, 1968b.

Ranney, H. M., Nagel, R. L., and Udem, L.: Some properties of the M-hemoglobins. In Arends, T., Bemski, G., and Nagel, R. L. (eds.): Proceedings of First Inter-American Symposium on Hemoglobins, Caracas, Venezuela, 1969. Basel, S. Karger, 1971, p. 143.

Raper, A. B., Black, A. J., Huntsman, R. G., and Pollack, M.: Sickling and steroid hormones. Trans. Roy. Soc. Trop. Med. Hyg. *64*:293, 1970.

Redetzki, J. E., Bickers, J. N., and Samuels, M. S.: Homozygous hemoglobin C disease: Clinical review of 15 patients. South. Med. J. *61*:238, 1968.

Reed, C. S., Hampson, R., Gordon, S., et al.: Erythrocytosis secondary to increased oxygen affinity of a mutant hemoglobin, Hemoglobin Kempsey. Blood *31*:623, 1968.

Reed, L. J., and Mollin, D. W.: Synthesis of hemoglobin A_2 in sideroblastic and megaloblastic anemias. Abstracts, XII Congress of the International Society of Hematology, New York, The Society, 1968, p. 63.

Reissmann, K. R., Ruth, W. E., and Nomura, T.: A human hemoglobin with lowered oxygen affinity and impaired heme-heme interactions. J. Clin. Invest. *40*:1826, 1961.

Reynolds, C. A., and Huisman, T. H. J.: Hemoglobin Russ or $\alpha_2^{51\ \mathrm{Arg}}\beta_2$. Biochim. Biophys. Acta *130*:541, 1966.

Reynolds, J.: Roentgenological features of sickle cell disease and related hemoglobinopathies. Springfield, Illinois, Charles C Thomas, 1965.

Reynolds, J. D. H.: Painful sickle cell crisis— successful treatment with hyperbaric oxygen therapy. JAMA *216*:1977, 1971.

Rickles, F. R., and O'Leary, D. S.: Role of coagulation system in pathophysiology of sickle cell disease. Arch. Intern. Med. *133*:635, 1974.
Rieder, R. F.: Hemoglobin stability: Observations on the denaturation of normal and abnormal hemoglobins by oxidant dyes, heat and alkali. J. Clin. Invest. *49*:2369, 1970.
Rieder, R. F.: Synthesis of hemoglobin Gun Hill: Increased synthesis of the heme-free β^{GH} globin chain and subunit exchange with a free α-chain pool. J. Clin. Invest. *50*:388, 1971.
Rieder, R. F.: Translation of β-globin mRNA in β-thalassemia and the S and C hemoglobinopathies. J. Clin. Invest. *51*:364, 1972.
Rieder, R. F.: Globin chain synthesis in Hb D (Punjab)-β-thalassemia. Blood *47*:113, 1976.
Rieder, R. F., and Bradley, T. B.: Hemoglobin Gun Hill: An unstable protein associated with chronic hemolysis. Blood *32*:355, 1968.
Rieder, R. F., and James, G. W., III: Imbalance in alpha and beta globin synthesis associated with a hemoglobinopathy. J. Clin. Invest. *54*:948, 1974.
Rieder, R. F., and Weatherall, D. J.: Studies on hemoglobin biosynthesis: asynchronous synthesis of hemoglobin A and hemoglobin A_2 by erythrocyte precursors. J. Clin. Invest. *44*:42, 1965.
Rieder, R. F., Zinkman, W. H., and Holtzman, N. A.: Hemoglobin Zürich: Clinical, chemical and kinetic studies. Am. J. Med. *39*:4, 1965.
Rieder, R. F., Oski, F. A., and Clegg, J. B.: Hemoglobin Philly (β35 Tyrosine→Phenylalanine): Studies in the molecular pathology of hemoglobin. J. Clin. Invest. *48*:1627, 1969.
Rieder, R. F., Wolf, D. J., Clegg, J. B., et al.: Hemoglobin Bushwick, β74 (E18) Gly→Val: Rapid postsynthetic destruction of an unstable hemoglobin. Blood *44*:946, 1974.
Rieder, R. F., Wolf, D. J., Clegg, J. B., et al.: Rapid postsynthetic destruction of unstable haemoglobin Bushwick. Nature *254*:725, 1975.
Rieder, R. F., Woodbury, D. H., and Rucknagel, D. L.: The interaction of α-thalassaemia and haemoglobin G Philadelphia. Br. J. Haematol. *32*:159, 1976.
Rifkind, R. A.: Heinz body anemia: an ultrastructural study. II. Red cell sequestration and destruction. Blood *26*:433, 1965.
Rifkind, R. A., and Danon, D.: Heinz body anemia—an ultrastructural study: I. Heinz body formation. Blood *25*:885, 1965.
Rigas, D. A., and Koler, R. D.: Decreased erythrocyte survival in hemoglobin H disease as a result of the abnormal properties of hemoglobin H: the benefit of splenectomy. Blood *18*:1, 1961.
Ringelhann, B.: Immunodeficiency in sickle-cell anemia. N. Engl. J. Med. *289*:326, 1973.
Ringelhann, B., and Konotey-Ahulu, F. I. D.: Immunological studies and sickle cell crises in Ghana. Afr. J. Med. Sci. *4*:17, 1973.
Ringelhann, B., Konotey-Ahulu, F. I. D., Talapatra, N. C., et al.: Haemoglobin K Woolwich ($\alpha_2\beta_2{}^{132}$ Lysine→Glutamine) in Ghana. Acta Haematol. (Basel) *45*:250, 1971.
Roberts, A. V., Weatherall, D. J., and Clegg, J. B.: The synthesis of human hemoglobin A_2 during erythroid maturation. Biochem. Biophys. Res. Commun. *47*:81, 1972.
Roberts, A. V., Clegg, J. B., Weatherall, D. J., et al.: Synthesis *in vitro* of anti-Lepore haemoglobin. Nature [New Biol.] *245*:23, 1973.
Robinson, M. G., and Halpern, C.: Infections, Escherichia coli and sickle cell anemia. JAMA *230*:1145, 1974.
Robinson, M. G., and Watson, R. J.: Pneumococcal meningitis in sickle-cell anemia. N. Engl. J. Med. *274*:1006, 1966.
Rodriguez, J. M., and Shahidi, N. T.: Erythrocyte 2,3-diphosphoglycerate in adaptive red-cell–volume deficiency. N. Engl. J. Med. *285*:479, 1971.
Rosa, J., Audart, J. C., Pagnier, J., et al.: A new abnormal hemoglobin: $\alpha_2{}^{112\ His \rightarrow Gly}\beta_2$ Hb Dakar. XII Congress of the International Society of Hematology, New York, The Society, 1968, p. 72.
Rosa, J., Labie, D., Wajcman, H., et al.: Haemoglobin I Toulouse: β66 (E1fl) Lys→Glu: A new abnormal haemoglobin with a mutation localized on the E10 porphyrin surrounding zone. Nature *223*:190, 1969.

Rosenzweig, A. I., Heywood, J. D., Motulsky, A. G., et al.: Hemoglobin H as an acquired defect of alpha-chain synthesis: report of two cases. Acta Haematol. (Basel) *39*:91, 1968.

Ross, J., Ikawa, Y., and Leder, P.: Globin mRNA induction during erythroid differentiation of cultured leukemic cells. Proc. Natl. Acad. Sci. USA *69*:3620, 1972b.

Rossi-Bernardi, L., Luzzana, M., Samaja, M., et al.: The functional properties of sickle cell blood. FEBS Lett. *59*:15, 1975.

Rossi-Fanelli, A., Antonini, E., and Povoledo, D.: Further study on myoglobin II. Chemical and biochemical properties of a new type of myoglobin in molluscs. In Neuberger, A. (ed.): Symposium on Protein Structure. London, Methuen, 1958b, p. 144.

Roth, E. F., Nagel, R. L., Bookchin, R. M., and Grayzel, A. L.: Nitrogen mustard: an "in vitro" inhibitor of erythrocyte sickling. Biochem. Biophys. Res. Commun. *48*:612, 1972.

Roth, E. F., Jr., Nagel, R. L., Bookchin, R. M., et al.: The effects of nitrogen and sulfur mustards on hemoglobin S and intact red cells. In Hercules, J. I., Schechter, A. N., Eaton, W. A., et al. (eds.): Proceedings of First National Symposium on Sickle Cell Disease, Washington, D.C. DHEW Pub. No. 75–723 (NIH), Bethesda, Md., 1974, p. 41.

Rotter, R., Luttgens, W. F., Peterson, W. L., et al.: Splenic infarction in sicklemia during airplane flight: pathogenesis, hemoglobin analysis and clinical features of six cases. Ann. Intern. Med. *44*:257, 1956.

Rowley, P. T., and Kosciolek, B.: Distinction between two types of beta-thalassemia by inducibility of the cell-free synthesis of beta-chains by non-thalassemic soluble fraction. Nature [New Biol.] *239*:234, 1972.

Rucknagel, D. L.: The genetics of sickle cell anemia and related syndromes. Arch. Intern. Med. *133*:595, 1974.

Rucknagel, D. L., and Rising, J. A.: A heterozygote for Hb_B^S, Hb_B^C and $Hb_\alpha^{G\ Philadelphia}$ in a family presenting evidence for heterogeneity of hemoglobin alpha chain loci. Am. J. Med. *59*:53, 1975.

Rucknagel, D. L., and Winter, W. P.: Duplication of structural genes for hemoglobin α and β chains in man. Ann. NY Acad. Sci. *241*:80, 1974.

Rucknagel, D. L., Spencer, H. H., and Brandt, N. J.: Hemoglobin Ann Arbor, a complex alpha chain abnormality. Abstracts, XII Congress of the International Society of Hematology, New York 1968. New York, The Society, 1968, p. 56.

Russell, M. O., Goldberg, H. I., Friedman, S., et al.: Reversal of cerebral arterial changes in sickle cell anemia with prolonged transfusion therapy. In Hercules, J. I., Schechter, A. N., Eaton, W. A., et al. (eds.): Proceedings of First National Symposium on Sickle Cell Disease, Washington, D.C. DHEW Pub. No. 75–723 (NIH), Bethesda, Md., 1974, p. 77.

Russell, M. O., Goldberg, H. I., Reis, L., et al.: Transfusion therapy for cerebrovascular abnormalities in sickle cell disease. J. Pediatr. *88*:382, 1976.

Russo, G., and Mollica, F.: Sickle-cell haemoglobin and two types of thalassaemia in the same family. Acta Haematol. (Basel) *28*:329, 1962.

Ryan, S. J., and Goldberg, M. F.: Anterior segment ischemia following scleral buckling in sickle cell hemoglobinopathy. Am. J. Ophthalmol. *72*:35, 1971.

Salhany, J. M.: The deoxygenation kinetics of hemoglobin Rainier ($\alpha_2\beta_2{}^{145\ Tyr \rightarrow Cys}$). Biochem. Biophys. Res. Commun. *47*:784, 1972.

Salhany, J. M., Osawa, S., and Shulman, R. G.: Spectral-kinetic heterogeneity in reactions of nitrosyl hemoglobin. Proc. Natl. Acad. Sci. USA *71*:3359, 1974.

Salhany, J. M., Ogawa, S., and Shulman, R. G.: Correlation between quaternary structure and ligand dissociation kinetics for fully liganded hemoglobin. Biochemistry *14*:2180, 1975.

Salvaggio, J. E., Arnold, C. A., and Banov, C. H.: Long-term anticoagulation in sickle-cell disease: a clinical study. N. Engl. J. Med. *269*:182, 1963.

Sansone, G., and Pik, C.: Familial haemolytic anaemia with erythrocyte inclusion bodies, bilifuscinuria and abnormal haemoglobin (haemoglobin Galliera Genova). Br. J. Haematol. *11*:511, 1965.

Sansone, G., Carrell, R. W., and Lehmann, H.: Haemoglobin Genova: β28 (B10) Leucine → Proline. Nature *214*:877, 1967.

Schlitt, L. E., and Keitel, H. G.: Renal manifestations of sickle cell disease. A review. Am. J. Med. Sci. *239*:773, 1960.

Schmid, R., Williams, G. Z., and Clemens, T., Jr.: Familial hemolytic anemia with spontaneous erythrocyte inclusion bodies. Proceedings of VI Congress of the International Society of Hematology, Boston, 1956. New York, Grune & Stratton, 1958.
Schmid, R., Brecher, G., and Clemens, T.: Familial hemolytic anemia with erythrocyte inclusion bodies and a defect in pigment metabolism. Blood *14*:991, 1959.
Schneider, R. G., Alperin, J. B., Beale, D., and Lehmann, H.: Hemoglobin I in an American Negro family: structural and hematologic studies. J. Lab. Clin. Med. *68*:940, 1966.
Schneider, R. G., Ueda, S., Alperin, J. B., et al.: Hemoglobin Sabine beta 91 (F7) Leu → Pro. An unstable variant causing severe anemia with inclusion bodies. N. Engl. J. Med. *280*:739, 1969.
Schneider, R. G., Takeda, I,, Gustavson, L. P., and Alperin, J. B.: Intraerythrocytic precipitations of haemoglobins S and C. Nature [New Biol.] *235*:88, 1972.
Schneider, R. G., Atkins, R. J., Hosty, T. S., et al.: Haemoglobin Titusville: α94 Asp → Asn. A new haemoglobin with a lowered affinity for oxygen. Biochim. Biophys. Acta *400*:365, 1975.
Schneiderman, L. J., Junga, I. G., and Fawley, D. E.: Effects of phosphate and non-phosphate buffers on thermolability of unstable haemoglobins. Nature *225*:1041, 1970.
Schnitzer, B., Rucknagel, D. L., Spencer, H. H., and Aikawa, M.: Erythrocytes: Pits and vacuoles as seen with transmission and scanning electron microscopy. Science *173*:251, 1971.
Schokker, R. C., Went, L. N., and Bok, J.: A new genetic variant of beta-thalassemia. Nature *209*:44, 1966.
Schroeder, W. A., Cua, J. T., Matsuda, G., and Fenninger, W. D.: Hemoglobin F_1, an acetyl-containing hemoglobin. Biochim. Biophys. Acta *63*:532, 1962.
Schroeder, W. A., Huisman, T. J. H., Shelton, J. R., et al.: Evidence for multiple structural genes for γ chain of human fetal hemoglobin. Proc. Natl. Acad. Sci. USA *60*:537, 1968.
Schroeder, W. A., Huisman, T. H. J., Shelton, J. R., et al.: An improved method for quantitative determination of human fetal hemoglobin. Anal. Biochem. *35*:235, 1970.
Schroeder, W. A., Shelton, J. R., Shelton, J. B., et al.: World-wide occurrence of nonallelic genes for the γ chain of human foetal haemoglobin in newborns. Nature [New Biol.] *240*:273, 1972.
Schroeder, W. A., Bannister, W. H., Grech, J. L., et al.: Nonsynchronized suppression of postnatal activity in nonallelic genes which synthesize the Gγ chain in human foetal haemoglobin. Nature [New Biol.] *244*:89, 1973.
Schulman, H. M.: Evidence supporting a physiological role for the hemin-controlled translational repressor of globin synthesis in reticulocytes. Biochim. Biophys. Acta *414*:161, 1975.
Schumacher, H. R., Andres, R., and McLaughlin, G.: Arthropathy in sickle-cell disease. Ann. Intern. Med. *78*:203, 1973.
Schwartz, A. D., and Pearson, H. A.: Impaired antibody response to intravenous immunization in sickle cell anemia. Pediatr. Res. *6*:145, 1972.
Schwartz, E.: The silent carrier of beta-thalassemia. N. Engl. J. Med. *281*:1327, 1969.
Schwartz, E.: Heterozygous beta thalassemia: balanced globin synthesis in bone marrow cells. Science *167*:1513, 1970.
Schwartz, E., and Atwater, J.: α-Thalassemia in the American Negro. J. Clin. Invest. *51*:412, 1972.
Schwartz, E., and McElfresh, A. E.: Treatment of painful crises of sickle cell disease: a double-blind study. J. Pediatr. *64*:132, 1964.
Seakins, M., Gibbs, W. N., Milner, P. F., and Bertles, J. F.: Erythrocyte Hb-S concentration; an important factor in the low oxygen affinity of blood in sickle cell anemia. J. Clin. Invest. *52*:422, 1973.
Searle, J. F.: Anaesthesia and sickle-cell haemoglobin. Br. J. Anaesth. *44*:1335, 1972.
Seeler, R. A.: Deaths in children with sickle cell anemia. Clin. Pediatr. (Philadelphia) *11*:634, 1972.
Seeler, R. A.: Intensive transfusion therapy for priapism in boys with sickle cell anemia. J. Urol. *110*:360, 1973.
Seeler, R. A., and Shwiaki, M. Z.: Acute splenic sequestration crisis (ASSC) in young children with sickle cell anemia. Clinical observations in 20 episodes in 14 children. Clin. Pediatr. (Philadelphia) *11*:701, 1972.

Seeler, R. A., Metzger, W., and Mufson, M. A.: Diplococcus pneumoniae infections in children with sickle cell anemia. Am. J. Dis. Child. *123*:8, 1972.

Seid-Akhavan, M., Winter, W. P., et al.: Hemoglobin Wayne: a frameshift variant occurring in two distinct forms. Blood *40*:927, 1972.

Seid-Akhavan, M., Winter, W. P., Abramson, R. K., et al.: Hemoglobin Wayne: A frameshift mutation detected in human hemoglobin alpha chains. Proc. Natl. Acad. Sci. USA *73*:882, 1976.

Serjeant, G. R.: Sickle cell anemia: clinical features in adulthood and old age. In Abramson, H., Bertles, J. F., and Wethers, D. L. (eds.): Sickle Cell Disease—Diagnosis, Management, Education and Research. St. Louis, The C. V. Mosby Co., 1973, p. 252.

Serjeant, G. R.: Leg ulceration in sickle cell anemia. Arch. Intern. Med. *133*:690, 1974.

Serjeant, G. R., and Ashcroft, M. T.: Shortening of the digits in sickle cell anaemia—A sequela of the hand-foot syndrome. Trop. Geogr. Med. *23*:341, 1971.

Serjeant, G. R., Richards, R., Barbor, P. R., et al.: Relatively benign sickle-cell anaemia in 60 patients aged over 30 in the West Indies. Br. Med. J. *3*:86, 1968.

Serjeant, G. R., Galloway, R. E., and Gueri, M. C.: Oral zinc sulfate in sickle cell ulcers. Lancet *2*:891, 1970.

Serjeant, G. R., Petch, M. C., and Serjeant, B. E.: The in vivo sickle phenomenon: a reappraisal. J. Lab. Clin. Med. *81*:850, 1973.

Shaeffer, J. R.: Evidence for soluble α chains as intermediates in hemoglobin synthesis in the rabbit reticulocyte. Biochem. Biophys. Res. Commun. *28*:647, 1967.

Shaeffer, J. R.: Structure and synthesis of the unstable hemoglobin Sabine (alpha 2 beta 2-91 Leu → Pro). J. Biol. Chem. *248*:7473, 1973.

Shaeffer, J. R., Trostle, P. K., and Evans, R. F.: Inhibition of the biosynthetic completion of rabbit hemoglobin by isolated human hemoglobin chains. J. Biol. Chem. *244*:4284, 1969.

Shaeffer, J. R., Desimone, J., and Kleve, L. J.: Hemoglobin synthesis studies of a family with alpha-thalassemia trait and sickle cell trait. Biochem. Genet. *13*:783, 1975a.

Shaeffer, J. R., Langley, M. A., DeSimone, J., and Kleve, L. J.: Patterns of hemoglobin assembly in reticulocytes of sickle cell trait individuals. J. Biol. Chem. *250*:8630, 1975b.

Shaeffer, J. R., Kleve, L. J.; and DeSimone, J.: β^S chain turnover in reticulocytes of sickle trait individuals with high or low concentrations of haemoglobin S. Br. J. Haematol. *32*:365, 1976.

Shappell, S. D., Murray, J. A., Nasser, M. G., et al.: Acute change in hemoglobin affinity for oxygen during angina pectoris. N. Engl. J. Med. *282*:1219, 1970.

Sharma, V. S., Noble, R. W., and Ranney, H. M.: Structure-function relationship in Hemoglobin Köln (β98 Val → Met). J. Mol. Biol. *82*:139, 1974.

Shchory, M., and Ramot, B.: Globin chain synthesis in the marrow and reticulocytes of beta thalassemia, hemoglobin H disease and beta-delta thalassemia. Blood *40*:105, 1972.

Shchory, M., and Weatherall, D. J.: Haemoglobin synthesis in human fetal liver maintained in short-term tissue culture. Br. J. Haematol. *30*:9, 1975.

Shen, S. C., Fleming, E. M., and Castle, W. B.: Studies on the destruction of red blood cells. V. Irreversibly sickled erythrocytes: The experimental production *in vitro*. Blood *4*:498, 1949.

Shepard, M. K., Weatherall, D. J., and Conley, C. L.: Semi-quantitative estimation of the distribution of fetal hemoglobin in red cell populations. Bull. Johns Hopkins Hosp. *110*:293, 1962.

Sherman, I. J.: The sickling phenomenon, with special reference to differentiation of sickle cell anemia from the sickle cell trait. Bull. Johns Hopkins Hosp. *67*:309, 1940.

Shibata, S., Miyaji, T., Iuchi, I., et al.: Substitution of tyrosine for histidine (87) in the α chain of hemoglobin M_{Iwate}. Acta Haematol. Jap. *27*:13, 1964.

Shibata, S., Miyaji, T., Iuchi, I., et al.: Hemoglobins M of the Japanese. Bull. Yamaguchi Med. Sch. *14*:141, 1967a.

Shibata, S., Miyaji, T., Karita, K., et al.: A new type of hereditary nigremia discovered in Akita—hemoglobin M Hyde Park disease. Proc. Jap. Acad. *43*:65, 1967b.

Shulman, S., Bartlett, J., Clyde, W. A., et al.: The unusual severity of mycoplasmal pneumonia in children with sickle-cell disease. N. Engl. J. Med. *287*:164, 1972.

Singer, K.: Pure (homozygous) hemoglobin C disease. Blood 9:1023, 1954.

Singer, K.: Hereditary hemolytic disorders associated with abnormal hemoglobins. Am. J. Med. *18*:633, 1955.

Singer, K., and Singer, L.: The gelling phenomenon of sickle cell hemoglobin: its biological and diagnostic significance. Blood *8*:1008, 1953.

Singer, K., Chernoff, A. I., and Singer, L.: Studies on abnormal hemoglobins. I. Their demonstration in sickle cell anemia and other hematologic disorders by means of alkali denaturation. Blood *6*:413, 1951.

Slater, L. M., Muir, W. A., and Weed, R. I.: Influence of splenectomy on insoluble hemoglobin inclusion bodies in β-thalassemic erythrocytes. Blood *31*:766, 1968.

Smith, C. H., Erlandson, M. E., Stern, G., and Hilgartner, M. W.: Postsplenectomy infection in Cooley's anemia. N. Engl. J. Med. *266*:737, 1962.

Smith, C. H., Erlandson, M. E., Stern, G., and Hilgartner, M. W.: Postsplenectomy infection in Cooley's anemia. Ann. NY Acad. Sci. *119*:748, 1964.

Smith, D. H., Clegg, J. B., Weatherall, D. J., et al.: Hereditary persistence of foetal haemoglobin associated with a $\gamma\beta$ fusion variant, haemoglobin Kenya. Nature [New Biol.] *246*:184, 1973.

Smith, E., Rosenblatt, P., and Bedo, A. V.: Sickle cell anemia crisis: report on seven patients treated with priscoline. J. Pediatr. *43*:655, 1953.

Smith, E. W., and Krevans, J. R.: Clinical manifestations of hemoglobin C disorders. Bull. Johns Hopkins Hosp. *104*:17, 1959.

Smith, E. W., and Torbert, J. V.: Two abnormal hemoglobins with evidence for a new genetic locus for hemoglobin formation. Bull. Johns Hopkins Hosp. *102*:38, 1958.

Smith, L. L., Barton, B. P., and Huisman, T. H. J.: Subunit dissociation of the unstable hemoglobin Bibba ($\alpha_2^{136\ \mathrm{Pro}}$ (H19)β_2). J. Biol. Chem. *245*:2185, 1970.

Smith, R. S.: Iron excretion in thalassaemia major after administration of chelating agents. Br. Med. J. *2*:1577, 1962.

Smith, R. S.: Chelating agents in the diagnosis and treatment of iron overload in thalassemia. Ann. NY Acad. Sci. *119*:776, 1964.

Smits, H. L., Oski, F. A., and Brody, J. I.: The hemolytic crisis of sickle cell disease: the role of glucose-6-phosphate dehydrogenase deficiency. J. Pediatr. *74*:544, 1969.

Smolin, M. F., Zanjani, E. D., Hoffman, R., and Wasserman, L. R.: Mechanism of androgen action on erythropoiesis. Clin. Res. *23*:583A, 1975.

Snyder, L. M., and Reddy, W. J.: Mechanism of action of thyroid hormones on erythrocyte 2,3-diphosphoglyceric acid synthesis. J. Clin. Invest. *49*:1993, 1970b.

Sofroniadou, K., Kaltsova, A., Loukopoulos, D., et al.: Hemoglobin "Athens": an alpha-chain variant with unusual properties. Abstracts, XII Congress of the International Society of Hematology, New York. N. Y., The Society, 1968, p. 56.

Sofroniadou, K., Wood, W. G., Nute, P. E., and Stamatoyannopoulos, G.: Globin chain synthesis in the Greek type ($^{A}\gamma$) of hereditary persistence of foetal haemoglobin. Br. J. Haematol. *29*:137, 1975.

Spaet, T. H., Alway, R. H., and Ward, G.: Homozygous type "C" hemoglobin. Pediatrics *12*:483, 1953.

Sproule, B. J., Halden, E. R., and Miller, W. F.: A study of cardiopulmonary alterations in patients with sickle cell disease and its variants. J. Clin. Invest. *37*:486, 1958.

Stamatoyannopoulos, G.: Gamma-thalassaemia. Lancet *2*:192, 1971.

Stamatoyannopoulos, G.: The molecular basis of hemoglobin disease. Ann. Rev. Genet. *6*:47, 1972.

Stamatoyannopoulos, G., Fessas, P., and Papayannopoulou, T.: F-thalassemia: a study of thirty-one families with simple heterozygotes and combinations of F-thalassemia with A_2-thalassemia. Am. J. Med. *47*:194, 1969a.

Stamatoyannopoulos, G., Parer, J. T., and Finch, C. A.: Physiologic implications of a hemoglobin with decreased oxygen affinity (Hemoglobin Seattle). N. Engl. J. Med. *281*:915, 1969b.

Stamatoyannopoulos, G., Bellingham, A. J., Lenfant, C., and Finch, C. A.: Abnormal hemoglobins with high and low oxygen affinity. Ann. Rev. Med. *22*:221, 1971.

Stamatoyannopoulos, G., Nute, P. E., Adamson, J. W., et al.: Hemoglobin Olympia (β20 Valine→Methionine): An electrophoretically silent variant associated with high oxygen affinity and erythrocytosis. J. Clin. Invest. *52*:342, 1973.

Stamatoyannopoulos, G., Woodson, R., Papayannopoulou, T., et al.: Inclusion body β-thalassemia trait. N. Engl. J. Med. *290*:939, 1974.

Stamatoyannopoulos, G., Wood, W. G., Papayannopoulou, T., et al.: A new form of hereditary persistence of fetal hemoglobin in Blacks and its association with sickle cell trait. Blood *46*:683, 1975.

Statius van Eps, L. W., Schouten, H., La Porte-Wijsman, L. W., and Struyker Boudier, A. M.: The influence of red blood cell transfusions on the hyposthenuria and renal hemodynamics of sickle cell anemia. Clin. Chim. Acta *17*:449, 1967.

Statius van Eps, L. W., Pinedo-Veels, C., DeVries, G. H., et al.: Nature of concentrating defect in sickle-cell nephropathy. Lancet *1*:450, 1970.

Stavem, P., Strömme, J., Lorkin, P. A., et al.: Haemoglobin M Saskatoon with slight constant haemolysis, markedly increased by sulfonamides. Scand. J. Haematol. *9*:566, 1972.

Steadman, J. H., Yates, A., and Huehns, E. R.: Idiopathic Heinz body anaemia: Hb Bristol (β67[E11] Val→Asp). Br. J. Haematol. *18*:435, 1970.

Stein, R. E., and Urbaniak, J. R.: Sickle cell disease and the tourniquet. Is there a risk? J. Bone Joint Surg. *57*:1027, 1975.

Steinberg, M. H., and Dreiling, B. J.: Glucose-6-phosphate dehydrogenase deficiency in sickle cell anemia. Ann. Intern. Med. *80*:217, 1974.

Steinberg, M. H., Dreiling, B. J., Morrison, F. S., et al.: Mild sickle cell disease. JAMA *224*:317, 1973.

Steinberg, M. H., Adams, J. G., and Dreiling, B. J.: Alpha-thalassemia in adults with sickle-cell trait. In Hercules, J. I., Schechter, A. N., Eaton, W. A., et al. (eds.): Proceedings of First National Symposium on Sickle Cell Disease, Washington, D.C. DHEW Pub. No. 75–723 (NIH), Bethesda, Md., 1974, p. 259.

Steiner, M., Baldini, M., and Dameshek, W.: Enzymatic defects of heme synthesis in thalassemia. Ann. NY Acad. Sci. *119*:548, 1964.

Stetson, C. A., Jr.: The state of hemoglobin in sickled erythrocytes. J. Exp. Med. *123*:431, 1966.

Stockman, J. A., Nigro, M. A., Mishkin, M. M., and Oski, F. A.: Occlusion of large cerebral vessels in sickle cell anemia. N. Engl. J. Med. *287*:846, 1972.

Stout, C., Holland, C. K., and Bird, R. M.: Hemoglobin D in an Oklahoma family. Arch. Intern. Med. *114*:296, 1964.

Sturgeon, P., Itano, H. A., and Bergren, W. R.: Clinical manifestations of inherited abnormal hemoglobins. II. Interaction of hemoglobin E and thalassemia trait. Blood *10*:396, 1955.

Sundin, O. H., and Williams, R. C.: Acceleration of gelation of hemoglobin S by erythrocyte membrane preparations. Fed. Proc. *35*:1524, 1976.

Suzuki, T., Hayashi, A., Yamamura, Y., et al.: Functional abnormality of hemoglobin M_{Osaka}. Biochem. Biophys. Res. Commun. *19*:691, 1965.

Suzuki, T., Hayashi, A., Shimizu, A., and Yamamura, Y.: The oxygen equilibrium of hemoglobin $M_{Saskatoon}$. Biochim. Biophys. Acta *127*:280, 1966.

Taketa, F., Mauk, A. G., and Lessard, J. L.: β chain amino termini of the cat hemoglobins and the response to 2,3-diphosphoglycerate and adenosine triphosphate. J. Biol. Chem. *246*:4471, 1971.

Tatsis, B., Dosik, H., Rieder, R., et al.: Hemoglobin Hasharon: severe hemolytic anemia and hypersplenism associated with a mildly unstable hemoglobin. Birth Defects *8*:25, 1972.

Taylor, J. M., Dozy, A., Kan, Y. W., et al.: Genetic lesion in homozygous α thalassaemia (hydrops foetalis). Nature *251*:392, 1974.

Tenhunen, R., Marver, H. S., and Schmid, R.: The enzymatic conversion of heme to bilirubin by microsomal heme oxygenase. Proc. Natl. Acad. Sci. USA *61*:748, 1968.

Terry, D. W., Motulsky, A. G., and Rath, C. E.: Homozygous hemoglobin C: a new hereditary hemolytic disease. N. Engl. J. Med. *251*:365, 1954.

Thomas, E. D., Storb, R., Clift, R. A., et al.: Bone-marrow transplantation. N. Engl. J. Med. *292*:832 and 895, 1975.

Thomas, H. M., Lefrak, S. S., Irwin, R. S., et al.: The oxyhemoglobin dissociation curve in health and disease. Am. J. Med. *57*:331, 1974.

Thompson, R. B., Warrington, R., Odom, J., and Bell, W. N.: Interaction between genes for delta thalassaemia and hereditary persistence of foetal haemoglobin. Acta Genet. Stat. Med. *15*:190, 1965a.

Thompson, R. B., Odom, J., and Bell, W. N.: Hb-S, beta thalassaemia, and Hb (β_2) in a family with evidence of a crossover between beta and delta loci. Acta Genet. Stat. Med. *15*:371, 1965b.

Thurmon, T. F., Boyer, S. H., Crosby, E. F., et al.: Hemoglobin switching in nonanemic sheep. III. Evidence for presumptive identity between the A → C factor and erythropoietin. Blood *36*:598, 1970.

Todd, D., Lai, M. C. S., and Braga, C. A.: Thalassaemia and hydrops foetalis—family studies. Br. Med. J. *3*:347, 1967.

Todd, D., Lai, M. C. S., Beaven, G. H., et al.: The abnormal haemoglobins in homozygous α-thalassaemia. Br. J. Haematol. *19*:27, 1970.

Tolstoschev, P., Mitchell, J., Lanyon, G., et al.: Presence of gene for β-globin in homozygous β^0 thalassaemia. Nature *259*:95, 1976.

Tomada, Y.: Demonstration of foetal erythrocyte by immunofluorescent staining. Nature *202*:910, 1964.

Torlontano, G., Tata, A., and Camagna, A.: A rapid screening test for thalassaemic trait. Acta Haematol. (Basel) *48*:234, 1972.

Tosteson, D. C., Carlsen, E., and Dunham, E. T.: The effects of sickling on ion transport. I. Effect of sickling on potassium transport. J. Gen. Physiol. *39*:31, 1956.

Trabuchet, G., Dahmane, M., Pagnier, J., et al.: Hb J Mexico in Algeria: arguments for an heterogeneous distribution of α genes. FEBS Lett. *61*:156, 1976.

Travis, S. F., Sugarman, H. J., Ruberg, R. L., et al.: Alterations of red-cell glycolytic intermediates and oxygen transport as a consequence of hypophosphatemia in patients receiving intravenous hyperalimentation. N. Engl. J. Med. *285*:763, 1971.

Tso, S. C.: Red cell survival studies in haemoglobin H disease using [^{51}Cr] chromate and [^{32}P] di-isopropyl phosphofluoridate. Br. J. Haematol. *23*:621, 1972.

Tuchinda, S., Rucknagel, D. L., Minnich, V., et al.: The coexistence of the genes for hemoglobin E and α thalassemia in Thais, with resultant suppression of hemoglobin E synthesis. Am. J. Hum. Genet. *16*:311, 1964.

Tyuma, I., Shimizu, K., and Imai, K.: Effect of 2,3-diphosphoglycerate on the cooperativity in oxygen binding of human adult hemoglobin. Biochem. Biophys. Res. Commun. *43*:423, 1971.

Udem, L., Ranney, H. M., Bunn, H. F., and Pisciotta, A.: Some observations on the properties of hemoglobin M-Milwaukee-1. J. Mol. Biol. *48*:489, 1970.

Valeri, C. R., and Hirsch, N. M.: Restoration in vivo of erythrocyte adenosine triphosphate, 2,3-diphosphoglycerate, potassium ion and sodium ion concentrations following the transfusion of acid-citrate-dextrose–stored human red blood cells. J. Lab. Clin. Med. *73*:722, 1969.

Valtis, D. J., and Kennedy, A. C.: Defective gas-transport function of stored red blood cells. Lancet *1*:119, 1954.

Van Enk, A., Lang, A., White, J. M., and Lehmann, H.: Benign obstetric history in women with sickle-cell anaemia associated with α-thalassaemia. Br. Med. J. *4*:524, 1972.

Van Vliet, G., and Huisman, T. H. J.: Changes in the haemoglobin types of sheep as a response to anaemia. Biochem. J. *93*:410, 1964.

Varat, M. A., Adolph, R. J., and Fowler, N. O.: Cardiovascular effects of anemia. Am. Heart J. *83*:415, 1972.

Veismold, H., Kohne, E., Riegel, K., et al.: Oxygen carrying functions of blood in hereditary methemoglobinemia: ambivalent effects of 2,3-diphosphoglycerate. In Gerlach, E., Moser, K., Deutsch, E., et al. (eds.): Erythrocytes, Thrombocytes, Leukocytes. Stuttgart, 1973, pp. 171–174. (Recent Advances in Membrane and Metabolic Research, 2nd International Symposium, Vienna, 1972.)

Vella, F., and Lehmann, H.: Haemoglobin D Punjab (D Los Angeles). J. Med. Genet. *11*:341, 1974.

Vella, F., Labossiere, A., Wiltshire, B., et al.: The occurrence of hemoglobins E and M Saskatoon in central Canada. Am. J. Clin. Pathol. *60*:314, 1973.

Vella, F., Kamuzora, H., Lehmann, H., et al.: A second family with hemoglobin M Saskatoon in Saskatchewan. Clin. Biochem. *7*:186, 1974.

Wade, L. J., and Stevenson, L. D.: Necrosis of the bone marrow with fat embolism in sickle cell anemia. Am. J. Clin. Pathol. *17*:47, 1941.

Wajcman, H., Byckova, V., Haidas, S., et al.: Consequences of heme loss in unstable hemoglobins: a study of hemoglobin Köln. FEBS Lett. *13*:145, 1971.

Wajcman, H., Belkhodja, O., and Labie, D.: Hb Setif: G1(94) α Asp → Tyr. A new α chain hemoglobin variant with substitution of the residue involved in hydrogen bond between unlike subunits. FEBS Lett. *27*:298, 1972.

Wajcman, H., Labie, D., and Schapira, G.: Two new hemoglobin variants with deletion: Hemoglobin Tours (Thr β87 [F3] deleted) and hemoglobin St. Antoine ([Gly→ Leu β74–75] [E18–19] deleted). Consequences for oxygen affinity and protein stability. Biochim. Biophys. Acta *295*:495, 1973a.

Wajcman, H., Leroux, A., and Labie, D.: Functional properties of hemoglobin Hammersmith. Biochimie *55*:119, 1973b.

Walker, B. R., and Alexander, F.: Uric acid excretion in sickle cell anemia. JAMA *215*:255, 1971.

Wapnick, A. A., Lynch, S. R., Charlton, R. W., et al.: The effect of ascorbic acid deficiency on desferrioxamine-induced urinary iron excretion. Br. J. Haematol. *17*:563, 1969.

Ward, J., and Smith, A. L.: Hemophilus influenzae bacteremia in children with sickle cell disease. J. Pediatr. *88*:261, 1976.

Wasi, C., Wasi, P., and Thongcharoen, P.: Serum-immunoglobulin levels in thalassaemia and the effect of splenectomy. Lancet *2*:237, 1971.

Wasi, P.: The alpha thalassaemia genes. J. Med. Assoc. Thai. *53*:677, 1970.

Wasi, P.: Streptococcal infection leading to cardiac and renal involvement in thalassaemia. Lancet *1*:949, 1971.

Wasi, P.: Is the human globin α-chain locus duplicated? Br. J. Haematol. *24*:267, 1973.

Wasi, P., Na-Nakorn, S., and Suingdumrong, A.: Hemoglobin H disease in Thailand: a genetical study. Nature *204*:907, 1964.

Wasi, P., Disthasongchan, P., and Na-Nakorn, S.: The effect of iron deficiency on the levels of hemoglobins A_2 and E. J. Lab. Clin. Med. *71*:85, 1968.

Wasi, P., Na-Nakorn, S., Pootrakul, S., et al.: Alpha- and beta-thalassemia in Thailand. Ann. NY Acad. Sci. *165*:60, 1969.

Watson, J. D.: Molecular Biology of the Gene. 2nd ed. Reading, Mass., W. A. Benjamin, 1970.

Watson-Williams, E. J.: Sickle-cell crisis treated with Rheomacrodex. Lancet *1*:1053, 1963.

Watson-Williams, E. J., Beale, D., Irvine, D., and Lehmann, H.: A new haemoglobin, D-Ibadan (β87 threonine→lysine), producing no sickle cell/haemoglobin D disease with haemoglobin S. Nature *205*:1273, 1965.

Weatherall, D. J.: Abnormal haemoglobins in the neonatal period and their relationship to thalassaemia. Br. J. Haematol. *9*:265, 1963.

Weatherall, D. J.: Biochemical phenotypes of thalassemia in the American Negro population. Ann. NY Acad. Sci. *119*:450, 1964a.

Weatherall, D. J.: Hemoglobin J (Baltimore) coexisting in a family with hemoglobin S. Bull. Johns Hopkins Hosp. *114*:1, 1964b.

Weatherall, D. J.: Recent advances in the haemoglobinopathies with special reference to the first months of life. Proc. Roy. Soc. Med. *65*:747, 1972.

Weatherall, D. J., and Clegg, J. B.: The Thalassaemia Syndromes. 2 ed. Oxford, Blackwell Scientific Publications, 1972.

Weatherall, D. J., and Clegg, J. B.: Hereditary persistence of fetal haemoglobin. Br. J. Haematol. *29*:191, 1975.

Weatherall, D. J., Clegg, J. B., and Naughton, M. A.: Globin synthesis in thalassemia: an *in vitro* study. Nature *208*:1061, 1965.

Weatherall, D. J., Edwards, J. A., and Donohoe, W. T. A.: Haemoglobin and red cell enzyme changes in juvenile myeloid leukaemia. Br. Med. J. *1*:679, 1968.

Weatherall, D. J., Clegg, J. B., Na-Nakorn, S., and Wasi, P.: The pattern of disordered haemoglobin synthesis in homozygous and heterozygous β-thalassaemia. Br. J. Haematol. *16*:251, 1969a.

Weatherall, D. J., Clegg, J. B., Blankson, J., and McNeil, J. R.: A new sickling disorder resulting from interaction of the genes for haemoglobin S and α-thalassaemia. Br. J. Haematol. *17*:517, 1969b.

Weatherall, D. J., Clegg, J. B., and Wong, H. B.: The haemoglobin constitution of infants with the haemoglobin Bart's hydrops foetalis syndrome. Br. J. Haematol. *18*:357, 1970.

Weatherall, D. J., Clegg, J. B., and Knox-Macaulay, A. H. M.: A genetically determined disorder with features of both thalassaemia and congenital dyserythropoietic anaemia. Br. J. Haematol. *24*:681, 1973.

Weatherall, D. J., Pembrey, M. E., and Pritchard, J.: Fetal haemoglobin. Clin. Haematol. *3*:467, 1974.

Weatherall, D. J., Cartner, R., Clegg, J. B., et al.: A form of hereditary persistence of foetal haemoglobin characterized by uneven cellular distribution of haemoglobin F and the production of haemoglobins A and A_2 in homozygotes. Br. J. Haematol. *29*:205, 1975a.

Weatherall, D. J., Clegg, J. B., Wood, W. G., et al.: Foetal erythropoiesis in human leukaemia. Nature *257*:710, 1975b.

Weed, R. I., LaCelle, P. L., and Merrill, E. W.: Metabolic dependence of red cell deformability. J. Clin. Invest. *48*:795, 1969.

Wennberg, E., and Weiss, L.: Splenic erythroclasia: an electronic microscopic study of hemoglobin H disease. Blood *31*:778, 1968.

Wheby, M. S., Thorup, O. A., and Leavell, B. S.: Homozygous hemoglobin C disease in siblings: further comments on intra-erythrocytic crystals. Blood *11*:266, 1956.

White, J. C., Ellis, M., Coleman, P. N., et al.: An unstable haemoglobin associated with cases of leukaemia. Br. J. Haematol. *6*:171, 1960.

White, J. G.: The fine structure of sickled hemoglobin in situ. Blood *31*:561, 1968.

White, J. M.: The synthesis of abnormal haemoglobins. Ser. Haematol. *4*:116, 1971.

White, J. M.: The synthesis of abnormal hemoglobins. Biochimie *54*:657, 1972.

White, J. M.: The unstable haemoglobin disorders. Clin. Haematol. *3*:333, 1974.

White, J. M., and Brain, M. C.: Defective synthesis of an unstable haemoglobin Köln (β^{98}Val → Met). Br. J. Haematol. *18*:195, 1970.

White, J. M., and Dacie, J. V.: In vitro synthesis of Hb Hammersmith (CD1 Phe → Ser). Nature *225*:860, 1970.

White, J. M., and Dacie, J. V.: The unstable hemoglobins—molecular and clinical features. Progr. Hematol. *7*:69, 1971.

White, J. M., Brain, M. C., Lorkin, P. A., et al.: Mild "unstable haemoglobin haemolytic anaemia" caused by haemoglobin Shepherds Bush (β74 [E18] Gly→Asp). Nature *225*:939, 1970.

White, J. M., Lang, A., Larkin, P. A., et al.: Synthesis of haemoglobin Lepore. Nature [New Biol.] *235*:208, 1972a.

White, J. M., Lang, A., and Lehmann, H.: Compensation of β chain synthesis by the single β chain gene in Hb Lepore trait. Nature [New Biol.] *240*:271, 1972b.

White, J. M., Szur, L., Gillies, I. D. S., et al.: Familial polycythaemia caused by a new haemoglobin variant: Hb Heathrow, β103 (G5) phenylalanine → leucine. Br. Med. J. *3*:665, 1973.

Williams, R. C.: Concerted formation of the gel of hemoglobin S. Proc. Natl. Acad. Sci. USA *70*:1506, 1973.

Wilson, J. B., Edwards, W. C., McDaniel, M., et al.: The structure of sheep hemoglobins. II. The amino acid composition of the tryptic peptides of the non-alpha chains of hemoglobins A, B, C and F. Arch. Biochem. Biophys. *115*:385, 1966.

Wilson, M. G., Schroeder, W. A., Graves, D. A., and Kach, V. D.: Hemoglobin variations in D-trisomy syndrome. N. Engl. J. Med. *277*:953, 1967.

Wilson, W. W., Luzzana, M. R., Penniston, J. T., and Johnson, C. S., Jr.: Pregelation aggregation of sickle cell hemoglobin. Proc. Natl. Acad. Sci. USA *71*:1260, 1974.

Wiltshire, B. G., Clark, K. G., Lorkin, P. A., et al.: Haemoglobin Denmark Hill 95 (G2) Pro → Ala, a variant with unusual electrophoretic and oxygen-binding properties. Biochim. Biophys. Acta *278*:459, 1972.

Winkelstein, J. A., and Drachman, R. H.: Deficiency of pneumococcal serum opsonizing activity in sickle cell disease. N. Engl. J. Med. *279*:459, 1968.

Winslow, R. M., Swenberg, M.-L., Gross, E., et al.: Hemoglobin McKees Rocks ($\alpha_2\beta_2{}^{145}{}_{Tyr \rightarrow Term}$): A human "nonsense" mutation leading to a shortened β-chain. J. Clin. Invest. *57*:772, 1976.

Winterbourn, C. C., and Carrell, R. W.: Characterization of Heinz bodies in unstable haemoglobin haemolytic anaemia. Nature *240*:150, 1972.

Winterbourn, C. C., and Carrell, R. W.: The attachment of Heinz bodies to the red cell membrane. Br. J. Haematol. *25*:585, 1973.

Winterbourn, C. C., and Carell, R. W.: Studies of hemoglobin denaturation and Heinz body formation in the unstable hemoglobins. J. Clin. Invest. *54*:678, 1974.

Winterhalter, K. H., and Colosimo, A.: Chromatographic isolation and characterization of isolated chains from hemoglobin after regeneration of sulfhydryl groups. Biochemistry *10*:621, 1971.

Winterhalter, K. H., and Deranleau, D. A.: The structure of a hemoglobin carrying only two hemes. Biochemistry *6*:3136, 1967.

Winterhalter, K. H., and Wüthrich, K.: Structural investigations of modified haemoglobins by nuclear magnetic resonance spectroscopy. J. Mol. Biol. *63*:477, 1972.

Winterhalter, K. H., Amiconi, G., and Antonini, E.: Functional properties of a hemoglobin carrying heme only on α chains. Biochemistry *7*:2228, 1968.

Wishner, B. C., and Love, W. E.: Crystals of deoxy sickle cell hemoglobin. In Hercules, J. I., Schechter, A. N., Eaton, W. A., et al. (eds.): Proceedings of First National Symposium on Sickle Cell Disease, Washington, D.C. DHEW Pub. No. 75–723 (NIH), Bethesda, Md., 1974, p. 85.

Wishner, B. C., Ward, K. B., Lattman, E. E., and Love, W. E.: Crystal structure of sickle-cell deoxyhemoglobin at 5 Å resolution. J. Mol. Biol. *98*:179, 1975.

Wishner, B. C., Hanson, J. C., Ringle, W. M., and Love, W. E.: Crystal structure of sickle cell deoxyhemoglobin. In Waterman, M., and Cottam, L. (eds.): Molecular and Cellular Aspects of Sickle Cell Disease. In press, 1976.

Wolff, J. A., and Luke, K. H.: Management of thalassemia: a comparative program. Ann. NY Acad. Sci. *165*:423, 1969.

Wolman, I. J.: Transfusion therapy in Cooley's anemia: growth and health as related to long-range hemoglobin levels, a progress report. Ann. NY Acad. Sci. *119*:736, 1964.

Wolman, I. J., and Ortolani, M.: Some clinical features of Cooley's anemia patients as related to transfusion schedules. Ann. NY Acad. Sci. *165*:407, 1969.

Wong, S. C., and Huisman, T. H. J.: Further evidence for non-linkage of the Hb α and Hb β structural loci in man. Clin. Chim. Acta *38*:473, 1972.

Wood, L., and Beutler, E.: The effect of ascorbate and dihydroxyacetone on the 2,3-diphosphoglycerate and ATP levels of stored human red cells. Transfusion *14*:272, 1974.

Wood, W. G., and Stamatoyannopoulos, G.: Globin synthesis in fractionated normoblasts of β-thalassemia heterozygotes. J. Clin. Invest. *55*:567, 1975.

Wood, W. G., and Weatherall, D. J.: Haemoglobin synthesis during human foetal development. Nature *244*:162, 1973.

Wood, W. G., Stamatoyannopoulos, G., Lim, G., and Nute, P. E.: F-cells in the adult: Normal values and levels in individuals with hereditary and acquired elevations of Hb F. Blood *46*:671, 1975.

Woodson, R. D., Heywood, J. D., and Lenfant, C.: Oxygen transport in hemoglobin Köln. Effect of increased oxygen affinity in absence of compensatory erythrocytosis. Arch. Intern. Med. *134*:711, 1974.

Wyatt, J. P., and Orrahood, M. D.: Massive fat embolism following marrow infarction in sickle cell anemia. Arch. Pathol. *53*:233, 1952.

Yamaoka, K., Cottman, G. L., and Waterman, M. R.: Spin-label studies at F9(93)β of deoxyhemoglobin S aggregation. Biochem. Biophys. Res. Commun. *58*:1058, 1974.

Yataganas, X., and Fessas, P.: The pattern of hemoglobin precipitation in thalassemia and its significance. Ann. NY Acad. Sci. *165*:270, 1969.

Yoffey, J. M.: The stem cell problem in the fetus. Isr. J. Med. Sci. *7*:825, 1971.

Zak, S. J., Brimhall, B., Jones, R. T., and Kaplan, M. E.: Hemoglobin Andrew-Minneapolis $\alpha_2^{A}\beta_2^{144\ Lys\rightarrow Asn}$: a new high-oxygen-affinity mutant human hemoglobin. Blood *44*:543, 1974.

Zalusky, R., Ross, J., and Katz, J. H.: Dissociation and exchange of α chains in an unstable haemoglobin. Proceedings of XIII Congress of the International Society of Hematology, Munich, 1970.

Zanjani, E. D., Mann, L. I., Burlington, H., et al.: Evidence for a physiologic role of erythropoietin in fetal erythropoiesis. Blood *44*:285, 1974a.

Zanjani, E. D., Peterson, E. N., Gordon, A. S., and Wasserman, L. R.: Erythropoietin production in the fetus: the role of the kidney and maternal anemia. J. Lab. Clin. Med. *83*:281, 1974b.

Zarkowsky, H. S., and Hochmuth, R. M.: Sickling times of individual erythrocytes at zero PO_2. J. Clin. Invest. *56*:1023, 1975.

Zipp, A., James, T. L., Kuntz, I. D., et al.: Water proton magnetic resonance studies of normal and sickle erythrocytes: temperature and volume dependence. Biochim. Biophys. Acta *428*:291, 1976.

Zucker, W., and Schulman, H.: The synthesis of globin dimers by a reticulocyte cell-free system. Biochim. Biophys. Acta *138*:400, 1967.

INDEX

Note: Page numbers in *italics* represent illustrations; those followed by (t) represent tables; those followed by *f* represent footnote text.